WORLD
POVERTY

ISSN 1930-3300

WORLD POVERTY

Sandra M. Alters

INFORMATION PLUS® REFERENCE SERIES
Formerly Published by Information Plus, Wylie, Texas

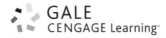

Detroit • New York • San Francisco • New Haven, Conn • Waterville, Maine • London

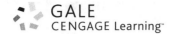
GALE
CENGAGE Learning

World Poverty

Sandra M. Alters

Kepos Media, Inc.: Paula Kepos and Janice Jorgensen, Series Editors

Project Editors: Elizabeth Manar, Kathleen J. Edgar

Rights Acquisition and Management: Margaret Abendroth

Composition: Evi Abou-El-Seoud, Mary Beth Trimper

Manufacturing: Cynde Lentz

Cover photograph: Image copyright Teoh Boon Thiam, 2010. Used under license from Shutterstock.com

Gale
27500 Drake Rd.
Farmington Hills, MI 48331-3535

ISBN-13: 978-0-7876-5103-9 (set)
ISBN-13: 978-1-4144-4124-5
ISBN-10: 0-7876-5103-6 (set)
ISBN-10: 1-4144-4124-X

ISSN 1930-3300

This title is also available as an e-book.
ISBN-13: 978-1-4144-7003-0 (set)
ISBN-10: 1-4144-7003-7 (set)
Contact your Gale sales representative for ordering information.

Printed in the United States of America
1 2 3 4 5 6 7 14 13 12 11 10

TABLE OF CONTENTS

PREFACE vii

CHAPTER 1

What Is Poverty? 1

International, regional, and local organizations and governmental bodies use complex definitions and calculations to measure poverty and create aid programs. This chapter explains how they determine who is and who is not poor.

CHAPTER 2

The Causes of Poverty and the Search for Solutions . . . 15

Many factors cause or contribute to poverty at the individual, family, community, or national level. Employment, health, education, housing, political opportunities, environmental factors, and trade policies all influence people's ability to secure basic human needs. Besides discussing these factors, this chapter considers the impact of globalization and trade agreements as well as international plans to eradicate poverty.

CHAPTER 3

Poverty in Underdeveloped Countries—The Poorest
of the Poor 33

Underdeveloped countries tend to have long histories of social, economic, and political instability; armed conflict; widespread government corruption; little or no infrastructure; and frequent natural disasters. This chapter shows how these factors combine to keep underdeveloped countries at the bottom of the global economy.

CHAPTER 4

Emerging and Transition Economies: Widening the
Poverty Gap 53

Since the 1990s several countries have moved from developing to emerging or transition economic status. Two in particular—China and India—have garnered much attention for their rapidly growing economies, but what effect does this unprecedented growth have on the poorest people living in these countries? This chapter seeks answers to this question.

CHAPTER 5

Poverty in the Developing World 69

Developing countries are those whose incomes (in terms of gross domestic product) place them between the least developed countries and industrialized nations. Developing countries often have pockets of both extreme poverty and great wealth. This chapter looks at examples of such countries around the world.

CHAPTER 6

The Poor in Developed Countries 87

What does it mean to be poor in a wealthy country? The causes and consequences of poverty in some of the world's richest nations are examined in this chapter.

CHAPTER 7

Women and Children in Poverty 103

Women and children make up the largest groups of poor people. Worldwide, women receive lower wages than men, have fewer educational opportunities, and lack equal political representation; in addition, women face gender-specific health issues related to childbearing. Because of their social and physical vulnerability, women and children can be kept poor by violence, kidnapping, and forced labor.

CHAPTER 8

Poverty and Environmental Hazards 123

Environmental hazards such as famines, earthquakes, and other natural and human-made disasters frequently arise in countries that are already poor. They can also, however, destroy local and regional economies in wealthier countries. This chapter explores the economic effects of some of the major environmental hazards of the past quarter century, including the Asian tsunami of 2004, Hurricane Katrina in 2005, the Java earthquake and tsunami in 2006, Cyclone Sidr in Bangladesh in 2007, Tropical Cyclone Nargis in Burma (Myanmar) in 2008, the Sumatra earthquake in 2009, and the Haiti and Chile earthquakes in 2010.

CHAPTER 9

Poverty and Violent Conflict. 137

Few events so brutally affect people's lives and livelihoods as war and violent conflict, which can keep an entire country in poverty for decades. Some of the most recent and extreme examples of the connection between war and poverty are cited in this chapter.

CHAPTER 10

Combating Poverty: Measuring Progress 147

This chapter analyzes progress toward the Millennium Development Goals by assessing gains already made toward targets for reducing economic poverty, improving child and maternal health, increasing universal primary schooling and gender parity in education, and broadening access to clean water and basic sanitation.

IMPORTANT NAMES AND ADDRESSES 159

RESOURCES 161

INDEX 163

PREFACE

World Poverty is part of the *Information Plus Reference Series*. The purpose of each volume of the series is to present the latest facts on a topic of pressing concern in modern American life. These topics include the most controversial and studied social issues in the 21st century: abortion, capital punishment, care for the elderly, crime, the environment, health care, immigration, minorities, social welfare, women, youth, and many more. Even though this series is written especially for high school and undergraduate students, it is an excellent resource for anyone in need of factual information on current affairs.

By presenting the facts, it is the intention of Gale, Cengage Learning to provide its readers with everything they need to reach an informed opinion on current issues. To that end, there is a particular emphasis in this series on the presentation of scientific studies, surveys, and statistics. These data are generally presented in the form of tables, charts, and other graphics placed within the text of each book. Every graphic is directly referred to and carefully explained in the text. The source of each graphic is presented within the graphic itself. The data used in these graphics are drawn from the most reputable and reliable sources, such as from the various branches of the U.S. government, from well-respected worldwide sources such as the United Nations, and from major organizations and associations. Every effort has been made to secure the most recent information available. Readers should bear in mind that many major studies take years to conduct and that additional years often pass before the data from these studies are made available to the public. Therefore, in many cases the most recent information available in 2010 is dated from 2006 or 2007. Older statistics are sometimes presented as well, if they are landmark studies or of particular interest and no more-recent information exists.

Even though statistics are a major focus of the *Information Plus Reference Series*, they are by no means its only content. Each book also presents the widely held positions and important ideas that shape how the book's subject is discussed in the United States. These positions are explained in detail and, where possible, in the words of their proponents. Some of the other material to be found in these books includes historical background, descriptions of major events related to the subject, relevant laws and court cases, and examples of how these issues play out in American life. Some books also feature primary documents or have pro and con debate sections that provide the words and opinions of prominent Americans on both sides of a controversial topic. All material is presented in an even-handed and unbiased manner; readers will never be encouraged to accept one view of an issue over another.

HOW TO USE THIS BOOK

It can be argued that poverty is the most widespread and serious problem confronting the modern world. Billions of people are so poor that they struggle, and sometimes fail, to meet their needs for sustenance, shelter, and security. Even among those who can meet these basic needs, there are many who cannot afford adequate medical care, a good education, and other aspects of a decent standard of living. The problems posed by poverty are especially acute in what is sometimes called the undeveloped world. When judged in relative terms, however, poverty afflicts substantial numbers of people in even the richest nations on Earth. This book examines the forms that poverty takes around the world, its many causes, the serious negative consequences that it has for individuals and societies, and the effort to eliminate it.

World Poverty consists of 10 chapters and 3 appendixes. Each chapter is devoted to a particular aspect of poverty throughout the world. For a summary of the information covered in each chapter, please see the synopses provided in the Table of Contents. Chapters generally begin with an overview of the basic facts and background information on the chapter's topic, then proceed to examine subtopics of particular interest. For example, Chapter 2: The Causes of Poverty and the Search for Solutions begins with a short explanation of the multidimensional nature of the causes of poverty. This section includes a discussion of the working poor, many of whom are employed in the informal labor sector where national and international regulatory guidelines do not exist to protect workers. Next explored is the relationship between poverty and level of education and literacy. Not only do rates of illiteracy correlate positively with poverty among regions and countries of the world but also income-based educational disparities exist within countries. Hunger is also a part of the multidimensional problem of poverty. Hunger's relation to poverty is reciprocal: Poverty usually results in hunger, but hunger is a factor that keeps people in poverty. The chapter concludes with a discussion of free trade and fair trade, and the impact of trade agreements on poor countries. Readers can find their way through a chapter by looking for the section and subsection headings, which are clearly set off from the text. They can also refer to the book's extensive index if they already know what they are looking for.

Statistical Information

The tables and figures featured throughout *World Poverty* will be of particular use to readers in learning about this issue. These tables and figures represent an extensive collection of the most recent and important statistics on poverty, hunger, and related issues—for example, graphics cover progress toward the elimination of world hunger, the link between illiteracy and poverty, links between poverty and school attendance, and the impact of war on poverty levels. Gale, Cengage Learning believes that making this information available to readers is the most important way to fulfill the goal of this book: to help readers understand the issues and controversies surrounding poverty around the world and reach their own conclusions.

Each table or figure has a unique identifier appearing above it, for ease of identification and reference. Titles for the tables and figures explain their purpose. At the end of each table or figure, the original source of the data is provided.

To help readers understand these often complicated statistics, all tables and figures are explained in the text. References in the text direct readers to the relevant statistics. Furthermore, the contents of all tables and figures are fully indexed. Please see the opening section of the index at the back of this volume for a description of how to find tables and figures within it.

Appendixes

Besides the main body text and images, *World Poverty* has three appendixes. The first is the Important Names and Addresses directory. Here, readers will find contact information for a number of government and private organizations that can provide further information on aspects of world poverty. The second appendix is the Resources section, which can also assist readers in conducting their own research. In this section, the author and editors of *World Poverty* describe some of the sources that were most useful during the compilation of this book. The final appendix is the detailed index, which facilitates reader access to specific topics in this book.

ADVISORY BOARD CONTRIBUTIONS

The staff of Information Plus would like to extend its heartfelt appreciation to the Information Plus Advisory Board. This dedicated group of media professionals provides feedback on the series on an ongoing basis. Their comments allow the editorial staff who work on the project to continually make the series better and more user-friendly. The staff's top priority is to produce the highest-quality and most useful books possible, and the Information Plus Advisory Board's contributions to this process are invaluable.

The members of the Information Plus Advisory Board are:

- Kathleen R. Bonn, Librarian, Newbury Park High School, Newbury Park, California

- Madelyn Garner, Librarian, San Jacinto College, North Campus, Houston, Texas

- Anne Oxenrider, Media Specialist, Dundee High School, Dundee, Michigan

- Charles R. Rodgers, Director of Libraries, Pasco-Hernando Community College, Dade City, Florida

- James N. Zitzelsberger, Library Media Department Chairman, Oshkosh West High School, Oshkosh, Wisconsin

COMMENTS AND SUGGESTIONS

The editors of the *Information Plus Reference Series* welcome your feedback on *World Poverty*. Please direct all correspondence to:

Editors
Information Plus Reference Series
27500 Drake Rd.
Farmington Hills, MI 48331-3535

CHAPTER 1
WHAT IS POVERTY?

Most people have an idea of what it means to be poor. Many think of conditions such as hunger, homelessness, preventable diseases, unemployment, and illiteracy as elements of poverty. These and other issues will be covered in this book. However, from a social and economic standpoint, poverty is a complex topic that can be difficult to describe in objective terms. Most governments and social service agencies have their own definitions of poverty, including how it is measured and who is considered poor. This chapter will explain the means used by the United States and the international community to define and measure poverty.

DEFINING AND MEASURING POVERTY INTERNATIONALLY

Income and Consumption: Absolute and Relative Poverty

Because being poor differs dramatically across countries, experts have had a difficult time establishing concrete terms to discuss it. A common way for governments and organizations to describe poverty is to focus on income and consumption habits and to describe poverty in terms of absolute poverty and relative poverty. Absolute poverty means that a person's basic subsistence needs (for food, clothing, sanitation, and shelter) are not being met. The measurement of absolute poverty considers whether a family can afford a specified amount of goods and services that are necessary for basic living in the country, city, or village in which the family lives, and this measurement rises only with inflation. By contrast, relative poverty means that a person's needs are not being met in comparison with others in his or her society. The measurement of relative poverty assesses a family's financial situation with what is customary for the rest of the population group to which it belongs. This measurement rises not only with inflation but also with the standard of living.

Critics suggest that the concepts of absolute poverty and relative poverty are not objective and depend too heavily on individual judgments of what it means to be poor. The idea of absolute poverty is particularly problematic, because a consensus list of "basic necessities" is difficult to develop and varies among countries and circumstances. For example, is an automobile a basic necessity? If adequate public transportation is available, a car is likely not a basic necessity. However, if adequate public transportation is not available and a family lives in a remote area, then a vehicle might be necessary for survival. Nonetheless, this may be true only in developed countries; in underdeveloped countries a donkey might be the necessary transportation for a family living in remote regions.

Additionally, definitions of poverty can change over time within a single country. Living conditions that were acceptable in previous centuries and even in previous decades may now be considered inhumane; most Americans would agree that indoor plumbing and electricity are basic necessities, yet as recently as the mid-20th century these things were luxuries to many Americans. Similarly, a person who is considered rich in one country might be seen as abysmally poor in a wealthier country.

Poverty Measurements Used by the World Bank

The World Bank is an international organization of member nations whose goal is to reduce poverty and increase development in poor countries. It is divided into two distinct groups: the International Bank for Reconstruction and Development, which focuses on middle-income countries and those with good credit, and the International Development Association, which focuses on the very poorest countries, many of which may be deeply in debt to other nations. The World Bank provides lines of credit, loans, and grants so that poor countries can improve infrastructure (e.g., roads, bridges, and waterways), communications, health care, and education.

Like many international institutions, the World Bank uses its own terminology to define and measure poverty:

- Incidence of poverty—the percentage of a country's population that cannot afford basic necessities (a "basket of goods and services"). This is also known as living below the poverty line—an income level below which a person is unable to meet basic needs.

- Depth of poverty—how far below the poverty line the poor population lives. This is also called the poverty gap.

- Poverty severity—measures how poor the poor are. In other words, poverty severity (also called the squared poverty gap) measures how far below the poverty line individuals and households are, with more consequence given to those at the very bottom.

VULNERABILITY TO POVERTY. An important facet of the World Bank's measurements is tracking how likely people are to fall into poverty or to fall deeper into poverty. A number of incidents can trigger a descent into poverty, and these incidents can occur at several socio-economic levels. At the individual level, unexpected events can occur such as a major illness or death of the main breadwinner, which can lead to financial ruin when medical bills cannot be paid. At the community level, external problems such as environmental damage due to pollution can cause unsuitable working conditions or local social problems such as rioting and crime. Larger trends at the macroeconomic level include national or international incidents such as natural disasters and war, which also affect people's level of vulnerability to poverty. A family that is already experiencing financial instability can easily fall into poverty under any of these circumstances, and the more people there are living on the brink of poverty, the less stable will become the local, national, and international economies.

Even though vulnerability to poverty is difficult to measure and track, the World Bank uses monetary indicators such as income and consumption, as well as nonmonetary indicators such as health status, weight (to determine whether minimum calorie requirements are being met), and how many financial and nonmonetary assets a person or family has.

POVERTY LINES. As mentioned previously in this chapter, a poverty line is a level of income below which a person cannot afford the bare minimum to exist—an amount of food sufficient to fuel the human body, clothing appropriate to a person's living and working conditions, and suitable shelter to be protected from the elements. Every government determines its country's national poverty line by calculating the annual average cost of basic necessities for an adult to function. Because these costs differ substantially across countries, it is impossible to set a single international poverty line.

National poverty lines are defined by identifying a minimally acceptable diet, meaning the most basic number of calories on which the human body can function. Once this number is determined, analysts calculate the cost of obtaining this minimum amount of food at the current market price. The cost of necessary items other than food is then added to the equation, the total of which forms the national poverty line of a particular country.

However, several factors complicate measurements using national poverty lines. It is difficult to compare national poverty across countries because wealthy, middle-income, and low-income countries have varying notions of what percentage of income is or should be spent on food and nonfood items. Also, what constitutes an "adequate diet" is a subject of debate. People living in poor countries tend to exist on a much less varied diet than those living in richer countries, where a reliance on more expensive prepackaged food is usually assumed.

The second problem with comparing national poverty lines is that countries may estimate two separate lines, one for urban households and one for rural households, which may skew measurements because of assumptions about how much each group spends on necessities. Other problems include disparities that result from countries basing their household surveys on income rather than on expenditures (income—how much people make—is considered more difficult to measure than expenditures—how much people spend), and adjustments for price changes are not always correctly applied to poverty lines, causing them to drift over time, which makes it more difficult to track changes in poverty.

THE $1.25-PER-DAY STANDARD. Besides the problems with comparing national poverty lines across countries, the calculation of national poverty lines depends in part on household surveys that are issued and analyzed by government agencies. These agencies may fail to take poverty surveys regularly, may use inadequate survey methodologies, and may analyze and present data in varying ways. Therefore, to measure poverty at the international level and to provide a single global measurement of poverty, the World Bank developed in *World Development Report 1990* (June 1990, http://www-wds.worldbank.org/) the $1-per-day standard (U.S. dollars), which assumed an income for those living in extreme poverty of $370 per year, or about $1 per day in 1985 U.S. dollars. To account for exchange rates and differences in prices and the gross domestic product (GDP; the total value of all goods and services produced by a country in a year), the World Bank had to set a level that would be relevant in underdeveloped, developing, and developed countries despite immense differences in the meaning of poverty around the world. In 2008 the World Bank updated this standard to $1.25 per day in 2005 dollars in *World Development Indicators 2008* (December 2008, http://siteresources.worldbank.org/DATASTATISTICS/Resources/WDI08supplement1216.pdf).

Generally speaking, earning $1.25 per day or less means that a person in any country is living in "extreme poverty," which means that that person cannot afford to buy even the most basic human necessities. However, "$1.25 per day" is not a literal amount of money. Rather, it means $1.25 per day at purchasing power parity (PPP) in 2005 prices. PPP is a way to measure the value of currency that allows economists and poverty researchers to compare the standards of living in different countries while accounting for differences in both wages and costs of living. In general, PPP refers to the goods and services that a currency has the power to buy, typically expressed as a basket or bundle of necessary items. PPP measures how much the same basket or bundle of goods and services costs around the world. By considering exchange rates, the PPP number in each country should allow people to purchase the same basket of goods and services that a U.S. dollar can purchase in the United States. As with absolute poverty, critics of PPP point out that one problem with this measure lies in the notion of what is and is not a necessity: A product or service considered a staple in one culture may be a luxury in others. Nevertheless, most researchers agree that PPP is the best way to examine poverty at the global level.

THE $2-PER-DAY STANDARD. To measure poverty—as distinguished from extreme poverty—the World Bank uses a US $2-per-day standard, meaning that anyone earning less than $2 per day is living in poverty. In this measurement the concept of PPP is the same, but the $2-per-day standard allows researchers to study the poor in slightly less impoverished countries while still using the PPP standard.

Table 1.1 shows the numbers of people by region at or below the $1.25-per-day and the $2-per-day poverty standards for 1997, 2002, and 2007. Worldwide, the numbers of the $1.25-per-day working poor decreased from 822 million in 1997 to 609.5 million in 2007. East Asia experienced the largest decrease, whereas South Asia, the Middle East, North Africa, and sub-Saharan Africa all experienced increases. In 2007 South Asia (278.8 million people) and sub-Saharan Africa (165.6 million people) had the highest number of working poor at the $1.25-per-day level.

Worldwide, the numbers of the $2-per-day working poor decreased from 1.4 billion in 1997 to 1.2 billion in 2007. (See Table 1.1.) The number of working poor dropped dramatically in East Asia. The numbers also dropped in central and southeastern Europe and the Commonwealth of Independent States (CIS; an alliance of 12 former Soviet republics: Armenia, Azerbaijan, Belarus, Georgia, Kazakhstan, Kyrgyzstan, Moldova, Russia,

TABLE 1.1

Working poor indicators, 1997, 2002, and 2007

	1997 (million)	2002 (million)	2007 (million)	1997 Share in total employment (%)	2002 Share in total employment (%)	2007 Share in total employment (%)
			United States Dollar (USD) 1.25 a day working poor			
World	822.0	787.2	609.5	32.7	29.0	20.6
Central and South Eastern Europe (non-EU) & CIS	12.2	10.4	8.2	8.2	6.8	5.1
East Asia	278.5	231.4	84.0	38.4	30.2	10.4
South-East Asia and the Pacific	80.3	66.1	44.7	35.6	26.8	16.4
South Asia	276.6	288.2	278.8	57.2	53.5	47.1
Latin America and the Caribbean	24.9	25.8	16.9	12.9	11.8	6.8
Middle East	3.9	5.0	5.3	9.7	10.1	9.0
North Africa	5.2	6.0	5.9	11.7	11.8	9.8
Sub-Saharan Africa	140.3	154.4	165.6	65.0	62.7	58.3
			United States Dollar (USD) 2 a day working poor			
World	1,361.5	1,350.9	1,201.0	54.2	49.7	40.6
Central and South Eastern Europe (non-EU) & CIS	32.1	27.4	22.6	21.5	17.9	13.9
East Asia	501.9	426.5	265.4	69.2	55.8	33.0
South-East Asia and the Pacific	142.6	145.1	127.0	63.2	58.8	46.6
South Asia	417.6	454.7	479.4	86.3	84.4	80.9
Latin America and the Caribbean	53.7	56.8	40.6	27.8	26.0	16.4
Middle East	10.6	12.9	14.3	25.8	26.1	24.0
North Africa	18.8	18.9	18.2	42.0	37.1	30.2
Sub-Saharan Africa	184.2	208.5	233.5	85.4	84.7	82.2

CIS = Commonwealth of Independent States. EU = European Union.

SOURCE: "Table A7. Working Poor Indicators, World and Regions," in *Global Employment Trends*, International Labour Organization, January 2009, http://www.ilo.org/wcmsp5/groups/public/--dgreports/--dcomm/documents/publication/wcms_101461.pdf (accessed November 24, 2009). Copyright © 2009 International Labour Organization. Data from International Labour Organization (ILO), Trends Econometric Models, December 2008; International Monetary Fund (IMF), World Economic Outlook, November 2008.

Tajikistan, Turkmenistan, Ukraine, and Uzbekistan), Southeast Asia and the Pacific, Latin America and the Caribbean, and North Africa but rose in all the other regions listed.

Composite Poverty Indicators

National and international agencies have recognized since the mid-1990s that poverty affects more than a person's income and consumption habits, which led to expanded definitions of poverty—also called composite indicators—used by the United Nations (UN) and others. Composite poverty indicators allow for a broader explanation and measurement of poverty, because they take into account factors not directly related to a family's income or larger economic forces such as a country's GDP. Even though the GDP is often used to measure a nation's standard of living (the quality and quantity of goods and services available to a country's people), many experts contend that it is not an adequate way to explain poverty because it measures only the consumption of material goods. Composite poverty indicators allow those who study and track poverty to consider a person's overall quality of life, rather than just income and possessions.

Since the publication of *Human Development Report 1997: Human Development to Eradicate Poverty* (1997, http://hdr.undp.org/en/reports/global/hdr1997/chapters/), the UN Development Programme (UNDP) has maintained that "human poverty is more than income poverty." The report added that, from a human development perspective, poverty means "the denial of choices and opportunities most basic to human development—to lead a long, healthy, creative life and enjoy a decent standard of living, freedom, self-esteem, and the respect of others." This definition takes into account nearly all aspects of human experience: financial, personal, political, and social.

The 1997 UNDP concept of poverty was still being used effectively by that organization more than a decade later. Moreover, in 2009 the World Bank reflected the UNDP's idea that poverty encompasses a majority of life aspects in "What Is Poverty?" (http://web.worldbank.org/). The World Bank expresses the concept as:

> Poverty is hunger. Poverty is lack of shelter. Poverty is being sick and not being able to see a doctor. Poverty is not having access to school and not knowing how to read. Poverty is not having a job, is fear for the future, living one day at a time. Poverty is losing a child to illness brought about by unclean water. Poverty is powerlessness, lack of representation and freedom.
>
> Poverty has many faces, changing from place to place and across time, and has been described in many ways.... Most often, poverty is a situation people want to escape. So poverty is a call to action—for the poor and the wealthy alike—a call to change the world so that many more may have enough to eat, adequate shelter, access to education and health, protection from violence, and a voice in what happens in their communities.

THE HUMAN POVERTY INDEX. In *Human Development Report 1997*, the UNDP developed a composite indicator called the Human Poverty Index (HPI) to measure the more-inclusive concept of poverty described in the report. The HPI is frequently divided into two measures: HPI-1 and HPI-2. HPI-1 is used to measure poverty in less-developed countries. It measures deprivations in three basic dimensions of human development: a long and healthy life, knowledge, and a decent standard of living. The HPI-2 includes these three dimensions but, in addition, includes a dimension of unemployment, which the UNDP called social exclusion.

The HPI worked well as a measure of poverty in 1997 and was still being used by the UNDP in 2009. Table 1.2 shows the data by country that are used to calculate the HPI-1: the percentage of the population that does not survive to the age of 40, the percentage of people aged 15 years and older who are illiterate, the percentage of the population that does not have sustainable access to an improved water source, and the percentage of children who are underweight for their age. The higher the value of the HPI-1, the higher the level of human and income poverty in that country. Data for various measures of income poverty are also shown in Table 1.2 in the far-right columns.

Table 1.2 lists less-developed countries grouped according to their level of human development (Human Development Index [HDI]), but the table also includes HPI-1 rank, HPI-1 values, and HPI-1 data for the factors that make up the HPI-1. Like the HPI, the HDI was devised by the UNDP, but its purpose is to measure the well-being of a country and how favorably it is progressing toward development, whereas the HPI measures deprivation (the level of poverty and suffering experienced in a country at any given time). The HDI measures development and well-being using a combination of factors, such as life expectancy, literacy, and amount of education, along with the domestic purchasing power of the GDP (how much citizens of a country are able to buy based on the country's GDP).

The HDI rankings in Table 1.2 range from 23 to 182; they are shown in the far-left column and determine the order in which countries are listed in the table. HDI rankings from 1 to 22 are shown in Table 1.3, which lists HDI rankings of countries in the Organization for Economic Cooperation and Development (OECD). Countries in the OECD are, in general, developed countries. A few countries are listed in both tables. The HPI-1, HPI-2, and HDI are each constructed differently, so rankings based on each may differ.

The HPI-1 rankings in Table 1.2 range from 1 to 135 and are listed in the second column. The country shown as number 1 in HPI-1 rankings and that has the lowest HPI-1 value is the Czech Republic. Among the less-developed countries, the Czech Republic is doing the best in terms of

TABLE 1.2

Human and income poverty, less developed countries, 2009

Human Development Index (HDI) rank	Human poverty index (HPI-1) Rank	Human poverty index (HPI-1) Value (%)	Probability of not surviving to age 40[a,†] (% of cohort) 2005–2010	Adult illiteracy rate[b,†] (% aged 15 and above) 1999–2007	Population not using an improved water source[†] (%) 2006	Children underweight for age (% aged under 5) 2000–2006[c]	Population below income poverty line (%) $1.25 a day 2000–2007[c]	Population below income poverty line (%) $2 a day 2000–2007[c]	Population below income poverty line (%) National poverty line 2000–2006[c]	HPI-1 rank minus income poverty rank[d]
Very high human development										
23 Singapore	14	3.9	1.6	5.6[i]	0[f]	3	—	—	—	—
24 Hong Kong, China (SAR)	—	—	1.4	—[k]	8[i]	—	<2[f,g]	<2[f,g]	—	—
26 Korea (Republic of)	—	—	1.9	—[e]	0	—	<2	<2	—	—
27 Israel	—	—	1.9	2.9[i]	—	—	—	—	—	—
29 Slovenia	—	—	1.9	0.3[e,i]	0	—	<2	<2	—	—
30 Brunei Darussalam	—	—	2.6	5.1[i]	—	10[g]	—	—	—	—
31 Kuwait	—	—	2.5	5.5[h]	0	—	—	—	—	—
32 Cyprus	—	—	2.1	2.3[i]	0	—	—	—	—	—
33 Qatar	19	5.0	3.0	6.9[h]	0	6[g]	—	—	—	—
35 United Arab Emirates	35	7.7	2.3	10.0[h]	0	14[g]	<2[g]	<2[g]	—	—
36 Czech Republic	1	1.5	2.0	—[e]	0	1[g]	<2[g]	<2[g]	—	0
37 Barbados	4	2.6	3.0	—[e,k]	0	6[g,m]	—	—	—	—
38 Malta	—	—	1.9	7.6[n]	0	—	—	—	—	—
High human development										
39 Bahrain	39	8.0	2.9	11.2[i]	0[f]	9[g]	—	—	—	—
40 Estonia	—	—	5.2	0.2[e,i]	0[f]	—	<2	<2	8.9[g]	—
41 Poland	—	—	2.9	0.7[e,i]	0[f]	—	<2[g]	<2[g]	14.8	—
42 Slovakia	3	2.2	2.7	—[e]	0	2[g,m]	<2	<2	17.3[g]	2
43 Hungary	10	3.2	3.1	1.1[i]	0	1	<2	<2	17.0[g]	6
44 Chile	2	1.9	3.1	3.5[i]	5	1[g]	<2	2.4	—	1
45 Croatia	—	—	2.6	1.3[i]	1	—	<2	<2	—	—
46 Lithuania	—	—	5.7	0.3[e,i]	9[g]	10[g,m]	<2	<2	—	—
47 Antigua and Barbuda	—	—	—	1.1[n]	1	—	—	—	—	—
48 Latvia	—	—	4.8	0.2[e,i]	4	—	<2	<2	5.9	—
49 Argentina	13	3.7	4.4	2.4[i]	0	4	4.5[i]	11.3[i]	—	-18
50 Uruguay	6	3.0	3.8	2.1[h]	0	5	<2[i]	4.2[i]	—	4
51 Cuba	17	4.6	2.6	0.2[e,i]	9	4	—	—	—	—
52 Bahamas	—	—	7.3	—[k]	3[i]	5	—	—	—	—
53 Mexico	23	5.9	5.0	7.2[h]	5	5	<2	4.8	17.6	16
54 Costa Rica	11	3.7	3.3	4.1[i]	2	5[g]	2.4	8.6	23.9	-13
55 Libyan Arab Jamahiriya	60	13.4	4.0	13.2[i]	29[g]	5[g]	—	—	—	—
56 Oman	64	14.7	3.0	15.6[i]	18[i]	18[g]	—	—	—	—
57 Seychelles	—	—	6.7	8.2[n]	13[i]	6[g,m]	—	—	—	—
58 Venezuela (Bolivarian Republic of)	28	6.6	4.7	4.8[h]	10[i]	5	3.5	10.2	—	-5
59 Saudi Arabia	53	12.1	5.9	15.0[i]	8	14[g]	—	—	—	—
60 Panama	30	6.7	3.8	6.6[i]	8	7[g]	9.5	17.8	37.3[g]	-15
61 Bulgaria	—	—	—	1.7[i]	1	—	<2	2.4	12.8	—
62 Saint Kitts and Nevis	—	—	4.3	2.2[o]	1	—	—	—	—	—
63 Romania	20	5.6	4.3	2.4[i]	12	3	<2	3.4	28.9	13
64 Trinidad and Tobago	27	6.4	8.4	1.3[i]	6	6	4.2[g]	13.5[g]	21.0[g]	-7
65 Montenegro	8	3.1	3.0	3.6[n,p]	2	3	<2	<2	—	—
66 Malaysia	25	6.1	3.7	8.1[i]	1	8	<2	7.8	—	17
67 Serbia	7	3.1	3.3	3.6[n,p]	1	2	—	—	—	—
68 Belarus	16	4.3	6.2	0.3[e,i]	0	1	<2	<2	18.5	11
69 Saint Lucia	26	6.3	4.6	5.2[q]	2	14[g,m]	20.9[g]	40.6[g]	—	-35

TABLE 1.2

Human and income poverty, less developed countries, 2009 [CONTINUED]

Human Development Index (HDI) rank	HPI-1 Rank	HPI-1 Value (%)	Probability of not surviving to age 40[a,†] (% of cohort) 2005–2010	Adult illiteracy rate[b,†] (% aged 15 and above) 1999–2007	Population not using an improved water source[†] (%) 2006	Children under weight for age (% aged under 5) 2000–2006[c]	Population below income poverty line (%) $1.25 a day 2000–2007[c]	$2 a day 2000–2007[c]	National poverty line 2000–2006[e]	HPI-1 rank minus income poverty rank[d]
70 Albania	15	4.0	3.6	1.0[e,i]	3	8	<2	7.8	25.4	10
71 Russian Federation	32	7.4	10.6	0.5[e,i]	3	3[g]	<2	<2	19.6	24
72 Macedonia (the Former Yugoslav Rep. of)	9	3.2	3.4	3.0[i]	0	6[g]	<2	3.2	21.7	5
73 Dominica	—	—	—	12.0[q]	3[i]	5[g,m]	—	—	—	—
74 Grenada	—	—	3.2	4.0[q]	6[i]	—	—	—	—	—
75 Brazil	43	8.6	8.2	10.0[h]	9	6[g]	5.2	12.7	21.5	1
76 Bosnia and Herzegovina	5	2.8	3.0	3.3[i]	1	2	<2	<2	19.5	3
77 Colombia	34	7.6	8.3	7.3[h]	7	7	16.0	27.9	64.0[o]	-21
78 Peru	47	10.2	7.4	10.4[h]	16	8	7.9	18.5	53.1	0
79 Turkey	40	8.3	5.7	11.3[h]	3	4	2.7	9.0	27.0	6
80 Ecuador	38	7.9	7.3	9.0[h]	5	9	4.7	12.8	46.0[o]	0
81 Mauritius	45	9.5	5.8	12.6[i]	0	15[g]	—	—	—	—
82 Kazakhstan	37	7.9	11.2	0.4[e,i]	4	4	3.1	17.2	15.4	3
83 Lebanon	33	7.6	5.5	10.4[h]	0	4	—	—	—	—
Medium human development										
84 Armenia	12	3.7	5.0	0.5[e,i]	2	4	10.6	43.4	50.9	-30
85 Ukraine	21	5.8	8.4	0.3[e,i]	3	1	<2	<2	19.5	14
86 Azerbaijan	50	10.7	8.6	0.5[e,h]	22	7	<2	<2	49.6	38
87 Thailand	41	8.5	11.3	5.9[i]	2	9	<2	11.5	13.6[o]	30
88 Iran (Islamic Republic of)	59	12.8	6.1	17.7[h]	6[i]	11[q]	<2	8.0	—	44
89 Georgia	18	4.7	6.7	0.0[e,s]	1	3[q]	13.4	30.4	54.5	-29
90 Dominican Republic	44	9.1	9.4	10.9[s]	5	5	5.0	15.1	42.2	3
91 Saint Vincent and the Grenadines	—	—	5.8	11.9[q]	—	—	—	—	—	—
92 China	36	7.7	6.2	6.7[i]	12	7	15.9[i]	36.3[i]	2.8	-19
93 Belize	73	17.5	5.6	24.9[q]	9[j]	7	—	—	—	—
94 Samoa	—	—	5.6	1.3[i]	12	—	—	—	—	—
95 Maldives	66	16.5	6.0	3.0[i]	17	30	—	—	—	—
96 Jordan	29	6.6	5.3	8.9[h]	2	4	<2	3.5	14.2	21
97 Suriname	46	10.1	10.0	9.6[i]	8	13	15.5[g]	27.2[g]	—	-9
98 Tunisia	65	15.6	4.1	22.3[i]	6	4	2.6	12.8	7.6[o]	26
99 Tonga	—	—	5.4	0.8[e,i]	0	—	—	—	—	—
100 Jamaica	51	10.9	9.9	14.0[h]	7	4	<2	5.8	18.7	39
101 Paraguay	49	10.5	8.9	5.4[h]	23	5	6.5	14.2	—	5
102 Sri Lanka	67	16.8	5.5	9.2[h]	18	29	14.0	39.7	22.7	7
103 Gabon	72	17.5	22.6	13.8[i]	13	12	4.8	19.6	—	24
104 Algeria	71	17.5	6.4	24.6[i]	15	4	6.8[g]	23.6[g]	22.6[g]	19
105 Philippines	54	12.4	5.7	6.6[i]	7	28	22.6	45.0	25.1[g]	-19
106 El Salvador	63	14.6	10.7	18.0[h]	16	10	11.0	20.5	37.2	8
107 Syrian Arab Republic	56	12.6	3.9	16.9[i]	11	10	—	—	—	—
108 Fiji	79	21.2	6.2	—[k]	53	8[g]	—	—	—	—
109 Turkmenistan	24	6.0	13.0	0.5[e,i]	11	11	24.8[g]	49.6[g]	—	—
110 Occupied Palestinian Territories	69	17.0	4.3	6.2[h]	11	3	—	—	—	—
111 Indonesia	61	13.7	6.7	8.0[h]	20	28	29.4	60.0	16.7	-3
112 Honduras	52	11.6	9.3	16.4[h]	16	11	18.2	29.7	50.7	-10
113 Bolivia	48	10.2	13.9	9.3[h]	14	8	19.6	30.3	65.2	2
114 Guyana	58	12.7	12.8	—[k]	7	14	7.7[g]	16.8[g]	35.0[o]	—
115 Mongolia	58	12.7	10.3	2.7[i]	28	6	22.4	49.0	36.1	-15
116 Viet Nam	55	12.4	5.8	9.7[h]	8	25	21.5	48.4	28.9	-13

TABLE 1.2

Human and income poverty, less developed countries, 2009 [CONTINUED]

Human Development Index (HDI) rank	Human poverty index (HPI-1) Rank	Human poverty index (HPI-1) Value (%)	Probability of not surviving to age 40[a,†] (% of cohort) 2005–2010	Adult illiteracy rate[a,†] (% aged 15 and above) 1999–2007	Population not using an improved water source[†] (%) 2006	Children under weight for age (% aged under 5) 2000–2006[c]	Population below income poverty line (%) $1.25 a day 2000–2007[c]	Population below income poverty line (%) $2 a day 2000–2007[c]	Population below income poverty line (%) National poverty line 2000–2006[c]	HPI-1 rank minus income poverty rank[d]
117 Moldova	22	5.9	6.2	0.8[e,i]	10	4	8.1	28.9	48.5	-21
118 Equatorial Guinea	98	31.9	34.5	13.0[f]	57	19	—	—	—	—
119 Uzbekistan	42	8.5	10.7	3.1[f]	12	5	46.3	76.7	27.5	-46
120 Kyrgyzstan	31	7.3	9.2	0.7[e,i]	11	3	21.8	51.9	43.1	-34
121 Cape Verde	62	14.5	6.4	16.2[i]	20[i]	14[g]	20.6	40.2	—	-6
122 Guatemala	76	19.7	11.2	26.8[i]	4	23	11.7	24.3	56.2	15
123 Egypt	82	23.4	7.2	33.6[h]	2	6	<2	18.4	16.7	58
124 Nicaragua	68	17.0	7.9	22.0[h]	21	10	15.8	31.8	47.9[g]	6
125 Botswana	81	22.9	31.2	17.1[i]	4	13	31.2[i]	49.4[i]	—	-8
126 Vanuatu	83	23.6	7.1	21.9[i]	41[i]	20[g,m]	—	—	44.4	—
127 Tajikistan	74	18.2	12.5	0.4[e,i]	33	17	21.5	50.8	—	-2
128 Namibia	70	17.1	21.2	12.0[i]	7	24	49.1[i]	62.2[i]	—	-29
129 South Africa	85	25.4	36.1	12.0[i]	7	12[g]	26.2	42.9	—	-2
130 Morocco	96	31.1	6.6	44.4[i]	17	10	2.5	14.0	—	50
131 Sao Tome and Principe	57	12.6	13.9	12.1[i]	14	9	—	—	—	—
132 Bhutan	102	33.7	14.2	47.2[h]	19	19[g]	26.2	49.5	—	13
133 Lao People's Democratic Republic	94	30.7	13.1	27.3[h]	40	40	44.0	76.8	33.0	-6
134 India	88	28.0	15.5	34.0[i]	11	46	41.6[i]	75.6[i]	28.6	-10
135 Solomon Islands	80	21.8	11.6	23.4[i]	30	21[g,m]	—	—	—	—
136 Congo	84	24.3	29.7	18.9[i]	29	14	54.1	74.4	35.0	-27
137 Cambodia	87	27.7	18.5	23.7[i]	35	36	40.2	68.2	—	-10
138 Myanmar	77	20.4	19.1	10.1[i]	20	32	—	—	—	—
139 Comoros	78	20.4	12.6	24.9[i]	15	25	46.1	65.0	41.8[g]	-20
140 Yemen	111	35.7	15.6	41.1[i]	34	46	17.5	46.6	32.6[g]	35
141 Pakistan	101	33.4	12.6	45.8[h]	10	38	22.6	60.3	—	16
142 Swaziland	108	35.1	47.2	20.4[i]	40	10	62.9	81.0	69.2	-15
143 Angola	118	37.2	38.5	32.6[i]	49	31	54.3	70.2	—	2
144 Nepal	99	32.1	11.0	43.5[i]	11	39	55.1[i]	77.6[i]	30.9	-16
145 Madagascar	113	36.1	20.8	29.3[i]	53	42	67.8	89.6	71.3[i]	-14
146 Bangladesh	112	36.1	11.6	46.5	20[u]	48	49.6[i]	81.3[i]	40.0	2
147 Kenya	92	29.5	30.3	26.4[i]	43	20	19.7	39.9	52.0[i]	16
148 Papua New Guinea	121	39.6	15.9	42.2[i]	60	35[g,m]	35.8[i]	57.4[i]	37.5[i]	23
149 Haiti	97	31.5	18.5	37.9[i,n]	42	22	54.9	72.1	—	-16
150 Sudan	104	34.0	23.9	39.1[i,w]	30	41	—	—	—	—
151 Tanzania (United Republic of)	93	30.0	28.2	27.7[i]	45	22	88.5	96.6	35.7	-37
152 Ghana	89	28.1	25.8	35.0[i]	20	18	30.0	53.6	28.5	0
153 Cameroon	95	30.8	34.2	32.1[i]	30	19	32.8	57.7	40.2	4
154 Mauritania	115	36.2	21.6	44.2[i]	40	32	21.2	44.1	46.3	32
155 Djibouti	86	25.6	26.2	—[k]	8	29	18.8	41.2	—	12
156 Lesotho	106	34.3	47.4	17.8[h]	22	20	43.4	62.2	68.0[i]	3
157 Uganda	91	28.8	31.4	26.4[i]	36	20	51.5	75.6	37.7	-17
158 Nigeria	114	36.2	37.4	28.0[i]	53	29	64.4	83.9	34.1[i]	-11
Low human development										
159 Togo	117	36.6	18.6	46.8[i]	41	26	38.7	69.3	—	18
160 Malawi	90	28.2	32.6	28.2[i]	24	19	73.9	90.4	65.3[i]	-35
161 Benin	126	43.2	19.2	59.5[i]	35	23	47.3	75.3	29.0[i]	19
162 Timor-Leste	122	40.8	18.0	49.9[x]	38	46	52.9	77.5	—	9
163 Côte d'Ivoire	119	37.4	24.6	51.3[i]	19	20	23.3	46.8	—	29

TABLE 1.2

Human and income poverty, less developed countries, 2009 [CONTINUED]

Human Development Index (HDI) rank	Human poverty index (HPI-1)		Probability of not surviving to age 40[a,†] (% of cohort) 2005–2010	Adult illiteracy rate[b,†] (% aged 15 and above) 1999–2007	Population not using an improved water source[†] (%) 2006	Children under weight for age[†] (% aged under 5) 2000–2006[c]	Population below income poverty line (%)			HPI-1 rank minus income poverty rank[d]
	Rank	Value (%)					$1.25 a day 2000–2007[c]	$2 a day 2000–2007[c]	National poverty line 2000–2006[c]	
164 Zambia	110	35.5	42.9	29.4[i]	42	20	64.3	81.5	68.0	-14
165 Eritrea	103	33.7	18.2	35.8[h]	40	40	—	—	53.0[g]	—
166 Senegal	124	41.6	22.4	58.1[h]	23	17	33.5	60.3	33.4[g]	28
167 Rwanda	100	32.9	34.2	35.1[i]	35	23	76.6	90.3	60.3	-28
168 Gambia	123	40.9	21.8	—[k]	14	20	34.3	56.7	61.3	26
169 Liberia	109	35.2	23.2	44.5[i]	36	26[g]	83.7	94.8	—	-24
170 Guinea	129	50.5	23.7	70.5[i]	30	26	70.1	87.2	40.0[g]	1
171 Ethiopia	130	50.9	27.7	64.1[h]	58	38	39.0	77.5	44.2	30
172 Mozambique	127	46.8	40.6	55.6[i]	58	24	74.7	90.0	54.1	-3
173 Guinea-Bissau	107	34.9	37.4	35.4[i]	43	19	48.8	77.9	65.7	-1
174 Burundi	116	36.4	33.7	40.7[i]	29	39	81.3	93.4	68.0[g]	-16
175 Chad	132	53.1	35.7	68.2[i]	52	37	61.9	83.3	64.0[g]	11
176 Congo (Democratic Republic of the)	120	38.0	37.3	32.8[i]	54	31	59.2	79.5	—	0
177 Burkina Faso	131	51.8	26.9	71.3[h]	28	37	56.5	81.2	46.4	12
178 Mali	133	54.5	32.5	73.8[h]	40	33	51.4	77.1	63.8[g]	22
179 Central African Republic	125	42.4	39.6	51.4[i]	34	29	62.4	81.9	—	3
180 Sierra Leone	128	47.7	31.0	61.9[i]	47	30	53.4	76.1	70.2	14
181 Afghanistan	135	59.8	40.7	72.0[i]	78	39	—	—	—	—
182 Niger	134	55.8	29.0	71.3[h]	58	44	65.9	85.6	63.0[g]	8
Other UN member states										
Iraq	75	19.4	10.0	25.9[r]	23	8	—	—	—	—
Kiribati	—	—	—	—	35	13[g]	—	—	—	—
Korea (Democratic People's Rep. of)	—	—	10.0	—	0	23	—	—	—	—
Marshall Islands	—	—	—	—	12[j]	—	—	—	—	—
Micronesia (Federated States of)	—	—	8.8	—	6	15[g]	—	—	—	—
Nauru	—	—	—	—	11	—	—	—	—	—
Palau	—	—	—	8.1[i,n]	71	—	—	—	—	—
Somalia	—	—	34.1	—	7	36	—	—	—	—
Tuvalu	—	—	—	—	7	—	—	—	—	—
Zimbabwe	105	34.0	48.1	8.8[i]	19	17	—	—	34.9[g]	—

† Denotes indicators used to calculate the human poverty index (HPI-1).
a Data refer to the probability at birth of not surviving to age 40, multiplied by 100.
b Data refer to national illiteracy estimates from censuses or surveys conducted between 1999 and 2007, unless otherwise specified. Due to differences in methodology and timeliness of underlying data, comparisons across countries and over time should be made with caution.
c Data refer to the most recent year available during the period specified.
d Income poverty refers to the share of the population living on less than $1.25 a day. All countries with an income poverty rate of less than 2% were given equal rank. The rankings are based on countries for which data are available for both indicators. A positive figure indicates that the country performs better in income poverty than in human poverty, a negative the opposite.
e For the purposes of calculating the HPI-1 a value of 1% was assumed.
f Estimates cover urban areas only.
g Data refer to an earlier year outside the range of years specified.
h Data are from a national household survey.
i UNESCO Institute for Statistics estimates based on its Global Age-specific Literacy Projections model, April 2009.
j Data refer to an earlier year than that specified.
k In the absence of recent data, estimates for 2005 from UNESCO Institute for Statistics (2003), based on outdated census or survey information, were used and should be interpreted with caution: Bahamas 4.2, Barbados 0.3, Djibouti 29.7, Fiji 5.6, Gambia 57.5, Guyana 1.0 and Hong Kong, China (SAR) 5.4.
l National estimate.
m UNICEF, The State of the World's Children 2006.

TABLE 1.2

Human and income poverty, less developed countries, 2009 [CONTINUED]

SOURCE: Jeni Klugman, "Table 1. Human and Income Poverty," in *Human Development Report 2009—Overcoming Barriers: Human Mobility and Development*, United Nations Development Programme (UNDP), published 2009, Palgrave Macmillan, http://hdr.undp.org/en/media/HDR_2009_EN_Complete.pdf (accessed November 22, 2009). Reproduced with permission of Palgrave Macmillan. Data in column 3 from the UN *World Population Prospects: The 2008 Revision*, 2009. Data in column 4 from the UNESCO Institute for Statistics, correspondence on adult and youth literacy rates, Montreal, February 2009. Data in columns 5 and 6 from the UN's *Millennium Development Goals Indicators Database*, 2009. Data in columns 7–9 from The World Bank's *World Development Indicators*, 2009.

Notes:

— = Data is not available.

UNESCO = United Nations Educational, Scientific and Cultural Organization.
UNICEF = United Nations Children's Fund.
UNDP = United Nations Development Programme

[a] Data are from a national census of population.
[o] Data are from the Secretariat of the Organization of Eastern Caribbean States, based on national sources.
[p] Data refer to Serbia and Montenegro prior to its separation into two independent states in June 2006. Data exclude Kosovo.
[q] Data are from the Secretariat of the Caribbean Community, based on national sources.
[s] UNICEF, *The State of the World's Children 2005.*
[t] Estimates are weighted averages of urban and rural values.
[u] Estimates have been adjusted for arsenic contamination levels based on national surveys conducted and approved by the government.
[v] Estimates are adjusted by spatial consumer price index information.
[w] Data refer to North Sudan only.
[x] UNDP, *Timor-Leste: Human Development Report 2006: The Path out of Poverty.*

HPI-1 Ranks for 135 countries and areas

1 Czech Republic	36 China	71 Algeria	106 Lesotho
2 Croatia	37 Kazakhstan	72 Gabon	107 Guinea-Bissau
3 Hungary	38 Ecuador	73 Belize	108 Swaziland
4 Barbados	39 Bahrain	74 Tajikistan	109 Liberia
5 Bosnia and Herzegovina	40 Turkey	75 Iraq	110 Zambia
6 Uruguay	41 Thailand	76 Guatemala	111 Yemen
7 Serbia	42 Uzbekistan	77 Myanmar	112 Bangladesh
8 Montenegro	43 Brazil	78 Comoros	113 Madagascar
9 Macedonia (the Former Yugoslav Rep. of)	44 Dominican Republic	79 Fiji	114 Nigeria
10 Chile	45 Mauritius	80 Solomon Islands	115 Mauritania
11 Costa Rica	46 Suriname	81 Botswana	116 Burundi
12 Armenia	47 Peru	82 Egypt	117 Togo
13 Argentina	48 Guyana	83 Vanuatu	118 Angola
14 Singapore	49 Paraguay	84 Congo	119 Côte d'Ivoire
15 Albania	50 Azerbaijan	85 South Africa	120 Congo (Democratic Republic of the)
16 Belarus	51 Jamaica	86 Djibouti	121 Papua New Guinea
17 Cuba	52 Bolivia	87 Cambodia	122 Timor-Leste
18 Georgia	53 Saudi Arabia	88 India	123 Gambia
19 Qatar	54 Philippines	89 Ghana	124 Senegal
20 Romania	55 Viet Nam	90 Malawi	125 Central African Republic
21 Ukraine	56 Syrian Arab Republic	91 Uganda	126 Benin
22 Moldova	57 Sao Tome and Principe	92 Kenya	127 Mozambique
23 Mexico	58 Mongolia	93 Tanzania (United Republic of)	128 Sierra Leone
24 Occupied Palestinian Territories	59 Iran (Islamic Republic of)	94 Lao People's Democratic Republic	129 Guinea
25 Malaysia	60 Libyan Arab Jamahiriya	95 Cameroon	130 Ethiopia
26 Saint Lucia	61 Honduras	96 Morocco	131 Burkina Faso
27 Trinidad and Tobago	62 Cape Verde	97 Haiti	132 Chad
28 Venezuela (Bolivarian Republic of)	63 El Salvador	98 Equatorial Guinea	133 Mali
29 Jordan	64 Oman	99 Nepal	134 Niger
30 Panama	65 Tunisia	100 Rwanda	135 Afghanistan
31 Kyrgyzstan	66 Maldives	101 Pakistan	
32 Russian Federation	67 Sri Lanka	102 Bhutan	
33 Lebanon	68 Nicaragua	103 Eritrea	
34 Colombia	69 Indonesia	104 Sudan	
35 United Arab Emirates	70 Namibia	105 Zimbabwe	

TABLE 1.3

Human and income poverty, OECD (developed) countries, 2009

Human Development Index (HDI) rank	Human poverty index (HPI-2)		Probability at birth of not surviving to age 60[a, †] (% of cohort) 2005–2010	People lacking functional literacy skills[b, †] (% aged 16–65) 1994–2003	Long-term unemployment[†] (% of labour force) 2007	Population living below 50% of median income[†] 2000–2005[c]	HPI-2 rank minus income poverty rank[d]
	Rank	Value (%)					
Very high human development							
1 Norway	2	6.6	6.6	7.9	0.2	7.1	−6
2 Australia	14	12.0	6.4	17.0[e]	0.7	12.2	−4
3 Iceland	—	—	5.4	—	0.1	—	—
4 Canada	12	11.2	7.3	14.6	0.4	13.0	−8
5 Ireland	23	15.9	6.9	22.6[e]	1.4	16.2	0
6 Netherlands	3	7.4	7.1	10.5[e]	1.3	4.9[f]	1
7 Sweden	1	6.0	6.3	7.5[e]	0.7	5.6	−3
8 France	8	11.0	7.7	—[g]	3.1	7.3	−1
9 Switzerland	7	10.6	6.4	15.9	1.5	7.6	−3
10 Japan	13	11.6	6.2	—[g]	1.2	11.8[f, h]	−4
11 Luxembourg	10	11.2	7.8	—[g]	1.3	8.8	−4
12 Finland	5	7.9	8.2	10.4[e]	1.5	6.5	−1
13 United States	22	15.2	9.7	20.0	0.5	17.3	−2
14 Austria	9	11.0	7.6	—[g]	1.2	7.7	−2
15 Spain	17	12.4	7.1	—[g]	2.0	14.2	−4
16 Denmark	4	7.7	9.2	9.6[e]	0.7	5.6	1
17 Belgium	15	12.2	8.0	18.4[e, i]	3.8	8.1	3
18 Italy	25	29.8	6.8	47.0	2.8	12.8	6
20 New Zealand	—	—	7.6	18.4[e]	0.2	—	—
21 United Kingdom	21	14.6	7.8	21.8[e]	1.3	11.6	5
22 Germany	6	10.1	7.6	14.4[e]	4.8	8.4	−7
25 Greece	18	12.5	7.0	—[g]	4.1	14.3	−4
26 Korea (Republic of)	—	—	8.1	—	0.0	—	—
34 Portugal	—	—	8.7	—	3.7	—	—
36 Czech Republic	11	11.2	10.2	—[g]	2.8	4.9[f]	10
High human development							
41 Poland	19	12.8	13.2	—[g]	4.4	11.5	4
42 Slovakia	16	12.4	13.3	—[g]	7.8	7.0[f]	9
43 Hungary	20	13.2	16.4	—[g]	3.5	6.4[f]	15
53 Mexico	24	28.1	13.0	43.2[i]	0.1	18.4	−1
79 Turkey	—	—	14.9	—	3.1	—	—

Notes:
—Data is not available.
OECD = Office of Economic Cooperation and Development
[†]Denotes indicators used to calculate the HPI-2.
[a]Data refer to the probability at birth of not surviving to age 60, multiplied by 100.
[b]Based on scoring at level 1 on the prose literacy scale of the IALS. Data refer to the most recent year available during the period specified.
[c]Data refer to the most recent year available during the period specified.
[d]Income poverty refers to the share of the population living on less than 50% of the median adjusted disposable household income. A positive figure indicates that the country performs better in income poverty than in human poverty, a negative the opposite.
[e]OECD and Statistics Canada, *Literacy in the Information Age: Final Report of the International Adult Literacy Survey*, 2000.
[f]Data refer to an earlier year than the period specified.
[g]For calculating HPI-2 an estimate of 16.4%, the unweighted average of countries with available data, was applied.
[h]Smeeding, "Financial Poverty in Developed Countries: The Evidence from the Luxembourg Income Study," in *Background Paper for UNDP, Human Development Report 1997*.
[i]Data refer to Flanders only.
[j]Data refer to the state of Nuevo Leon only.

SOURCE: Jeni Klugman, "Table 2. Human and Income Poverty: OECD Countries," in *Human Development Report 2009—Overcoming Barriers: Human Mobility and Development*, United Nations Development Programme (UNDP), published 2009, Palgrave Macmillan, http://hdr.undp.org/en/media/HDR_2009_EN_Complete.pdf (accessed November 22, 2009). Reproduced with permission of Palgrave Macmillan. Data in column 3 from the UN *World Population Prospects: The 2008 Revision*, 2009. Data in column 4 from the OECD and Statistics Canada, *Learning a Living: First Results of the Adult Literacy and Life Skills Survey*, 2005, unless otherwise stated. Data in column 5 calculated using data from OECD Stat Extracts database, http://stats.oecd.org/index.aspx, accessed July 2009. Data in column 6 from the Luxembourg Income Study (LIS), *Key Figures*, 2009.

human and income poverty. That is, poverty-related conditions in this country are not as severe as in the other less-developed countries. The poverty-related conditions in the country ranked as 135 (Afghanistan) are more severe than in any other of the less-developed countries and it has the highest HPI-1 value. Some of the less-developed countries are not ranked due to missing data.

HPI-2 is used to measure relative poverty in industrialized (more developed) countries. (See Table 1.3.) It focuses on similar variables as HPI-1, but with adjustments to the conditions of the poor living in wealthier countries. The factors that go into determining the value of the HPI-2 are the percentage of people likely to die before the age of 60, the percentage of adults living with functional illiteracy (a degree of illiteracy that does not allow people to function at a basic level in reading and writing), and the proportion of people living with long-term unemployment and below the poverty line, which is set at 50% of the median (average) disposable household income. Additionally, HPI-2 examines the social alienation that can accompany persistent unemployment and poverty.

Table 1.3 shows that Sweden is doing the best in terms of human and income poverty among the OECD (developed or industrialized) countries listed and ranked. That is, the conditions of human and income poverty are the least severe in Sweden (rank 1 and the lowest HPI-2 value) among the developed countries shown. The conditions of human and income poverty are the most severe in Italy (rank 25) among the developed countries shown. The rank of the United States is 22, meaning that it has more severe conditions of human and income poverty than 21 other developed nations. A few of the developed countries are not ranked due to missing data.

OTHER COMPOSITE INDICATORS. Other less-commonly used composite poverty indicators are the Human Suffering Index and the Physical Quality of Life Index. The Human Suffering Index ranks the levels of suffering experienced by poor people in the areas of life expectancy, caloric intake, supply of clean water, child immunization, enrollment in secondary school, GDP per capita (per person), inflation rate, access to communications systems, technological development, civil rights, and political freedoms. The Physical Quality of Life Index combines measurements of life expectancy, infant mortality, and literacy rates.

POVERTY THRESHOLDS AND GUIDELINES IN THE UNITED STATES

Governmental agencies in the United States tend to avoid using the term *poverty line* because they consider it ambiguous. Instead, these agencies divide poverty measurement tools into two categories: thresholds and guidelines. The U.S. Census Bureau issues poverty thresholds,

which are statistical measurements used to track the total number of people living in poverty in the United States. By contrast, poverty guidelines are issued by the U.S. Department of Health and Human Services (HHS). They are used for the administrative purpose of determining eligibility for certain federal social programs and services, including Head Start, Medicare, the AIDS Drug Assistance Program, the National School Lunch Program, and the Special Supplemental Nutrition Program for Women, Infants, and Children, among many others.

Poverty thresholds are calculated and issued by the Census Bureau in September or October of the year following the year in which they are measured. This arrangement occurs because they are based on the Consumer Price Index (a measure of price changes in consumer goods) and the Current Population Survey, the results of which are not known until the end of the year in question or the beginning of the following year. The 2008 poverty thresholds are shown in Table 1.4. "Weighted average thresholds" means that the averages vary by family size, for one- and two-person units, and whether elderly people are part of the one- or two-person unit. Poverty thresholds are the same in all 50 states and the District of Columbia.

Table 1.4 shows that for 2008 the poverty threshold for a family of two adults and two children was an annual income of $21,834. If that family of four was composed of one adult and three children, the poverty threshold was $21,910. The poverty threshold for an individual under 65 years of age in 2008 was an annual income of $11,201.

Poverty guidelines are published early in the year in the *Federal Register* by the HHS. They are based on price changes over the preceding year. The guidelines are a simplified version of the thresholds, even though

TABLE 1.4

United States poverty thresholds, 2008

Size of family unit	Weighted average thresholds	Related children under 18 years								
		None	One	Two	Three	Four	Five	Six	Seven	Eight or more
One person (unrelated individual)	10,991									
Under 65 years	11,201	11,201								
65 years and over	10,326	10,326								
Two people	14,051									
Householder under 65 years	14,489	14,417	14,840							
Householder 65 years and over	13,030	13,014	14,784							
Three people	17,163	16,841	17,330	17,346						
Four people	22,025	22,207	22,570	21,834	21,910					
Five people	26,049	26,781	27,170	26,338	25,694	25,301				
Six people	29,456	30,803	30,925	30,288	29,677	28,769	28,230			
Eight people	37,220	39,640	39,990	39,270	38,639	37,744	36,608	35,426	35,125	
Nine people or more	44,346	47,684	47,915	47,278	46,743	45,864	44,656	43,563	43,292	41,624

SOURCE: "Poverty Thresholds for 2008 by Size of Family and Number of Related Children under 18 Years," in *Poverty*, U.S. Census Bureau, 2009, http://www.census.gov/hhes/www/poverty/threshld/thresh08.html (accessed November 24, 2009)

TABLE 1.5

United States poverty guidelines, 2009

2009 Poverty guidelines for the 48 contiguous states and the District of Columbia

Persons in family	Poverty guideline
1	$10,830
2	14,570
3	18,310
4	22,050
5	25,790
6	29,530
7	33,270
8	37,010

For families with more than 8 persons, add $3,740 for each additional person.

2009 poverty guidelines for Alaska

Persons in family	Poverty guideline
1	$13,530
2	18,210
3	22,890
4	27,570
5	32,250
6	36,930
7	41,610
8	46,290

For families with more than 8 persons, add $4,680 for each additional person.

2009 poverty guidelines for Hawaii

Persons in family	Poverty guideline
1	$12,460
2	16,760
3	21,060
4	25,360
5	29,660
6	33,960
7	38,260
8	42,560

For families with more than 8 persons, add $4,300 for each additional person.

SOURCE: "2009 Poverty Guidelines for the 48 Contiguous States and the District of Columbia," "2009 Poverty Guidelines for Alaska," and "2009 Poverty Guidelines for Hawaii," in "Annual Update of the HHS Poverty Guidelines," *Federal Register*, vol. 74, no. 14, January 23, 2009, http://www.cdphe.state.co.us/pp/womens/PovertyGuidelines/2009PovertyGuidelines_FedRegistrar.pdf (accessed November 24, 2009)

at the time of their respective publications thresholds and guidelines are considered equally accurate.

Table 1.5 shows the 2009 poverty guidelines. Unlike the poverty thresholds, the poverty guidelines for Alaska and Hawaii are separate from those for the 48 contiguous states and the District of Columbia. In addition, the poverty guidelines do not consider the makeup of the family in terms of numbers of adults, children, or elderly.

Comparing the 2008 poverty thresholds and the 2009 poverty guidelines (which were released within a few months of one another) shows that the values are close. The 2008 poverty threshold for an individual under 65 years of age was $11,201, whereas the 2009 poverty guideline for such an individual living in the continental United States

was $10,830. For a family of four, the poverty threshold was between $21,834 and $22,570. The poverty guideline for such a family was $22,050.

Controversies over U.S. Poverty Measurements

In "U.S. Needs Better Way Measure Poverty" (*Salt Lake Tribune*, October 24, 2009), Terry Haven discusses problems with the use of thresholds and guidelines, noting three commonly cited failures of the measurements:

- The method of measuring poverty in the United States does not take into account all forms of income—specifically, the federal poverty threshold does not count noncash forms of aid, such as food stamps, Medicaid, school lunch programs, housing assistance, and the State Children's Health Insurance Program. It also does not recognize the Earned Income Tax Credit, the monetary value of assets such as houses, or income brought into a household by nonfamily members, such as a mother's boyfriend.

- The current poverty threshold calculation that assumes spending on food accounts for one-third of a household's budget most likely fails to reflect more contemporary household spending patterns. In the first few years of the first decade of the 21st century food spending was estimated to be one-seventh of a household's income. Additionally, the calculation has not been accurately updated to reflect the costs of other current needs such as child care, housing, transportation, and higher taxes.

- The poverty threshold is measured in the same way across all states except Alaska and Hawaii, yet the cost of living across states differs.

Haven notes that the National Academy of Sciences (NAS) developed a measure of poverty that takes these three issues into account. The NAS model was recommended in the Measuring American Poverty Act of 2009, which was introduced to the U.S. House of Representatives (H.R. 2909) in June 2009 by Representative Jim McDermott (1936–; D-WA) and to the U.S. Senate (S. 1625) in August 2009 by Senator Christopher J. Dodd (1944–; D-CT). This legislation seeks to change how the United States measures poverty by using the NAS model and would be the first change in approximately 50 years. As of January 2010, this bill was in the first stage of the legislative process in both houses of Congress.

CLASSIFYING COUNTRIES BY LEVEL OF ECONOMIC DEVELOPMENT

In global determinations of poverty, countries are classified by how "developed" they are economically. During the Cold War (the period of escalating tensions between the United States and the Soviet Union that lasted from the 1950s until 1991) the terms *first world*, *second world*, and *third world* came into use. Originally, third-world countries were those that did not align themselves with either the first-world United States and its Western allies, or the second-world Soviet Union and other Eastern bloc countries, such as Bulgaria, Czechoslovakia, East Germany, Hungary, Poland, and Romania. Over time, however, the term *first world* came to refer to those countries that were industrialized and relatively wealthy, whereas *third world* was used to describe countries that were poor, indebted to other nations, and not industrialized.

With the end of the Cold War and the dissolution of the Soviet Union in 1991, the term *second world* was abandoned. *First world* came to refer to all countries that are industrially and technologically developed, whereas *third world* described poor countries that are largely undeveloped. However, the idea of a third world was considered derogatory—as if poor countries were hopelessly removed from the rest of the world when their people make up at least two-thirds of the world's population.

Instead, academics and researchers began using the terms *developed*, *developing*, and *underdeveloped* to describe industrialized countries, countries whose economies are expanding, and those that remain poor and without large-scale industry or technology, respectively. Still others prefer the terms *least developed countries*, *majority world*, or *two-thirds world* when discussing countries that belong to the poorest segment of the global economy. The term *fourth world* is sometimes used to describe either the very poorest social or economic groups within underdeveloped countries or indigenous or marginalized people within any country.

There is still no widespread consensus about which terms to use. This book discusses countries using the following designations and groupings:

- Chapter 3, underdeveloped countries, including sub-Saharan Africa and the least developed countries of Asia (Afghanistan and Timor-Leste)

- Chapter 4, emerging and transition countries, including East Asia and India

- Chapter 5, developing countries, including Latin America, Caribbean, and central Asia (the CIS and North Korea)

- Chapter 6, developed countries, including the United States, western Europe, and the Russian Federation

CHAPTER 2
THE CAUSES OF POVERTY AND THE SEARCH FOR SOLUTIONS

Massive poverty and obscene inequality are such terrible scourges of our times—times in which the world boasts breathtaking advances in science, technology, industry and wealth accumulation—that they have to rank along-side slavery and apartheid as social evils.

—Nelson Mandela, Speech in Trafalgar Square (London, England), February 3, 2005

Poverty is a multidimensional human problem with many causes and contributing factors. It is experienced on every continent (except Antarctica, only because it does not have permanent human residents) and by all races. It is directly related to health, education, housing, political opportunities, and other issues. Likewise, poverty worsens people's social status and diminishes their involvement in their communities and in the larger sphere. These human development factors are critical to understanding poverty. They are also critical to solving the immense problem of poverty.

UNEMPLOYMENT

Many people throughout the world are in poverty because they are unemployed or underemployed and live in areas where economic opportunities are severely limited. Natural disasters, war, and other factors contribute to regional economic difficulties, but poor health and nutrition coupled with low education compound the cycle of poverty. The United Nations' (UN) International Labour Office (ILO) estimates in *Global Employment Trends* (January 2009, http://www.ilo.org/wcmsp5/groups/public/—dgreports/—dcomm/documents/publication/wcms_101461.pdf) that in 2008 there were approximately 190.2 million unemployed people in the world, an all-time high. (See Figure 2.1.) The global unemployment rate in 2008 was 6%, which approximately equaled the unemployment rate of 2000 to 2002, but was higher than the rates of 1999 and 2003 to 2005. (The unemployment rate is the percentage of the labor force that actively seeks work but cannot find it.)

Figure 2.2 shows that the number of employed people rose to an all-time high in 2008 to approximately 3 billion, but increases in the world's working-age population (those aged 15 years and older) caused the employment-to-population ratio to fall to 61.2%. That is, approximately 61.2% of the working-age population of the world was employed in 2008.

The unemployed are not the only people who live in poverty, however. The *working poor* are those whose low earnings prevent them from lifting themselves and their families above the poverty threshold (either the international threshold of US $1.25 or US $2 per day or the national poverty threshold of their individual country). The ILO reports that in 2007 approximately 1.2 billion people were working but earning only $2 per day; of that group, 609.5 million were working and living on $1.25 per day. (See Table 1.1 in Chapter 1.)

These figures address a common misconception about poverty: that poor people do not work. Regional rates of unemployment further illustrate the falsity of this assumption because global unemployment rates are relatively low. The ILO indicates in *Global Employment Trends* that the unemployment rate in sub-Saharan Africa, the overall poorest region in the world, was 7.9% in 2008; in Southeast Asia and the Pacific, which contains some of the poorest and most populous countries in the world, the unemployment rate was 5.7%; and in Latin America and the Caribbean the rate was 7.3%. By comparison, the unemployment rate in developed economies and the European Union was 6.4% in 2008.

In *A Profile of the Working Poor, 2007* (March 2009, http://www.bls.gov/cps/cpswp2007.pdf), the U.S. Bureau of Labor Statistics (BLS) defines the working poor in the United States as those people who participate at least 27 weeks per year in the labor force, either working or actively looking for work, but still live below the U.S. poverty threshold. The U.S. poverty thresholds for 2008

FIGURE 2.1

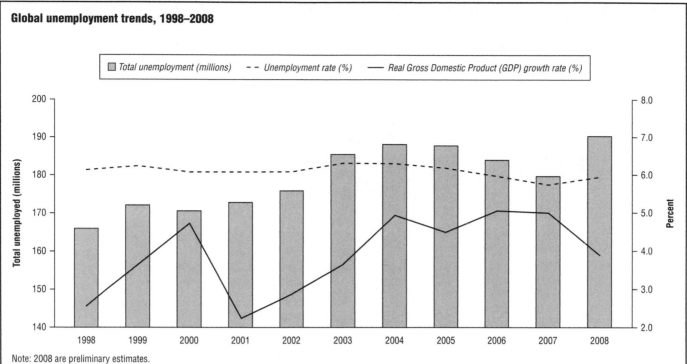

Global unemployment trends, 1998–2008

☐ Total unemployment (millions) – – Unemployment rate (%) —— Real Gross Domestic Product (GDP) growth rate (%)

Note: 2008 are preliminary estimates.

SOURCE: "Figure 1. Global Unemployment Trends, 1998–2008," in *Global Employment Trends*, International Labour Organization, January 2009, http://www.ilo.org/wcmsp5/groups/public/--dgreports/--dcomm/documents/publication/wcms_101461.pdf (accessed November 24, 2009). Copyright © 2009 International Labour Organization. Data from International Labour Organization (ILO) Trends Econometric Models, December 2008; International Monetary Fund (IMF), World Economic Outlook, November 2008.

FIGURE 2.2

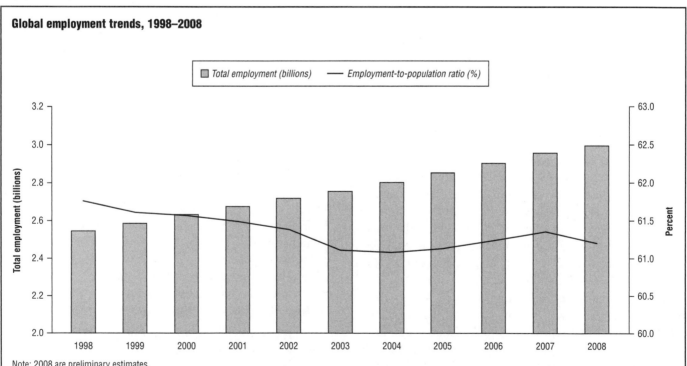

Global employment trends, 1998–2008

☐ Total employment (billions) —— Employment-to-population ratio (%)

Note: 2008 are preliminary estimates.

SOURCE: "Figure 2. Global Employment Trends, 1998–2008," in *Global Employment Trends*, International Labour Organization, January 2009, http://www.ilo.org/wcmsp5/groups/public/--dgreports/--dcomm/documents/publication/wcms_101461.pdf (accessed November 24, 2009). Copyright © 2009 International Labour Organization. Data from International Labour Organization (ILO) Trends Econometric Models, December 2008; International Monetary Fund (IMF), World Economic Outlook, November 2008.

are shown in Table 1.4 in Chapter 1. The BLS notes that more than 7.5 million Americans were classified as working poor in 2007. (See Table 2.1.)

Table 2.1 shows the poverty status of people in the labor force in the United States from 2004 to 2007. The category "total persons" means all the people in the labor force who worked 27 weeks or more during that year, regardless of their relationship to anyone else in the labor force. The category "unrelated individuals" means all the people in the labor force who were not living with relatives. "Primary families" include a "reference person"

and all the people living in the household who are related to the reference person by birth, marriage, or adoption. Thus, many people in the primary family may work, but in this category the family is counted as a unit.

The 7.5 million people who were classified as working poor in 2007 made up 5.1% of the U.S. labor force. (See Table 2.1.) This rate decreased from 5.6% in 2004. Figure 2.3 tracks working poor individuals across a longer period, from 1987 to 2007. The percentage of working poor individuals has risen and fallen over time, with the highest rate, 6.7%, registered in 1993, and the lowest rate, 4.7%, achieved in 2000.

Looking at the problem on the family level, 6.4% of working families were among the working poor in 2007. (See Table 2.1.) Women are more likely than men to be classified among the working poor. In 2007, 4.6% of the working male population 16 years and older were living in poverty, whereas 5.8% of the working female population 16 years and older were living in poverty. (See Table 2.2.) Men 16 to 19 years of age were more likely to be members of the working poor than were older individuals. Women 20 to 24 years of age were more likely to be members of the working poor than were older individuals. Of young people of both sexes who worked in the labor force for 27 weeks or more in 2007, 10.2% of the 16- to 19-year-olds and 10.6% of the 20- to 24-year-olds were living in poverty. Workers aged 35 to 44 (5%) were less than half as likely as younger workers to be among the working poor, and workers 55 to 64 years old (2.6%) were about one-fourth as likely.

African-American and Hispanic workers were more likely to be in poverty in 2007 than were Asian American and white workers of a comparable age. (See Table 2.2.)

TABLE 2.1

Poverty status of total persons, unrelated individuals, and primary families in the labor force for 27 weeks or more, United States, 2004–07

(Numbers in thousands)

Characteristic	2004	2005	2006	2007
Total persons[a]	140,908	142,824	145,229	146,567
In poverty	7,836	7,744	7,427	7,521
Poverty rate	5.6	5.4	5.1	5.1
Unrelated individuals	30,694	31,422	31,887	33,226
In poverty	2,742	2,846	2,741	2,558
Poverty rate	8.9	9.1	8.6	7.7
Primary families[b]	63,912	64,360	65,388	65,158
In poverty	4,261	4,094	3,960	4,169
Poverty rate	6.7	6.4	6.1	6.4

[a]Includes persons in families, not shown separately.
[b]Primary families with at least one member in the labor force for more than half the year.

SOURCE: "Table A. Poverty Status of Persons and Primary Families in the Labor Force for 27 Weeks or More, 2004–07," in *A Profile of the Working Poor, 2007*, U.S. Department of Labor, U.S. Bureau of Labor Statistics, March 2009, http://www.bls.gov/cps/cpswp2007.pdf (accessed November 24, 2009)

FIGURE 2.3

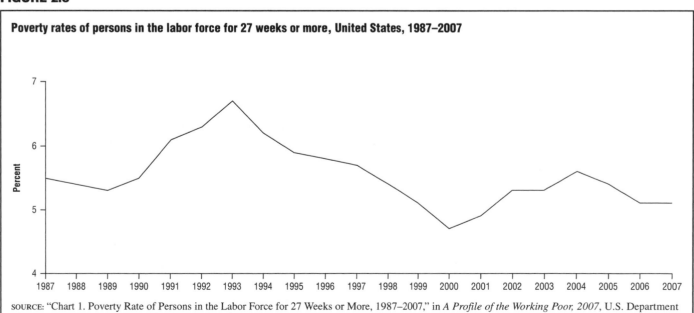

Poverty rates of persons in the labor force for 27 weeks or more, United States, 1987–2007

SOURCE: "Chart 1. Poverty Rate of Persons in the Labor Force for 27 Weeks or More, 1987–2007," in *A Profile of the Working Poor, 2007*, U.S. Department of Labor, U.S. Bureau of Labor Statistics, March 2009, http://www.bls.gov/cps/cpswp2007.pdf (accessed November 24, 2009)

TABLE 2.2

Poverty rate of persons in the labor force for 27 weeks or more by age, sex, race, and Hispanic or Latino ethnicity, United States, 2007

Age and sex	Total	White	Black or African American	Asian	Hispanic or Latino ethnicity
			Rate[a]		
Total, 16 years and older	**5.1**	**4.5**	**9.7**	**3.9**	**10.5**
16 to 19 years	10.2	9.4	17.0	9.2	14.9
20 to 24 years	10.6	9.7	17.4	4.5	12.9
25 to 34 years	6.7	5.8	12.9	3.8	11.5
35 to 44 years	5.0	4.4	9.1	3.5	10.9
45 to 54 years	3.3	3.0	5.4	3.5	8.5
55 to 64 years	2.6	2.1	5.9	5.1	6.1
65 years and older	1.7	1.4	5.0	1.3	3.7
Men, 16 years and older	**4.6**	**4.2**	**7.5**	**3.9**	**10.3**
16 to 19 years	10.0	9.1	18.0	(b)	14.1
20 to 24 years	8.2	7.5	12.6	2.0	11.6
25 to 34 years	5.7	5.5	8.1	3.1	11.6
35 to 44 years	4.7	4.3	8.0	3.5	10.3
45 to 54 years	3.4	3.1	5.0	4.0	8.9
55 to 64 years	2.4	2.0	4.3	6.2	5.8
65 years and older	1.5	1.3	3.3	1.9	4.0
Women, 16 years and older	**5.8**	**4.8**	**11.6**	**3.9**	**10.7**
16 to 19 years	10.4	9.7	16.3	(b)	16.1
20 to 24 years	13.5	12.2	22.5	7.3	14.9
25 to 34 years	7.8	6.1	17.0	4.7	11.3
35 to 44 years	5.4	4.6	10.1	3.5	11.8
45 to 54 years	3.3	2.8	5.8	2.9	7.8
55 to 64 years	2.8	2.1	7.1	3.9	6.4
65 years and older	2.0	1.6	6.5	0.6	3.2

[a]Number below the poverty level as a percent of the total in the labor force for 27 weeks or more.
[b]Data not shown where base is less than 80,000.
Note: Estimates for the above race groups (white, black or African American, and Asian) do not sum to totals because data are not presented for all races. Persons whose ethnicity is identified as Hispanic or Latino may be of any race.

SOURCE: Adapted from "Table 2. People in the Labor Force for 27 Weeks or More: Poverty Status by Age, Sex, Race, and Hispanic or Latino Ethnicity, 2007," in *A Profile of the Working Poor, 2007*, U.S. Department of Labor, U.S. Bureau of Labor Statistics, March 2009, http://www.bls.gov/cps/cpswp2007.pdf (accessed November 24, 2009)

Asian-Americans aged 16 to 44 and 65 years and older were less likely to be members of the working poor than whites of the same age groups. Asian-Americans aged 45 to 64 were more likely to be members of the working poor than whites of the same age group. Among teenage workers, 17% of African-Americans and 14.9% of Hispanics were living in poverty, compared with 9.4% of whites and 9.2% of Asian-Americans.

In *Profile of the Working Poor*, the BLS explains that those having higher levels of education are much less likely to be a part of the working poor. Those most likely to be a part of the working poor were people with less than a high school education, whereas those least likely to be a part of the working poor were college graduates.

The Working Poor in the Informal Economy

The ILO reports in "Training and the Informal Economy" (2008, http://www.ilo.org/public/english/region/ampro/cinterfor/temas/informal/about.htm) that many of the world's working poor are employed in the informal labor sector, or informal economy. The term *informal economy* refers to the exchange of goods and services outside of national and international regulatory guidelines, meaning that the people who work in the informal economy do not receive legal protection or employer-sponsored benefits and do not have official means by which to better their working situations. The ILO notes that the informal sector is the main type of employment in Latin American countries, where more than 53% of workers are a part of this sector.

Work in the informal economy is more common in developing than in developed countries, although informal labor does exist in wealthier countries, mostly in the form of self-employment and part-time and temporary work (the latter two are known as nonstandard wage employment). In the United States informal workers include casual laborers, as well as some employees with nonstandard pay arrangements, including those who work "under the table" (i.e., they are paid in cash). According to the ILO, in *The Informal Economy* (March 2007, http://www.ilo.org/public/english/standards/relm/gb/docs/gb298/pdf/esp-4.pdf), the formal segment of the economy in sub-Saharan Africa employs no more than 10% of the workforce. Thus, the rest of the working population in this developing region is employed in the informal economy. The ILO notes that "widespread underemployment and informality have therefore become structural characteristics of the developing countries' economies and not a peripheral problem that can be addressed in isolation from the mainstream development strategies. Curbing the spread of informality means first and foremost making employment a central concern of economic and social policies, promoting employment-friendly macroeconomic frameworks and making the productive sectors of the economy a priority target of poverty reduction strategies."

The ILO indicates that even though women have less of a presence in the overall labor force, they account for a greater percentage of informal workers. Children also make up a large proportion of the informal economy, especially in developing countries. The informal economy is not necessarily equated with the criminal economy, but children (most notably girls) working in informal employment are particularly vulnerable to the abuses and exploitation of unregulated work. Child laborers may end up being sold

or tricked into the world of human trafficking, prostitution, slavery, and debt bondage. This kind of forced labor is found not only in developing countries but also in developed countries. (See Figure 2.4.)

Working conditions in the informal sector vary greatly. Some enterprises exist in the informal economy simply because they cannot afford to abide by the bureaucratic regulations of the formal economy, whereas others deliberately avoid providing their workers with even the most reasonable legal protections. Furthermore, working in the informal economy does not necessarily mean living in poverty or even earning low wages. Nonetheless, in *Decent Work and the Transition to Formalization: Recent Trends, Policy Debates, and Good Practices* (December 2008, http://www.ilo.org/public/english/employment/policy/events/informal/download/report.pdf), the ILO's Tripartite Interregional Symposium on the Informal Economy points out the

FIGURE 2.4

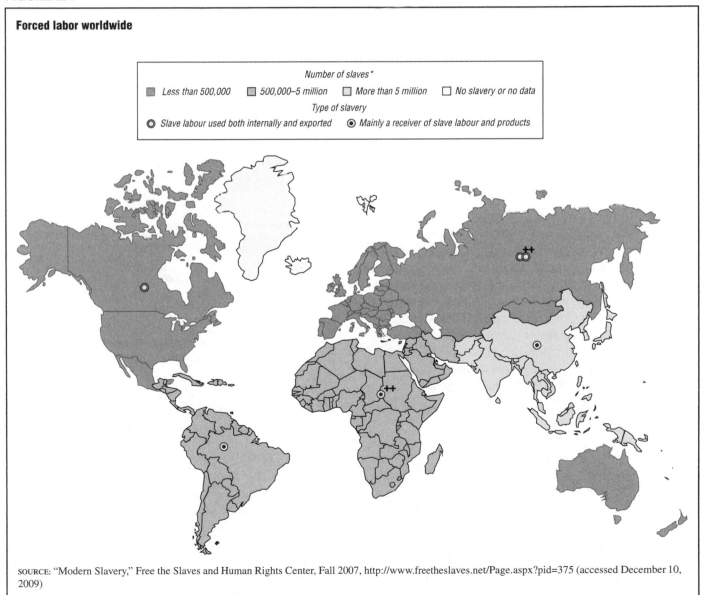

Forced labor worldwide

SOURCE: "Modern Slavery," Free the Slaves and Human Rights Center, Fall 2007, http://www.freetheslaves.net/Page.aspx?pid=375 (accessed December 10, 2009)

following serious problems with the informal economy and suggests that countries must therefore work toward the formalization of their workforces:

- Work in the informal economy is often characterized by small or undefined work places, unsafe and unhealthy working conditions, low level of skills and productivity, low or irregular incomes, long working hours and lack of access to information, markets, finance, training and technology.

- Workers in the informal economy are not recognized, registered, regulated or protected under labor legislation and social protection.

- Workers and economic units in the informal economy are generally characterized by poverty leading to powerlessness, exclusion and vulnerability.

- Most workers and economic units in the informal economy do not enjoy secure property rights, which does deprive them access to both capital and credit.

- They have difficulty accessing the legal and judicial system to enforce contracts and have limited or no access to public infrastructure and benefits.

- Women, young persons, migrants and all the workers are especially vulnerable to the most serious decent work deficits in the informal economy.

POVERTY, EDUCATION, AND LITERACY

As mentioned previously, the BLS describes in *Profile of the Working Poor* the inverse relationship between poverty and level of educational attainment: those with higher levels of educational attainment are less likely to be a part of the working poor, and those with lower levels of educational attainment are more likely to be a part of the working poor. In *Education for All Global Monitoring Report 2006: Literacy for Life* (2005, http://unesdoc.unesco.org/images/0014/001416/141639e.pdf), the UN Educational, Scientific, and Cultural Organization (UNESCO) names literacy as a basic human right and affirms its role in improving the human condition.

According to UNESCO, in *Education for All Global Monitoring Report 2009: Overcoming Inequality—Why Governance Matters* (2008, http://unesdoc.unesco.org/images/0017/001776/177683e.pdf), an illiterate person is someone who cannot read or write a simple statement in his or her national language and understand it. Figure 2.5 shows the countries with the greatest numbers of adult illiterates from 2000 to 2006. India and China, the leaders in the number of adult illiterates, also have large populations. However, comparing the gross national income

FIGURE 2.5

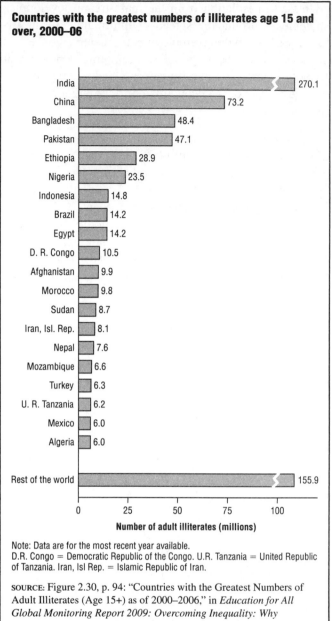

Countries with the greatest numbers of illiterates age 15 and over, 2000–06

Number of adult illiterates (millions)

Country	Value
India	270.1
China	73.2
Bangladesh	48.4
Pakistan	47.1
Ethiopia	28.9
Nigeria	23.5
Indonesia	14.8
Brazil	14.2
Egypt	14.2
D. R. Congo	10.5
Afghanistan	9.9
Morocco	9.8
Sudan	8.7
Iran, Isl. Rep.	8.1
Nepal	7.6
Mozambique	6.6
Turkey	6.3
U. R. Tanzania	6.2
Mexico	6.0
Algeria	6.0
Rest of the world	155.9

Note: Data are for the most recent year available.
D.R. Congo = Democratic Republic of the Congo. U.R. Tanzania = United Republic of Tanzania. Iran, Isl Rep. = Islamic Republic of Iran.

SOURCE: Figure 2.30, p. 94: "Countries with the Greatest Numbers of Adult Illiterates (Age 15+) as of 2000–2006," in *Education for All Global Monitoring Report 2009: Overcoming Inequality: Why Governance Matters*, United Nations Educational, Scientific and Cultural Organization (UNESCO), 2008, http://unesdoc.unesco.org/images/0017/001776/177683e.pdf (accessed November 24, 2009). Copyright © UNESCO, 2008. Used by permission of UNESCO.

(GNI; the total value produced within a country plus income from other countries minus payments made to other countries) per capita (per person) of the countries on this figure to countries not on this figure reveals a huge discrepancy in financial wealth. For example, the UN Children's Fund notes in "Information by Country and Programme" (2009, http://www.unicef.org/infobycountry/) that the GNI per capita of Bangladesh, India, and China in 2007 was $470, $950, and $2,360, respectively. In comparison, the GNI per capita that same year for France, the United States, and Norway was $38,500, $46,040, and $76,450, respectively.

TABLE 2.3

Estimated number of illiterates age 15 and over, worldwide by region, 1985–94 and 2000–06, with projections to 2015

	1985–1994*		2000–2006*		2015		Percentage change	
	Total (000)	Female (%)	Total (000)	Female (%)	Total (000)	Female (%)	1985–1994 to 2000–2006	2000–2006 to 2015
World	871,096	63	775,894	64	706,130	64	−11	−9
Developing countries	858,680	63	766,716	64	698,332	64	−11	−9
Developed countries	8,686	64	7,660	62	7,047	59	−12	−8
Countries in transition	3,730	84	1,519	71	752	59	−59	−51
Sub-Saharan Africa	133,013	61	161,088	62	147,669	60	21	−8
Arab States	55,311	63	57,798	67	53,339	69	4	−9
Central Asia	960	74	784	68	328	50	−18	−58
East Asia and the Pacific	229,172	69	112,637	71	81,398	71	−51	−28
East Asia	227,859	69	110,859	71	79,420	71	−51	−28
Pacific	1,313	56	1,778	55	1,979	52	35	11
South and West Asia	394,719	61	392,725	63	380,256	63	−1	−3
Latin America and the Caribbean	39,575	55	36,946	55	31,225	54	−7	−15
Caribbean	2,870	50	2,803	48	2,749	45	−2	−2
Latin America	36,705	55	34,142	56	28,476	55	−7	−17
North America and Western Europe	6,400	63	5,682	61	5,115	59	−11	−10
Central and Eastern Europe	11,945	78	8,235	80	6,801	79	−31	−17

*Data are for the most recent year available.

SOURCE: Table 2.11, p. 93: "Estimated Number of Adult Illiterates (Age 15+) in 1985–1994 and 2000–2006, with Projections to 2015, by Region," in *Education for All Global Monitoring Report 2009: Overcoming Inequality: Why Governance Matters*, United Nations Educational, Scientific and Cultural Organization (UNESCO), 2008, http://unesdoc.unesco.org/images/0017/001776/177683e.pdf (accessed November 24, 2009). Copyright © UNESCO, 2008. Used by permission of UNESCO.

UNESCO notes that the number of illiterate people worldwide declined somewhat from 871.1 million adults in 1985–94 to 775.9 million adults in 2000–06. (See Table 2.3.) The number is projected to decline further to 706.1 million adults by 2015. In most regions of the world, more than 50% of the illiterate population is female, even in developed countries. UNESCO explains in *Education for All Global Monitoring Report 2009* that this disparity reflects educational disadvantages of women over men from the past. Women are catching up with men in access to education worldwide. As this occurs, disparities in literacy are reduced or disappear altogether. UNESCO also notes that 80% of adult illiterates live in the 20 less-developed countries shown in Figure 2.5.

Table 2.4 shows the percent of adults who are literate worldwide and by region. The literacy rate rose from 76% in 1985–94 to 84% in 2000–06, and is projected to increase to 87% in 2015. Developed countries and countries in transition had 99% literacy rates in 2000–06, compared with a 79% literacy rate in developing countries. In North America and western Europe in 2000–06, the Gender Parity Index showed that females and males in that region had equal numbers who were literate. That is, for every 100 literate males there were 100 literate females in the population. That was not the case in sub-Saharan Africa and the Arab states, however. Only 75 females were literate for every 100 males in those regions of the world. In the Caribbean the ratio was reversed; for every 100 literate males there were 105 literate females.

How can Table 2.3, which shows that 62% of the adult illiterates were female in developed countries in 2000–06, be reconciled with Table 2.4, which shows that the Gender Parity Index for literacy rates in developed countries during this same period was 1.00? The explanation is that the illiterate population in developed countries is relatively small and consists primarily of older adults. In this older, illiterate population females outnumber males for two reasons: the male-female educational disparities of the past are reflected in older populations, and women, on average, outlive men. UNESCO points out in *Education for All Global Monitoring Report 2009* that the most dramatic increases in global literacy rates occurred in youths between the ages of 15 and 24. In 1985–94 only 84% of the world's youth were literate. By 2000–06 this number had risen to 89% most notably in South and West Asia, sub-Saharan Africa, the Caribbean, and the Arab states. The regions with low youth literacy rates (under 80%) were sub-Saharan Africa and South and West Asia.

Not only do rates of illiteracy correlate positively with poverty among regions and countries of the world but also income-based educational disparities exist within countries. Table 2.5 shows the differences in average years of education attained by the poorest 20% and the richest 20% of people aged 17 to 22 in a list of selected countries. In Mozambique, for example, someone in the poorest 20% of the 17- to 22-year-old population had on average 1.9 years of education in 2003, compared with 5 years of education for someone from the richest 20%. In

TABLE 2.4

Estimated rates of literacy for persons 15 and over, worldwide by region, 1985–94 and 2000–06, with projections to 2015

| | 1985–1994* | | 2000–2006* | | Projected 2015 | |
| | Literacy rates (%) | GPI | Literacy rates (%) | GPI | Literacy rates (%) | GPI |
	Total	(F/M)	Total	(F/M)	Total	(F/M)
World	76	0.85	84	0.89	87	0.92
Developing countries	68	0.77	79	0.85	84	0.90
Developed countries	99	0.99	99	1.00	99	0.99
Countries in transition	98	0.98	99	1.00	100	1.00
Sub-Saharan Africa	53	0.71	62	0.75	72	0.86
Arab States	58	0.66	72	0.75	79	0.81
Central Asia	98	0.98	99	0.99	99	1.00
East Asia and the Pacific	82	0.84	93	0.94	95	0.96
East Asia	82	0.84	93	0.94	96	0.96
Pacific	94	0.99	93	0.99	93	1.00
South and West Asia	48	0.57	64	0.71	71	0.78
Latin America and the Caribbean	87	0.98	91	0.98	93	0.99
Caribbean	66	1.02	74	1.05	78	1.07
Latin America	87	0.97	91	0.98	94	0.99
North America and Western Europe	99	0.99	99	1.00	99	1.00
Central and Eastern Europe	96	0.96	97	0.97	98	0.98

*Data are for the most recent year available.
GPI = Gender Parity Index, the ratio of females to males.

SOURCE: Table 2.12, p. 95: "Estimated Adult Literacy Rates (Age 15+) in 1985–1994 and 2000–2006, with Projections to 2015, by Region," in *Education for All Global Monitoring Report 2009: Overcoming Inequality: Why Governance Matters*, United Nations Educational, Scientific and Cultural Organization (UNESCO), 2008, http://unesdoc.unesco.org/images/0017/001776/177683e.pdf (accessed November 24, 2009). Copyright © UNESCO, 2008. Used by permission of UNESCO.

TABLE 2.5

Average years of education for poorest and richest 20% of 17- to 22-year-olds, selected countries, 2001–05

| | Poorest 20% | Richest 20% |
	(years)	
Bangladesh, 2004	3.7	8.1
Burkina Faso, 2003	0.8	5.6
Ethiopia, 2005	1.6	7.4
Ghana, 2003	3.2	9.2
Guatemala, 1999	1.9	8.3
India, 2005	4.4	11.1
Mali, 2001	0.4	4.8
Mozambique, 2003	1.9	5.0
Nicaragua, 2001	2.5	9.2
Nigeria, 2003	3.9	9.9
Peru, 2000	6.5	11.1
Philippines, 2003	6.3	11.0
U.R. Tanzania, 2004	3.9	8.1
Zambia, 2001	4.0	9.0

SOURCE: "Table 1.1. Average Years of Education for Poorest and Richest 20% of 17- to 22-Year-Olds, Selected Countries, Most Recent Year," in *Education for All Global Monitoring Report 2009: Overcoming Inequality: Why Governance Matters*, United Nations Educational, Scientific and Cultural Organization (UNESCO), 2008, http://unesdoc.unesco.org/images/0017/001776/177683e.pdf (accessed November 24, 2009). Data from Demographic and Health Surveys.

Bangladesh the gap between the rich and poor was 4.4 years of schooling in 2004, and in India the educational gap was 6.7 years in 2005.

HUNGER AND MALNUTRITION

Hunger's relation to poverty is reciprocal: poverty usually results in hunger, but hunger is a factor that keeps people in poverty. Deficiencies in nutrients such as iodine, vitamin A, iron, and zinc contribute to weakened immune systems, anemia, learning disabilities, complications in pregnancy and childbirth, and many childhood diseases. These conditions result in poverty-causing problems such as absenteeism and poor performance at school and work, unemployment, illiteracy, and the continuing cycle of poverty. (See Figure 2.6.)

In *The State of Food Insecurity in the World 2009: Economic Crises—Impacts and Lessons Learned* (2009, ftp://ftp.fao.org/docrep/fao/012/i0876e/i0876e.pdf), the Food and Agriculture Organization (FAO) of the UN notes that there were about 1 billion people suffering from undernourishment in 2009. Figure 2.7 shows the global distribution of undernourishment. Most undernourished individuals live in developing countries. The FAO indicates in *Feeding the World, Eradicating Hunger* (November 2009, ftp://ftp.fao.org/docrep/fao/Meeting/018/k6077e.pdf) that one out of three children under the age of five in developing countries is stunted due to chronic malnutrition and that 148 million children in these countries are underweight. Sub-Saharan Africa is the region with the highest prevalence of undernourishment.

Development Goals

On September 8, 2000, 189 member countries of the UN adopted the Millennium Declaration (http://www.un.org/millennium/declaration/ares552e.htm), an agreement to increase the state of human development, including reducing poverty. The declaration includes a commitment to

FIGURE 2.6

Relationship of hunger and malnutrition to other problems of poverty

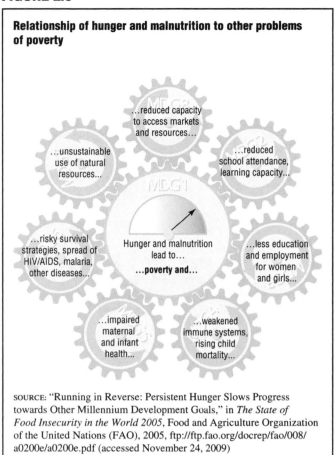

SOURCE: "Running in Reverse: Persistent Hunger Slows Progress towards Other Millennium Development Goals," in *The State of Food Insecurity in the World 2005*, Food and Agriculture Organization of the United Nations (FAO), 2005, ftp://ftp.fao.org/docrep/fao/008/a0200e/a0200e.pdf (accessed November 24, 2009)

reduce the number of nuclear weapons, protect the environment, and focus attention on Africa. However, a significant section of the declaration outlines the Millennium Development Goals (MDGs; http://www.undp.org/mdg/basics.shtml), a list of eight human development goals to be reached by 2015:

1. Eradicate extreme poverty and hunger

2. Achieve universal primary education

3. Promote gender equality and empower women

4. Reduce child mortality

5. Improve maternal health

6. Combat HIV/AIDS, malaria, and other diseases

7. Ensure environmental sustainability

8. Develop a global partnership for development

All eight MDGs involve poverty indicators directly, or they are linked to the problem of poverty in some way. The MDGs have become a standard way to gauge human development progress in all countries and regions of the world. Whether a country is "on target" to reach the goals by the 2015 deadline is a telling indicator in itself of the standard of living in that country. Since the adoption of the MDGs, some progress has been made toward achieving the goals. However, as the UN concedes, progress has been slow and uneven, with some regions moving forward and some falling behind. Table 2.6 presents specific targets for each goal and indicators for monitoring the progress of those targets.

As Table 2.6 shows, Target 1.C is "halve, between 1990 and 2015, the proportion of people who suffer from hunger." Figure 2.8 shows the number of undernourished people in the world from 1969–71 to 2008 and projected to 2009. The number of undernourished people fell from 1990–92 to 1995–97, but then began to rise, with a dramatic increase projected from 2008 to 2009.

The FAO indicates in *State of Food Insecurity in the World 2009* that the current crisis in undernutrition is "historically unprecedented" and notes that several factors have converged to bring this crisis about. Food prices began to rise after 2000 and reached a high in mid-2008 in conjunction with the food and fuel crisis that occurred between 2006 and 2008. The food crisis began in 2006 with price spikes due to droughts in grain-producing nations, diminishing food reserves worldwide, and rising oil prices. The rise in oil prices made agriculture and food transportation more expensive. In addition, it resulted in an increased use of biofuels, which resulted in some crops being used for biofuel production rather than for food production. This global food crisis resulted in great hardship for poor families. In many cases they had to eat less because they could not afford to buy enough food to adequately feed themselves and their families. The global economic crisis that had its roots in 2007 made matters worse. The FAO notes that the number of food-insecure people was expected to increase worldwide from 17% in 2008 to 19% in 2009.

Looking at undernourishment regionally, Figure 2.9 shows that the largest number of undernourished was in Asia and the Pacific from 1990–92 to 2008. Even though the number of undernourished fell from 1990–92 to 1995–97, the number began to rise again, almost reaching the 1990–92 level by 2008. The number of undernourished in sub-Saharan Africa was below the number in Asia and the Pacific, but it began to rise after 1990–92.

Figure 2.10 shows the proportion of undernourished people in the developing world from 1969–71 to 2008 and projected to 2009. The proportion of undernourished people declined in the developing world from 34% in 1969–71 to 16% in 2004–06, which means the developing world reached the MDG Target 1.C. This was accomplished by investments in agriculture in the developing world, which led to increased yields of grain and lower cereal prices. Nevertheless, the proportion of undernourished began to rise after 2004–06 as development assistance devoted to agriculture declined and the economic crisis took hold,

FIGURE 2.7

Percent undernourished worldwide, by country, 2009

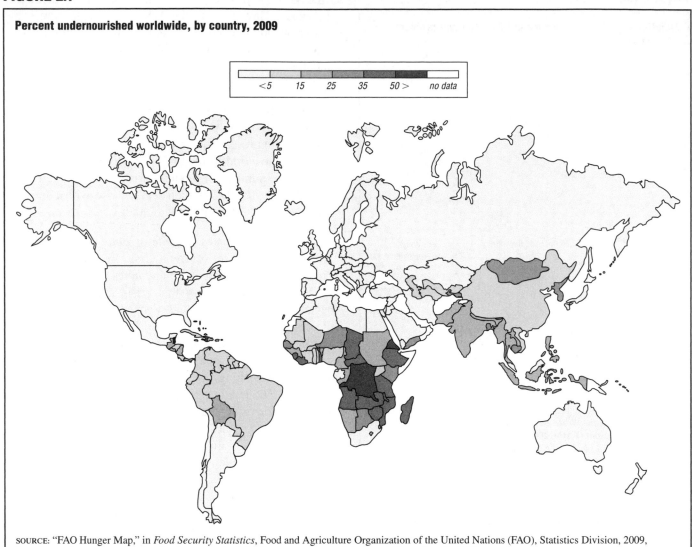

SOURCE: "FAO Hunger Map," in *Food Security Statistics*, Food and Agriculture Organization of the United Nations (FAO), Statistics Division, 2009, http://www.fao.org/economic/ess/food-security-statistics/fao-hunger-map/en/ (accessed November 25, 2009)

making it more difficult for families to afford adequate nutrition.

Hunger and Mortality

Rich countries have much greater purchasing power than poor countries. The strength of a country's purchasing power is definitely correlated with the health of its people—the difference in the health of people living in rich countries and those living in poor countries is dramatic. For example, in 2005 the death rate of children under five years old in middle-income countries was five times higher than in high-income countries. Figure 2.11 shows that in high-income countries 8 children per 1,000 live births died in 2005, compared with 40 children per 1,000 live births in middle-income countries. The difference in the death rate of children under five years old between low-income and high-income countries was even more dramatic. In low-income countries 110 children per 1,000 live births died in 2005. This was an

under-five mortality rate (U5MR) of approximately 15 times that of high-income countries in that year.

Another measure of the difference in the health of people living in rich countries compared with those living in poor countries is reflected in their life expectancy. The life expectancy at birth in 2005 of people living in high-income countries was nearly 80 years. (See Figure 2.12.) The life expectancy at birth in 2005 of people living in low-income countries was barely 60 years—a gap of 20 years. Even though progress was made between 1990 and 2005 in both reducing the U5MR and in extending life expectancy in low-income, developing, middle-income, and high-income countries, an enormous health gap between the rich and the poor still remains.

Money and the strength of purchasing power are not the only reasons why a high proportion of the human population is undernourished and unhealthy. As with other aspects of poverty, another reason involves global,

TABLE 2.6

Goals and targets from the Millennium Declaration and indicators for monitoring progress

Goal 1 Eradicate extreme poverty and hunger

Target 1.A Halve, between 1990 and 2015, the proportion of people whose income is less than $1 a day

1.1 Proportion of population below $1 purchasing power parity (PPP) a day[a]
1.2 Poverty gap ratio [incidence × depth of poverty]
1.3 Share of poorest quintile in national consumption

Target 1.B Achieve full and productive employment and decent work for all, including women and young people

1.4 Growth rate of (GDP) per person employed
1.5 Employment to population ratio
1.6 Proportion of employed people living below $1 (PPP) a day
1.7 Proportion of own-account and contributing family workers in total employment

Target 1.C Halve, between 1990 and 2015, the proportion of people who suffer from hunger

1.8 Prevalence of underweight children under five years of age
1.9 Proportion of population below minimum level of dietary energy consumption

Goal 2 Achieve universal primary education

Target 2.A Ensure that by 2015 children everywhere, boys and girls alike, will be able to complete a full course of primary schooling

2.1 Net enrollment ratio in primary education
2.2 Proportion of pupils starting grade 1 who reach last grade of primary education
2.3 Literacy rate of 15- to 24-year-olds, women and men

Goal 3 Promote gender equality and empower women

Target 3.A Eliminate gender disparity in primary and secondary education, preferably by 2005, and in all levels of education no later than 2015

3.1 Ratios of girls to boys in primary, secondary, and tertiary education
3.2 Share of women in wage employment in the nonagricultural sector
3.3 Proportion of seats held by women in national parliament

Goal 4 Reduce child mortality

Target 4.A Reduce by two-thirds, between 1990 and 2015, the under-five mortality rate

4.1 Under-five mortality rate
4.2 Infant mortality rate
4.3 Proportion of one-year-old children immunized against measles

Goal 5 Improve maternal health

Target 5.A Reduce by three-quarters, between 1990 and 2015, the maternal mortality ratio

Target 5.B Achieve by 2015 universal access to reproductive health

5.1 Maternal mortality ratio
5.2 Proportion of births attended by skilled health personnel
5.3 Contraceptive prevalence rate
5.4 Adolescent birth rate
5.5 Antenatal care coverage (at least one visit and at least four visits)
5.6 Unmet need for family planning

Goal 6 Combat HIV/AIDS, malaria, and other diseases

Target 6.A Have halted by 2015 and begun to reverse the spread of HIV/AIDS

6.1 HIV prevalence among population ages 15–24 years
6.2 Condom use at last high-risk sex
6.3 Proportion of population ages 15–24 years with comprehensive, correct knowledge of HIV/AIDS
6.4 Ratio of school attendance of orphans to school attendance of nonorphans ages 10–14 years
6.5 Proportion of population with advanced HIV infection with access to antiretroviral drugs

Target 6.B Achieve by 2010 universal access to treatment for HIV/AIDS for all those who need it

Target 6.C Have halted by 2015 and begun to reverse the incidence of malaria and other major diseases

6.6 Incidence and death rates associated with malaria
6.7 Proportion of children under age five sleeping under insecticide-treated bednets
6.8 Proportion of children under age five with fever who are treated with appropriate antimalarial drugs
6.9 Incidence, prevalence, and death rates associated with tuberculosis
6.10 Proportion of tuberculosis cases detected and cured under directly observed treatment short course

Goal 7 Ensure environmental sustainability

Target 7.A Integrate the principles of sustainable development into country policies and programs and reverse the loss of environmental resources

Target 7.B Reduce biodiversity loss, achieving, by 2010, a significant reduction in the rate of loss

7.1 Proportion of land area covered by forest
7.2 Carbon dioxide emissions, total, per capita and per $1 GDP (PPP)
7.3 Consumption of ozone-depleting substances
7.4 Proportion of fish stocks within safe biological limits
7.5 Proportion of total water resources used
7.6 Proportion of terrestrial and marine areas protected
7.7 Proportion of species threatened with extinction

Target 7.C Halve by 2015 the proportion of people without sustainable access to safe drinking water and basic sanitation

Target 7.D Achieve by 2020 a significant improvement in the lives of at least 100 million slum dwellers

7.8 Proportion of population using an improved drinking water source
7.9 Proportion of population using an improved sanitation facility
7.10 Proportion of urban population living in slums[b]

Goal 8 Develop a global partnership for development

Target 8.A Develop further an open, rule-based, predictable, nondiscriminatory trading and financial system (Includes a commitement to good governance, development, and poverty reduction—both nationally and internationaly.)

Target 8.B Address the special needs of the least developed countries (Includes tariff and quota-free access for the least developed countries' exports; enhanced program of debt relief for heavily indebted poor countries (HIPC) and cancellation of official bilateral debt; and more generous ODA for countries committed to poverty reduction.)

Some of the indicators listed below are monitored separately for the least developed countries (LDCs), Africa, landlocked developing countries, and small island developing states.

Official development assistance (ODA)

8.1 Net ODA, total and to the least developed countries, as percentage of OECD/DAC donors' gross national income
8.2 Proportion of total bilateral, sector-allocable ODA of OECD/DAC donors to basic social services (basic education, primary health care, nutrition, safe water, and sanitation)
8.3 Proportion of bilateral official development assistance of OECD/DAC donors that is untied
8.4 ODA received in landlocked developing countries as a proportion of their gross national incomes
8.5 ODA received in small island developing states as a proportion of their gross national incomes

Target 8.C Address the special needs of landlocked developing countries and small island developing states (through the Programme of Action for the Sustainable Development of Small Island Developing States and the outcome of the 22nd special session of the General Assembly)

Target 8.D Deal comprehensively with the debt problems of developing countries through national and international measures in order to make debt sustainable in the long term

Target 8.E In cooperation with pharmaceutical companies, provide access to affordable essential drugs in developing countries

Target 8.F In cooperation with the private sector, make available the benefits of new technologies, especially information and communications

Market access

8.6 Proportion of total developed country imports (by value and excluding arms) from developing countries and least developed countries, admitted free of duty

8.7 Average tariffs imposed by developed countries on agricultural products and textiles and clothing from developing countries

8.8 Agricultural support estimate for OECD countries as a percentage of the GDP

8.9 Proportion of ODA provided to help build trade capacity

Debt sustainability

8.10 Total number of countries that have reached their HIPC decision points and number that have reached their HIPC completion points cumulative)

8.11 Debt relief committed under HIPC Initiative and Multilateral Debt Relief Initiative (MDRI)

8.12 Debt service as a percentage of exports of goods and services

8.13 Proportion of population with access to affordable essential drugs on a sustainable basis

8.14 Telephone lines per 100 populaiton

8.15 Cellular subscribers per 100 population

8.16 Internet users per 100 population

aWhere available, indicators based on national poverty lines should be used for monitoring country poverty trends.
bThe proportion of people living in slums is measured by a proxy, represented by the urban population living in households with at least one of these characteristics: lack of access to improved water supply, lack of access to improved sanitation, overcrowding (3 or more persons per room), and dwellings made of nondurable material.
Notes: GDP = Gross Domestic Product, PPP = Purchasing Power Parity, OECD = Organisation for Economic Cooperation and Development, DAC = Development Assistance Committee, HIPC = Highly Indebted Poor Countries
The Millennium Development Goals and targets come from the Millennium Declaration, signed by 189 countries, including 147 heads of state and government, in September 2000 (www .un.org/millennium/declaration/ares552e.htm) as updated by the 60th UN General Assembly in September 2005. The revised Millennium Development Goal (MDG) monitoring framework shown here, including new targets and indicators, was presented to the 62nd General Assembly, with new numbering as recommended by the Inter-agency and Expert Group on MDG Indicators at its 12th meeting on 14 November 2007. The goals and targets are interrelated and should be seen as a whole. They represent a partnership between the developed countries and the developing countries "to create an environment—at the national and global levels alike—which is conducive to development and the elimination of poverty." All indicators should be disaggregated by sex and urban-rural location as far as possible.

SOURCE: "Millennium Development Goals: Goals and Targets from the Millennium Declaration and Indicators for Monitoring Progress," in *World Development Indicators 2009*, The International Bank for Reconstruction and Development/The World Bank, April 2009, http://siteresources.worldbank.org/ DATASTATISTICS/Resources/wdi09introch1.pdf (accessed November 25, 2009). Copyright © The International Bank for Reconstruction and Development/ World Bank 2007.

regional, and local politics—in this case the politics of agricultural subsidies, trade, and food aid.

Agricultural Subsidies, Trade, and Food Aid

Agricultural subsidies are often cited as a factor in either causing or worsening the problem of hunger. The governments of wealthy countries routinely pay farmers— mostly the owners of large farms—billions of dollars each year to produce too much or not enough of certain crops to control the prices of crops for export or import.

Farm subsidies in Europe, Japan, and the United States are designed to work in conjunction with trade barriers such as quotas (limitations of imports) and tariffs (taxes on imported goods). When farmers in developed countries are paid to overproduce certain foods (e.g., rice and corn), those countries export, or "dump," their surplus supplies to poor countries for extremely low prices or sometimes for free as aid. At the same time, trade barriers prevent poor countries from exporting crops and other goods to wealthy countries (this is sometimes called protectionism). Food dumping from wealthy countries floods the markets, which drives down the value of crops in poor countries so low that it is often more economical for them to import the food or accept it as foreign aid than to invest in their own agricultural development. However, this also makes them more vulnerable to international economic factors and inhibits their ability to sustain themselves.

International aid in the form of food seems like a straightforward way to deal with the worldwide crisis of hunger, yet many detractors claim that it actually makes the problem worse. Poverty researchers note that there is a difference between the kind of emergency aid that calls for the direct exportation of food to an area and the practice of simply sending food to a poor region not experiencing an emergency situation. Very often, nonemergency food aid is actually just food dumping, which causes dependence on a foreign food source and prevents a poor country's farmers from competing in the international market.

In addition, when developed countries in North America, Europe, and elsewhere give aid in the form of food, they do not typically give it directly to hungry people (except in emergency cases, when food may be dropped from low-flying airplanes). Rather, they give it to the federal governments of poor countries, who distribute it to local governments, who in many cases sell it to the hungry at prices so low that local food producers, if any exist, cannot compete and may be forced out of business. Furthermore, an underdeveloped or developing country that depends on food imports will often use its land to produce crops such as cut flowers or livestock feed for export to developed countries rather than growing food for local consumption. When small farms shut down or are forced out of business, people often migrate to urban areas to work in manufacturing operations (typically sweatshops), leaving rural regions even more vulnerable to economic depression.

The FAO finds in *State of Food Insecurity in the World 2009* a direct link between growth in a developing country's agricultural sector and a reduction in hunger and poverty. It also notes that growth in urban and industrial sectors or overall growth in the gross domestic product (the total value of all goods and services produced by a country in a year) does not necessarily translate into a reduction in hunger and poverty. Therefore, the FAO suggests that

economic growth itself is not enough to change patterns in hunger, but that the healthy development of farming, both for export and for domestic use, is essential.

Other Factors of Hunger

Besides economic, trade, and farming issues, other diverse factors affect the complex situation of world hunger, undernutrition, and malnutrition, and the related problems of high child mortality rates and poor health. These factors include governance, natural disasters, poor sanitation, and a lack of nutritional and health education.

In *State of Food Insecurity in the World 2009*, the FAO includes a country's system of governance as a factor affecting hunger rates. The World Bank, through its Worldwide Governance Indicators research project, has compiled several hundred variables to develop indicators that measure six dimensions of a country's governance. Four governance indicators in particular—political stability and absence of violence, government effectiveness, rule of law, and control of corruption—are necessary to achieve hunger reduction in a country. Hunger worsens and per capita food production drops, for example, in countries experiencing violent conflict and/or political instability. Daniel Kaufmann, Aart Kraay, and Massimo Mastruzzi provide in *Governance Matters VIII: Aggregate and Individual Governance Indicators 1996–2008* (June 29, 2009, http://papers.ssrn.com/sol3/papers.cfm?abstract_id=1424591) an update that covers 212 countries and territories.

Natural disasters, such as droughts, excess rainfall, earthquakes, and other environmental events, also cause food crises by slowing food production or halting it altogether. These occurrences have far more serious consequences in

FIGURE 2.8

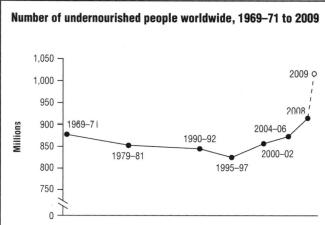

Number of undernourished people worldwide, 1969–71 to 2009

SOURCE: "Figure 5. Learning from the Past: Number of Undernourished in the World, 1969–71 to 2009," in *The State of Food Insecurity in the World 2009: Economic Crises—Impacts and Lessons Learned*, Food and Agriculture Organization of the United Nations (FAO), 2009, ftp://ftp.fao.org/docrep/fao/012/i0876e/i0876e.pdf (accessed November 25, 2009)

FIGURE 2.9

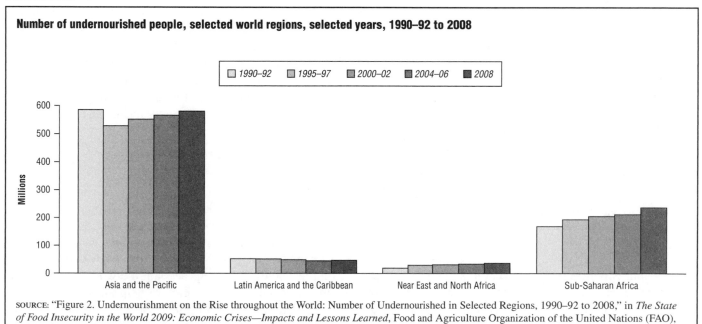

Number of undernourished people, selected world regions, selected years, 1990–92 to 2008

SOURCE: "Figure 2. Undernourishment on the Rise throughout the World: Number of Undernourished in Selected Regions, 1990–92 to 2008," in *The State of Food Insecurity in the World 2009: Economic Crises—Impacts and Lessons Learned*, Food and Agriculture Organization of the United Nations (FAO), 2009, ftp://ftp.fao.org/docrep/fao/012/i0876e/i0876e.pdf (accessed November 25, 2009)

FIGURE 2.10

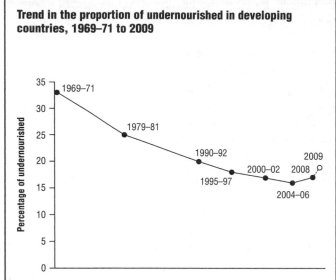

Trend in the proportion of undernourished in developing countries, 1969–71 to 2009

SOURCE: "Figure 6. The Declining Trend in the Proportion of Undernourished in Developing Countries Has Been Reversed," in *The State of Food Insecurity in the World 2009: Economic Crises—Impacts and Lessons Learned*, Food and Agriculture Organization of the United Nations (FAO), 2009, ftp://ftp.fao.org/docrep/fao/012/i0876e/i0876e .pdf (accessed November 25, 2009)

FIGURE 2.12

Life expectancy at birth by country income level, 1990 and 2005

SOURCE: "2f. A Health Gap Becomes a Life Gap," in *World Development Indicators 2007*, The International Bank for Reconstruction and Development/The World Bank, April 2007, http:// siteresources.worldbank.org/DATASTATISTICS/Resources/ WDI07section2-intro.pdf (accessed November 25, 2009). Copyright © The International Bank for Reconstruction and Development/ World Bank 2007.

FIGURE 2.11

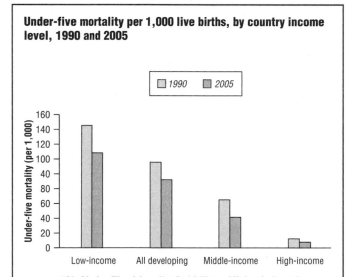

Under-five mortality per 1,000 live births, by country income level, 1990 and 2005

SOURCE: "2b. Under-Five Mortality Is 15 Times Higher in Low-Income Countries Than in High-Income Countries," in *World Development Indicators 2007*, The International Bank for Reconstruction and Development/The World Bank, April 2007, http://siteresources .worldbank.org/DATASTATISTICS/Resources/WDI07section2- intro.pdf (accessed November 25, 2009). Copyright © The International Bank for Reconstruction and Development/World Bank 2007. Data from WHO, UNICEF, and World Bank.

poor countries, where food production is already low. Displacement is another consequence of natural disasters that increases the incidence of hunger in poor countries. When people are forced to flee after major disasters such as earthquakes or migrate because of severe weather conditions, pressure to produce enough food to support them is placed on the areas in which they settle.

According to the World Bank, in *Repositioning Nutrition as Central to Development: A Strategy for Large-Scale Action* (2006, http://siteresources.worldbank.org/NUTRIT ION/Resources/281846-1131636806329/NutritionStrategy .pdf), a lack of food is just one of several factors contributing to malnutrition and undernutrition. Additional causes of severe malnutrition, especially in children, include a poor understanding of nutritional needs, insufficient knowledge about women's health in particular, and poor sanitation (which is the source of waterborne viruses and bacteria that cause diarrheal diseases). This suggests that investment in health education in general and nutrition education in particular would help reduce hunger and malnutrition, as would investment in infrastructure to improve sanitation and provide water free from disease-causing microbes.

GLOBALIZATION, FREE TRADE, AND FAIR TRADE

Globalization is the term used to refer to the growing economic interdependence of nations. Proponents of globalization maintain that opening markets across national borders provides opportunities for both large and small economies. They suggest that freer exchange of money and technology can help develop the world's smaller and poorer economies and therefore help alleviate poverty in developing regions while increasing the wealth of developed ones. Opponents of globalization argue that it puts the welfare of multinational corporations above the welfare of poor and indigenous people. They also claim globalization increases instances of unjust labor practices that take advantage of the poor, such as sweatshops and child labor.

In "How to End Poverty: Making Poverty History and the History of Poverty" (May 11, 2005, http://www.mail-archive.com/friends@sffreaks.org/msg00092.html), Vandana Shiva (1952–), an Indian physicist, ecofeminist, and environmental activist, contends that the globalization movement's focus on consumerism (selling products to people through international trade) denies people in traditional cultures the ability to support themselves by growing their own food, making their own clothing, and otherwise providing for themselves. Shiva further maintains that when corporations and industries take land from self-sustaining cultures, they actually push those people into poverty by depriving them of the resources they need to survive. In "Globalization and Poverty" (December 16, 2008, http://www.stwr.org/food-security-agriculture/globalization-and-poverty-an-interview-with-dr-vandana-shiva.html), an interview by Gary Null of the Progressive Radio Network, Shiva suggests that "India is a good test case to see how globalization increases real poverty even while measurements of growth make it look like the country is booming. India's growth these last few years has been 9 percent and it is seen as one of the fastest growing economies. And yet in this decade of high growth under free market globalization India has the largest number of hungry people in the world."

A major facet of globalization is the forging of free trade agreements (FTAs), which are arrangements between countries that allow the exchange of goods and labor across borders without governmental tariffs or other trade barriers. Two of the best-known FTAs are the North American Free Trade Agreement (NAFTA; among Canada, Mexico, and the United States) and the Central American Free Trade Agreement (CAFTA; among Costa Rica, El Salvador, Guatemala, Honduras, Nicaragua, and the United States). Despite the increasing number of FTAs, poor countries are often subject to higher import tariffs and other unfavorable circumstances when they export goods to developed countries. Oxfam International notes in *Signing away the Future: How Trade and Investment Agreements between Rich and Poor Countries Undermine Development* (March 2007, http://www.oxfam.org/sites/www.oxfam.org/files/Signing%20Away%20the%20Future.pdf) that "around 25 developing countries have now signed free trade agreements with developed countries, and more than 100 are engaged in negotiations." The problem with this plethora of bilateral and regional treaties, suggests Oxfam, is that the agreements are signed outside of the auspices of the World Trade Organization, "where developing countries can band together and hold out for more favourable rules." Rules that are favorable to rich countries often prevail under such circumstances, binding poor countries into long-term commitments "with

grave implications for the environment and development." Instead, fair trade should eliminate trade barriers to poor countries and develop healthy, sustainable, trade-based employment opportunities within them. As low-income countries gain fair access to markets, investment is stimulated, which in turn promotes employment opportunities at the local level and economic growth at the national level.

International Debt

Lending and debt relief to underdeveloped and developing nations is another controversial issue. Many low-income countries became heavily indebted to wealthy nations during the 1970s, when banks around the world began lending money to developing countries that were rich in resources such as oil. The money, however, was often mismanaged—particularly in the countries of sub-Saharan Africa—and spent on projects to expand the wealth of the upper classes rather than on infrastructure and social investments such as roadways, safe water, education, and health care. When interest rates on the loans rose and the prices of their resources dropped during the 1980s, the indebted countries were unable to repay the loans. Many of these nations turned to the World Bank or the International Monetary Fund (IMF) for help. These organizations underwrote more loans, but required that the poor countries agree to undergo structural adjustment programs (SAPs).

In essence, the World Bank and the IMF demanded that poor countries restructure their economies by cutting spending and revaluing their currency so that they could begin to repay their loans and emerge from debt. Most low-income countries met the restructuring criteria by limiting their social spending (e.g., on education, health care, and social services), lowering wages, cutting jobs, and taking land from subsistence farmers to grow crops for export. This focus on increasing trade has generated the most severe criticism from opponents of SAPs, who argue that the United States and other wealthy countries encourage such measures to improve their own trading opportunities, which destroys the ability of poor countries to support themselves because they become dependent on imports of food and other basic necessities. However, supporters of SAPs point out that this economic system allows poor countries to participate more fully in the global market and that the benefits of restructuring will eventually "trickle down" to the poor.

In 1996 the World Bank and the IMF created the Heavily Indebted Poor Countries (HIPC) Initiative. The initiative was intended to reduce the debt of the most heavily indebted poor countries to levels that were manageable for them. In 2005 the HIPC Initiative was supplemented by the Multilateral Debt Relief Initiative (MDRI) to help countries make progress toward the UN MDGs.

The MDRI cancels the debt of countries that meet the HIPC Initiative criteria, which include implementing agreed-on reforms and developing a Poverty Reduction Strategy Paper (PRSP; the paper describes the policies and programs that a country will pursue over several years to encourage economic growth and reduce poverty). As a country makes progress toward these goals, a decision point is reached, whereby the International Development Association of the World Bank and the IMF determine whether the country should receive debt relief. If the country will receive relief, it may begin receiving interim debt relief at the decision point. Once the PRSP has been adopted and implemented for at least one year, and when other criteria have been met, the country is said to have reached its completion point, and full debt relief is given.

The IMF explains in "Factsheet: The Multilateral Debt Relief Initiative (MDRI)" (June 2009, http://www.imf.org/external/np/exr/facts/mdri.htm) that "all countries with per-capita income of $380 a year or less (whether HIPCs or not) will receive MDRI debt relief financed by the IMF's own resources through the MDRI-I Trust. HIPCs with per capita income above that threshold will receive MDRI relief from bilateral contributions administered by the IMF through the MDRI-II Trust." Table 2.7 shows the countries that have benefited from the MDRI as of May 15, 2009, and the countries that will be eligible once they reach the completion point. Table 2.8 shows the amount of debt relief. The special drawing right (SDR) is not a currency but an IMF unit of account. More specifically, it is the value of the debt relief. Note that the amount of U.S. dollars given in debt relief can vary based on the exchange rate between the SDR and the U.S. dollar at the time debt relief is given.

TABLE 2.7

Country eligibility for debt relief under the Multilateral Debt Relief Initiative, 2009

	Eligible under the "MDRI-I Trust" (per-capita income at or below $380)	Eligible under the "MDRI-II Trust" (per-capita income above $380)
Countries that have benefited from MDRI as of May 15, 2009		
"Completion point" HIPCs: 24 countries that have reached the completion point under the Enhanced HIPC Initiative	Burkina Faso, Burundi, Ethiopia, The Gambia, Ghana, Madagascar, Malawi, Mali, Mozambique, Niger, Rwanda, São Tomé and Príncipe, Sierra Leone, Tanzania, Uganda	Benin, Bolivia, Cameroon, Guyana, Honduras, Mauritania, Nicaragua, Senegal, Zambia
Non-HIPC countries (2) with per capita income below $380 and outstanding debt to the IMF	Cambodia, Tajikistan	
Countries that will be eligible once they reach the completion point under the Enhanced HIPC Initiative		
"Decision point" HIPCs: 11 countries that have reached the decision point under the Enhanced HIPC Initiative	Afghanistan, Central African Republic, Chad, Democratic Republic of the Congo, Guinea-Bissau, Togo Liberia*	Côte d'Ivoire, Guinea, Haiti, Republic of Congo
5 additional countries may wish to be considered for HIPC debt relief. They met the income and indebtedness criteria based on end-2004 data.	Eritrea Precise data on the per capita income of Somalia are not available at this juncture.	Comoros, Kyrgyz Republic, Sudan

*Liberia has no MDRI-eligible debt to the International Monetary Fund (IMF) but is expected to receive additional beyond-HIPC debt relief from the IMF to fully cover its remaining eligible debt outstanding at the completion point.
Notes: MDRI = Multilateral debt relief, HIPC = Heavily indebted poor countries

SOURCE: "Table 1. Country Coverage of the MDRI," in *Factsheet: The Multilateral Debt Relief Initiative (MDRI)*, International Monetary Fund (IMF), June 2009, http://www.imf.org/external/np/exr/facts/mdri.htm (accessed November 25, 2009)

TABLE 2.8

Amount of debt relief to qualifying countries under the Multilateral Debt Relief Initiative, 2009[a]

	SDR million	US$ million[b]
HIPC completion point countries	**2,185**	**3,168**
Benin	34	49
Bolivia	155	224
Burkina Faso	57	82
Burundi	9	13
Cameroon	149	219
Ethiopia	80	115
The Gambia	7	12
Ghana	220	318
Guyana	32	46
Honduras	98	142
Madagascar	128	186
Malawi	15	22
Mali	62	90
Mauritania	30	45
Mozambique	83	120
Nicaragua	92	133
Niger	60	86
Rwanda	20	29
São Tomé and Príncipe	1	2
Senegal	95	137
Sierra Leone	77	115
Tanzania	207	299
Uganda	76	110
Zambia	398	576
Non-HIPCs	**126**	**182**
Cambodia	57	82
Tajikistan	69	100
Total	**2,312**	**3,350**

[a]For HIPCs, the amount of relief includes only MDRI assistance and excludes undisbursed HIPC assistance not yet delivered.
[b]Using the SDR/US$ exchange rates at the time of debt relief.
Notes: MDRI = Multilateral Debt Relief Initiative.
HIPC = Heavily Indebted Poor Countries.
SDR = Special Drawing Right, the unit of account of the International Monetary Fund.
US$ = United States dollars

SOURCE: "Table 2. Debt Relief to Qualifying Countries under the MDRI (in Millions and as of May 15, 2009)," in *Factsheet: The Multilateral Debt Relief Initiative (MDRI)*, International Monetary Fund (IMF), June 2009, http://www.imf.org/external/np/exr/facts/mdri.htm (accessed November 25, 2009)

CHAPTER 3
POVERTY IN UNDERDEVELOPED COUNTRIES—THE POOREST OF THE POOR

Underdeveloped countries are at the very bottom of the global economy, with widespread extreme poverty and dire living conditions. They usually have little or no infrastructure—that is, public structures, facilities, and services, such as paved roads, bridges, schools, hospitals, sewer systems, and water purification. Many underdeveloped countries have experienced long-term political unrest in the form of civil war (a war between different factions within a country) or armed conflict with other nations, or have been subject to unstable governments, dictatorships, and/or corruption. In addition, they may frequently suffer environmental events and natural disasters with which they cannot cope well or recover from easily. These events and disasters usually result in dire situations, such as famine, destruction of whatever they do have, and displacement of large segments of their populations.

THE UNITED NATIONS' LIST OF LEAST DEVELOPED COUNTRIES

Many scholars and researchers refer to nations whose economies are almost completely lacking in infrastructure, industry, and technology as least developed countries (LDCs). In "The Criteria for the Identification of the LDCs" (February 22, 2006, http://www.un.org/special-rep/ohrlls/ldc/ldc%20criteria.htm), the Economic and Social Council of the United Nations (UN) indicates that this term has a specific meaning according to whether countries meet certain criteria:

- A low-income criterion, based on a three-year average estimate of the gross national income (GNI) per capita (under $750 for inclusion, above $900 for graduation).

- A human resource weakness criterion, involving a composite Human Assets Index (HAI) based on indicators of: (a) nutrition; (b) health; (c) education; and (d) adult literacy.

- An economic vulnerability criterion, involving a composite Economic Vulnerability Index (EVI) based on indicators of: (a) the instability of agricultural production; (b) the instability of exports of goods and services; (c) the economic importance of nontraditional activities (share of manufacturing and modern services in GDP); (d) merchandise export concentration; and (e) the handicap of economic smallness (as measured through the population in logarithm); and the percentage of population displaced by natural disasters.

Of the UN's list of LDCs in 2009, 33 were in Africa, 15 were in Asia, and 1 was in Latin America and the Caribbean. (See Table 3.1.) Because the list automatically excludes large economies—which necessarily have certain advantages over smaller economies—not all countries where large percentages of the population are extremely poor are represented on the list. (Africa is notable as a continent with many large economies that is nonetheless almost uniformly underdeveloped and impoverished.) The list is maintained and reviewed every three years by the Economic and Social Council. To be removed from the list, a country must meet at least two of the criteria for two three-year reviews in a row.

AFRICA: THE POOREST CONTINENT

Africa is the second-largest continent (after Asia) in both land area and population—with 1 billion people living in 53 countries. With a total land area of more than 11 million square miles (28.5 million sq km), Africa accounts for 20% of the land on Earth, and its population accounts for almost 15% of the global population.

Africa is typically discussed as two distinct regions: northern Africa—the area in and around the Sahara, which is inhabited mostly by Arabic-speaking people whose ancestors come from the Middle East—and sub-Saharan Africa—the area south of the Sahara, in which many different tribes

TABLE 3.1

United Nations' list of least developed countries, 2009

Africa (33)

1 Angola	18 Madagascar
2 Benin	19 Malawi[b]
3 Burkina Faso[b]	20 Mali[b]
4 Burundi[b]	21 Mauritania
5 Central African Republic[b]	22 Mozambique
6 Chad[b]	23 Niger[b]
7 Comoros[a]	24 Rwanda[b]
8 Democratic Republic of the Congo	25 São Tomé and Príncipe[a]
9 Djibouti	26 Senegal
10 Equatorial Guinea	27 Sierra Leone
11 Eritrea	28 Somalia
12 Ethiopia[b]	29 Sudan
13 Gambia	30 Togo
14 Guinea	31 Uganda[b]
15 Guinea-Bissau[a]	32 United Republic of Tanzania
16 Lesotho[b]	33 Zambia[b]
17 Liberia	

Asia (15)

1 Afghanistan[b]	9 Nepal[b]
2 Bangladesh	10 Samoa[a]
3 Bhutan[b]	11 Solomon Islands[a]
4 Cambodia	12 Timor-Leste[a]
5 Kiribati[a]	13 Tuvalu[a]
6 Lao People's Democratic Republic[b]	14 Vanuatu[a]
7 Maldives[a]	15 Yemen
8 Myanmar	

Latin America and the Caribbean (1)

1 Haiti[a]

[a]Also SIDS
[b]Also LLDCs
LLDCs = Landlocked developing countries. SIDS = Small island developing states.

SOURCE: "Least Developed Countries: Country Profiles," © UN Office of the High Representative for the Least Developed Countries, Landlocked Developing Countries, and Small Island Developing States (UN-OHRLLS), 2009, http://www.unohrlls.org/en/ldc/related/62/ (accessed November 25, 2009). The United Nations is the author of the original material. Reproduced with permission.

FIGURE 3.1

Trend in human development worldwide, by region, 1975–2004

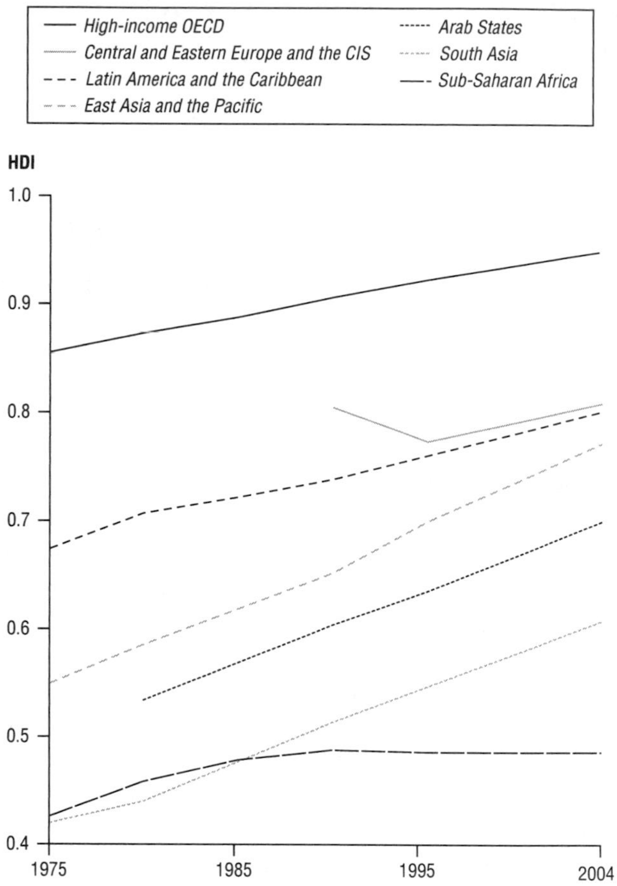

HDI = Human Development Index.
OECD = Office of Economic Cooperation and Development.
CIS = Commonwealth of Independent States.

SOURCE: Kevin Watkins, "Figure 2. The Human Development Trend—Upwards but Uneven," in *Human Development Report 2006*, United Nations Development Programme (UNDP), published 2006, Palgrave Macmillan, http://hdr.undp.org/en/media/HDR06-complete.pdf (accessed November 25, 2009). Reproduced with permission of Palgrave Macmillan.

and nationalities live. The Sahara, the world's largest non-arctic desert, is located primarily in the countries of Algeria, Libya, and Egypt, and occupies the northern portion of Mauritania. The countries south of the Sahara are sub-Saharan. The UN lists seven territories as North African (Algeria, Egypt, Libya, Morocco, Sudan, Tunisia, and the Moroccan-occupied Western Sahara) and the rest of the continent's countries as sub-Saharan Africa. Of the continent's 53 countries, 33—all typically considered to be part of sub-Saharan Africa—are on the UN's list of LDCs, making Africa the continent that suffers from the overall highest rate of poverty in the world.

SUB-SAHARAN AFRICA: THE POOREST REGION OF THE CONTINENT

The UN tracks trends in poverty worldwide using its Human Development Index (HDI; see Chapter 1), which measures the overall well-being of countries. In *Human Development Report 2006—Beyond Scarcity: Power, Poverty, and the Global Water Crisis* (2006, http://hdr.undp.org/en/media/HDR06-complete.pdf), Kevin Watkins of the UN

Development Programme (UNDP) indicates that the HDI has risen since the 1990s at variable rates across almost all regions except for sub-Saharan Africa. (See Figure 3.1; central and eastern Europe and the Commonwealth of Independent States recovered and progressed after a severe decline from 1990 to 1995.) Watkins also notes that most of the 18 countries that have experienced significant reversals in their HDIs since 1990 are in sub-Saharan Africa. In 2009, 22 of the 24 low human development countries were in sub-Saharan Africa. (See Table 1.2 in Chapter 1.) The main indicators on the HDI include health and life expectancy, literacy and educational attainment, and income.

Health and Life Expectancy

HUNGER AND UNDERNUTRITION. Hunger, malnutrition, and undernutrition severely affect the health of a

FIGURE 3.2

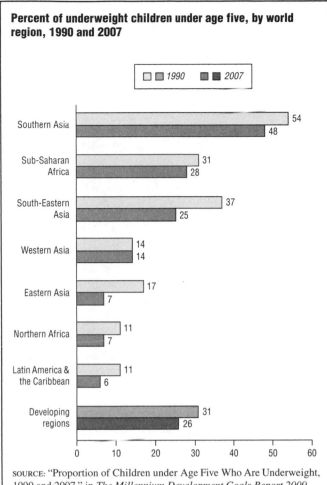

Percent of underweight children under age five, by world region, 1990 and 2007

☐ *1990* ■ *2007*

Region	1990	2007
Southern Asia	54	48
Sub-Saharan Africa	31	28
South-Eastern Asia	37	25
Western Asia	14	14
Eastern Asia	17	7
Northern Africa	11	7
Latin America & the Caribbean	11	6
Developing regions	31	26

SOURCE: "Proportion of Children under Age Five Who Are Underweight, 1990 and 2007," in *The Millennium Development Goals Report 2009*, © United Nations, 2009, http://www.un.org/millenniumgoals/pdf/ MDG_Report_2009_ENG.pdf (accessed December 5, 2009). The United Nations is the author of the original material. Reproduced with permission.

population. In children especially, adequate nutrition is essential for the development of their growing bodies, most particularly for building the immune system and for development of the brain and musculature. However, a huge proportion of children in sub-Saharan Africa are undernourished and, as a result, underweight.

Figure 3.2 compares child hunger and undernutrition in sub-Saharan Africa with that in northern Africa. In 1990, 31% of children under the age of five were underweight in sub-Saharan Africa, whereas 11% were underweight in northern Africa. By 2007 both regions of Africa had reduced the proportion of children under the age of five who were underweight, but a huge gap between these two regions still remained: 28% of children under the age of five were underweight in sub-Saharan Africa, whereas 7% were underweight in northern Africa.

The Center for International Earth Science Information Network (CIESIN) of Columbia University shows the regions of most severe child undernutrition in its most recent hunger map of Africa (May 2006, http://www.ciesin .columbia.edu/repository/povmap/maps/atlas/chp3.pdf). The region on the southern border of the Sahara, from Senegal to Ethiopia, was the region of the most severe hunger in 2000. In addition, countries on the coastline generally (but not always) had a less severe hunger problem than inland countries, and countries closer to South Africa generally had a less severe problem than countries farther away from South Africa.

The problem of undernutrition is extremely severe in sub-Saharan Africa and extends beyond children. Stacey Rosen and Shahla Shapouri of the U.S. Department of Agriculture's (USDA) Economic Research Service (ERS) note in "Global Economic Crisis Threatens Food Security in Lower Income Countries" (*Amber Waves*, December 2009) that sub-Saharan Africa is the most food-insecure region of the world. Food insecurity means that individuals or families do not always have access to enough food for proper nutrition and health. Rosen and Shapouri indicate that in sub-Saharan Africa the average food intake is the lowest in the world. Moreover, the severe global economic recession that began in 2007 threatened food security in many lower income countries, including sub-Saharan Africa, because they lacked the necessary funds to import the quantities of food they needed to supplement what they could grow.

In *Food Security Assessment, 2008–09* (June 2009, http://www.ers.usda.gov/Publications/GFA20/GFA20.pdf), Shahla Shapouri et al. of the ERS report that food production increased in sub-Saharan Africa from 1999 to 2008 (except for a reduction in grain production in 2004), but that the population of this region grew as well, from slightly over 600 million in 1999 to about 770 million in 2008. Figure 3.3 shows not only this trend in population growth but also how the number of hungry people in this region changed from year to year during this period. From 1999 to 2004 the number of food-insecure people in sub-Saharan Africa was relatively static at about 400 million. The number of food-insecure people dropped in 2005 and 2006 due to high rates of food production, commercial imports, and food aid. Nonetheless, as the global economic recession took hold, the number of food-insecure people rose in 2007 and 2008 despite accelerated food production in 2008.

Figure 3.4 shows a country-specific picture of hunger not only in Africa but also worldwide. Disparities in the number of calories consumed per capita (per person) per day are visible among countries. During the period 2003– 05 the Democratic Republic of the Congo and Somalia had the lowest per capita consumption of calories at less than 1,800 per day. The countries of Angola, Chad, the Central African Republic, Ethiopia, and Zambia all had a per capita consumption of calories at less than 2,000

FIGURE 3.3

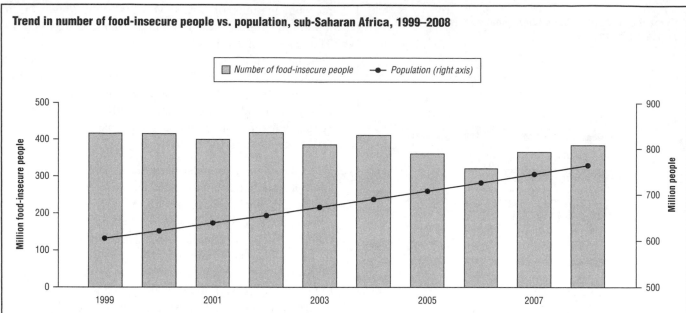

Trend in number of food-insecure people vs. population, sub-Saharan Africa, 1999–2008

☐ Number of food-insecure people   ●— Population (right axis)

SOURCE: Shahla Shapouri et al., "SSA: Trend in Number of Food-Insecure People vs. Population," in *Food Security Assessment, 2008–09*, U.S. Department of Agriculture (USDA), Economic Research Service (ERS), June 2009, http://www.ers.usda.gov/Publications/GFA20/GFA20.pdf (accessed November 25, 2009)

FIGURE 3.4

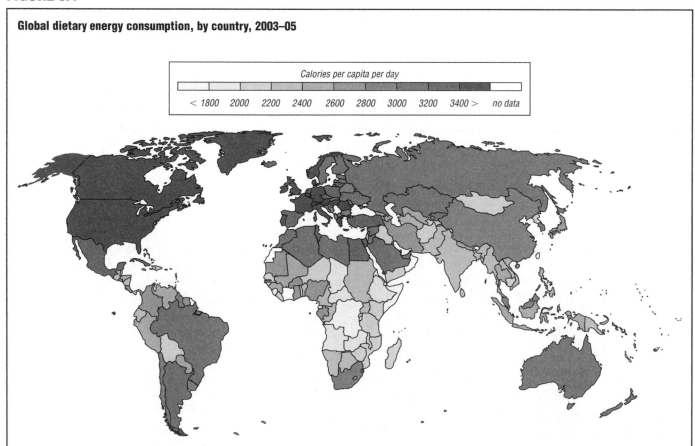

Global dietary energy consumption, by country, 2003–05

Calories per capita per day

< 1800   2000   2200   2400   2600   2800   3000   3200   3400 >   no data

SOURCE: "Dietary Energy Consumption," in *FAO Statistical Yearbook 2007–2008*, Food and Agriculture Organization of the United Nations (FAO), 2009, http://www.fao.org/fileadmin/templates/ess/documents/publications_studies/statistical_yearbook/FAO_statistical_yearbook_2007-2008/ybk_2007-2008_map07.pdf (accessed December 11, 2009) calories per day. Both amounts are fewer calories than the body needs to function properly and maintain its weight. In *Dietary Guidelines for Americans, 2005* (January 2005, http://www.health.gov/dietaryguidelines/dga2005/document/pdf/DGA2005.pdf), the most recent publication as of February 2010, the U.S. Department of Health and Human Services and the USDA estimate the number of calories needed to keep the body healthy. Moderately active females aged 19 to 30 require 2,000 to 2,200 calories per day, whereas moderately active males of the same age require 2,600 to 2,800 calories per day. Small children and older people require less. Except for South Africa, the countries of sub-Saharan Africa do not meet these guidelines.

LIFE EXPECTANCY AND THE HIV EPIDEMIC. According to the World Bank, in *The World Bank's Commitment to HIV/AIDS in Africa: Our Agenda for Action 2007–2011* (March 2008, http://siteresources.worldbank.org/

INTAFRREGTOPHIVAIDS/Resources/WB_HIV-AIDS-AFA_2007-2011_Advance_Copy.pdf), life expectancy has fallen dramatically in sub-Saharan Africa since 1990, when it saw a brief increase. In 1990 life expectancy in sub-Saharan Africa had reached 49 years, but by 2005 it had dropped to 46 years. This decrease in life expectancy is largely due to the spread of the human immunodeficiency virus (HIV) and the acquired immunodeficiency syndrome (AIDS) on the continent, and life expectancy varies within each country depending on the level of HIV prevalence.

Figure 3.5 shows the changes in life expectancy at birth in selected African countries with high and low HIV prevalence from 1965 to 2005. Life expectancy at birth was rising in all these countries until the HIV epidemic began in the early 1980s. By the mid- to late-1980s, in countries with a high prevalence of HIV infection and AIDS, such as Botswana, South Africa, and Zimbabwe,

FIGURE 3.5

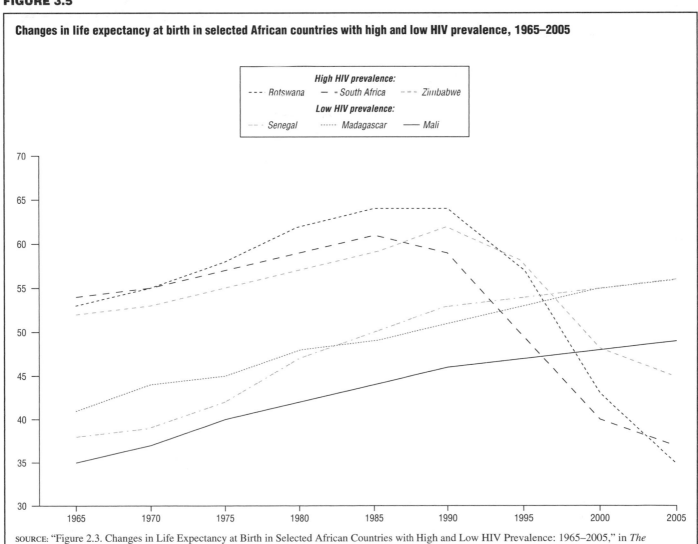

Changes in life expectancy at birth in selected African countries with high and low HIV prevalence, 1965–2005

SOURCE: "Figure 2.3. Changes in Life Expectancy at Birth in Selected African Countries with High and Low HIV Prevalence: 1965–2005," in *The World Bank's Commitment to HIV/AIDS in Africa: Our Agenda for Action 2007–2011*, The World Bank, March 2008, http://siteresources.worldbank.org/INTAFRREGTOPHIVAIDS/Resources/WB_HIV-AIDS-AFA_2007-2011_Advance_Copy.pdf (accessed November 25, 2009). Copyright © International Bank for Reconstruction and Development/The World Bank 2008.

life expectancy began to fall. For example, in Botswana life expectancy dropped from 64 years in 1990 to 35 years in 2005. In countries with a low prevalence of HIV infection and AIDS, such as Senegal, Madagascar, and Mali, life expectancy at birth continued to rise, although not quite as sharply as previously. For example, Senegal's life expectancy rose from 42 years in 1975 to 53 in 1990, a difference of 11 years, but rose only 3 more years to 56 during the next 15 years from 1990 to 2005.

The Joint UN Programme on HIV and AIDS and the World Health Organization (WHO) note in *AIDS Epidemic Update* (November 2009, http://data.unaids.org/pub/Report/2009/2009_epidemic_update_en.pdf) that in 2008 deaths due to HIV/AIDS in sub-Saharan Africa accounted for 72% of all AIDS-related deaths globally. Figure 3.6 shows that in 2008 between 1.1 million and 1.7 million sub-Saharan Africans died from the effects of HIV/AIDS and that between 20.8 million and 24.1 million

were living with the disease. Even though the number of sub-Saharan Africans newly infected with HIV has been slowly declining since the late 1990s, between 1.6 million and 2.2 million individuals in sub-Saharan Africa were newly infected in 2008. That same year, approximately 5.2% of the region's 15- to 49-year-old population was living with HIV infection.

More specific HIV statistics for countries in sub-Saharan Africa are shown in Table 3.2. In 2006 the countries with the highest HIV prevalence in the 15 to 49 age group were Swaziland (33.4%), Botswana (24.1%), Lesotho (23.2%), and Zimbabwe (20.1%). These statistics mean that between one-fifth and one-third of all people aged 15 to 49 in these countries were infected with HIV.

Even though HIV infection rates are high in sub-Saharan Africa, access to treatment is generally poor. (See Table 3.2.) In Swaziland, the country with the highest prevalence of HIV, less than one-third (31%) of

FIGURE 3.6

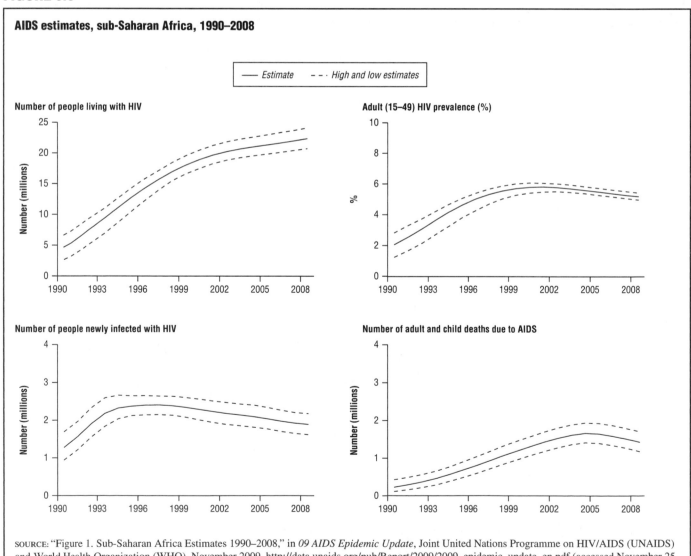

SOURCE: "Figure 1. Sub-Saharan Africa Estimates 1990–2008," in *09 AIDS Epidemic Update*, Joint United Nations Programme on HIV/AIDS (UNAIDS) and World Health Organization (WHO), November 2009, http://data.unaids.org/pub/Report/2009/2009_epidemic_update_en.pdf (accessed November 25, 2009)

TABLE 3.2

Gross domestic product (GDP) per capita, HIV prevalence, and access to health care, sub-Saharan Africa, 2006

Country	GDP per capita (U.S.$)	HIV prevalence, ages 15–49 (percent)	Access to treatment (percent)	Population per physician (units)	Population per nurse (units)	PLWH per physician (units)	PLWH per nurse (units)
Angola	1,873	3.7	6	12,993	871	363	24
Benin	595	1.8	33	22,244	1,195	280	15
Botswana	5,829	24.1	85	2,510	378	378	57
Burkina Faso	438	2	24	16,975	2,427	190	27
Burundi	107	3.3	14	35,340	5,243	750	111
Cameroon	952	5.4	22	5,216	626	163	20
Central African Republic	336	10.7	3	11,819	3,293	755	210
Chad	601	3.5	17	25,664	3,709	522	75
Congo	1,751	5.3	17	5,050	1,040	159	33
Côte d'Ivoire	850	7.1	17	8,120	1,660	360	74
Dem. Republic of Congo	119	3.2	4	9,339	1,890	172	35
Equatorial Guinea	5,934	3.2	0	3,314	2,224	58	39
Eritrea	206	2.4	5	19,986	1,715	274	24
Ethiopia	153	0.9–3.5	7	36,507	4,746	n.a.	n.a.
Gabon	6,538	7.9	23	3,420	194	152	9
Gambia	304	2.4	10	9,141	830	128	12
Ghana	512	2.3	7	6,598	1,085	99	16
Guinea	355	1.5	9	8,734	1,812	86	18
Guinea-Bissau	181	3.8	1	8,181	1,483	170	31
Kenya	574	6.1	24	7,195	874	289	35
Lesotho	537	23.2	14	20,247	1,605	3,034	240
Madagascar	263	0.5	0	3,442	3,162	9	9
Malawi	161	14.1	20	46,380	1,698	3,534	129
Mali	421	1.7	32	12,734	2,051	123	20
Mauritius	5,058	0.6	n.a.	946	271	3	1
Mozambique	346	16.1	9	37,319	4,851	3,502	455
Namibia	2,870	19.6	71	3,363	327	385	37
Niger	278	1.1	5	32,931	4,571	210	29
Nigeria	678	3.9	7	3,551	590	83	14
Rwanda	242	3.1	39	21,150	2,360	474	53
Senegal	715	0.9	47	17,406	3,145	103	19
Sierra Leone	219	1.6	2	30,762	2,807	286	26
South Africa	5,100	18.8	21	1,298	245	158	30
Sudan	783	1.6	1	n.a.	n.a.	n.a.	n.a.
Swaziland	2,323	33.4	31	6,333	159	1,287	32
Togo	378	3.2	27	12,086	1,646	50	7
Uganda	326	6.7	51	44,131	2,729	1,217	75
United Republic of Tanzania	324	6.5	7	22,298	2,343	6,222	654
Zambia	609	17	27	8,642	575	870	58
Zimbabwe	383	20.1	8	6,199	1,302	815	182

PLWH = Person living with HIV.

SOURCE: "Table A2.1. HIV Prevalence, Income, Access to Treatment and Quality of Health Services in Sub-Saharan Africa, 2006," in *The World Bank's Commitment to HIV/AIDS in Africa: Our Agenda for Action 2007–2011*, The World Bank, March, 2008, http://siteresources.worldbank.org/ INTAFRREGTOPHIVAIDS/Resources/WB_HIV-AIDS-AFA_2007-2011_Advance_Copy.pdf (accessed November 25, 2009). Copyright © International Bank for Reconstruction and Development/The World Bank 2008. Data from M. Haacker, "HIV/AIDS, Public Policy, and Development in the 'New Age' of Expanded Access to Treatment," unpublished manuscript, International Monetary Fund, 2007.

the population had access to treatment in 2006. In Equatorial Guinea there was no access to treatment. By contrast, Botswana, the country with the second-highest prevalence of HIV infection in sub-Saharan Africa, had the highest percentage (85%) of people having access to treatment. Nonetheless, this relatively high availability to treatment is unusual throughout sub-Saharan Africa. Table 3.2 also shows the number of people living with HIV (PLWH) per physician and per nurse in each country. Most numbers are in the hundreds, and some are in the thousands. This means that for a few hundred or, in some cases, a few thousand infected people, there is only one doctor available to provide medical care. There are more nurses than doctors, so their availability is greater.

MALARIA. Even though AIDS is certainly the most notable factor contributing to Africa's low life expectancy, it is not the only disease that takes tens of thousands of African lives per year, threatens the continent's economic stability, and leaves families even deeper in poverty. Table 3.3 shows that even though HIV/AIDS accounted for 20.4% of the deaths in sub-Saharan Africa in 2000, malaria accounted for 10.1% of all deaths.

Malaria is a highly infectious but preventable disease that is spread through tropical regions by mosquitoes. Countries with high rates of malarial infection are known to have a significantly lower gross domestic product (GDP; the total value of all goods and services produced by a country in a year), slower rates of economic growth,

TABLE 3.3

Ten most common causes of death in sub-Saharan Africa, 2000

The 10 most common causes of death	% of total deaths in 2000
HIV/AIDS	20.4
Malaria	10.1
Lower respiratory infections	9.8
Diarrheal diseases	6.5
Perinatal conditions	5.1
Measles	4.1
Cerebrovascular disease	3.3
Ischemic heart disease	3.1
Tuberculosis	2.8
Road traffic accidents	1.8

SOURCE: Adapted from "Table 2.1. Ten Most Common Causes of Mortality and Morbidity in Sub-Saharan Africa," in *The World Bank's Commitment to HIV/AIDS in Africa: Our Agenda for Action 2007–2011*, The World Bank, March 2008, http://siteresources.worldbank.org/INTAFRREGTOPHIVAIDS/Resources/WB_HIV-AIDS-AFA_2007-2011_Advance_Copy.pdf (accessed November 25, 2009). Copyright © International Bank for Reconstruction and Development/The World Bank 2008.

and higher rates of poverty than those without. In the case of sub-Saharan Africa, the disease has had a significant impact on labor force participation and school attendance; children who suffer from repeat infections often develop permanent neurological damage that cuts short their education and hampers their ability to participate fully in the labor force as adults.

In the early 21st century poverty researchers began to recognize malaria's role in increasing impoverishment at the family and community levels and diminishing economic advancement at the national and global levels in countries prone to epidemics of the disease. Aside from the obvious difficulties facing poor families who cannot afford treatment or prevention, the wider effects of frequent epidemics include impeded market activity and tourism industries as traders and potential tourists avoid areas with heavy infection rates. Even agricultural trends can shift with malaria rates; farmers dependent on the availability of workers during harvest seasons will be less likely to plant labor-intensive cash crops, instead relying on subsistence crops.

According to the WHO, in *World Malaria Report, 2009* (2009, http://whqlibdoc.who.int/publications/2009/9789241563901_eng.pdf), there were 243 million cases of malaria worldwide in 2008, with 208 million (86%) of these cases in the African region. Approximately 863,000 people died from malaria that year, with 767,000 (89%) of the deaths in the African region. Children are particularly vulnerable to the disease. According to the UN Children's Fund (UNICEF; September 29, 2009, http://www.unicef.org/health/index_malaria.html), approximately 20% of all deaths in children in Africa are directly attributable to malaria. Considerably more deaths are believed to be indirectly related to the disease because repeated malarial infections can lead to severe anemia, which in

turn makes children more susceptible to other illnesses. Additionally, the infection of pregnant women raises the rate of infant mortality because it can cause low birth weight and other complications.

Malaria is particularly common in sub-Saharan Africa due to the prevalence of *Plasmodium falciparum*—the most deadly of the four species of the *Plasmodium* parasite that causes malaria. In addition, Anopheles mosquitoes, which spread the parasite from person to person when they bite an infected individual and then bite an uninfected one, are prevalent in sub-Saharan Africa. Another complicating factor is the high level of HIV infection in sub-Saharan Africa and its effect on contracting malaria. People with HIV infections have suppressed immune systems, so they are more susceptible to being infected with malaria. HIV infection also appears to lower the effectiveness of malarial drugs.

In the past the most effective and affordable antimalarial drug was chloroquine. However, the malaria parasite in sub-Saharan Africa developed resistance to this drug, so the WHO no longer recommends chloroquine use. Since 2003 nearly all sub-Saharan countries have shifted to artemisinin-based combination drugs, which are effective in treating multidrug-resistant strains of the malaria parasite. Xiaochun Chen et al. examine in "Fumagillin and Fumarranol Interact with *P. falciparum* Methionine Aminopeptidase 2 and Inhibit Malaria Parasite Growth in Vitro and In Vivo" (*Chemistry and Biology*, vol. 16, no. 2, February 27, 2009) the results on the use of the chemical compound fumarranol in treating drug-resistant malaria. Fumarranol kills the parasite in mice, and the researchers believe it is a promising beginning for the development of new antimalarial drugs.

UNICEF notes in *Malaria and Children: Progress in Intervention Coverage—Summary Update 2009* (2009, http://www.unicef.org/health/files/WMD_optimized_reprint.pdf) that one of the most effective ways to prevent the spread of malaria is the use of insecticide-treated mosquito nets (ITNs), which are draped over beds at night, when most disease-carrying mosquitoes bite. Spraying living and sleeping spaces with insecticidal spray helps as well. With funding and support from a number of agencies, the number of ITNs produced worldwide more than tripled from 30 million in 2004 to 100 million in 2008.

Remarkable progress has been made in the use of ITNs in many sub-Saharan countries due to the rapid rise in their manufacture, efforts to increase their distribution, and governmental educational campaigns to promote their use. Some countries, such as Côte d'Ivoire, have not made as much progress as other countries, such as Rwanda. (See Figure 3.7.) In 2000 ITNs were used by 1% of children in Côte d'Ivoire; in 2006 ITNs were used by only 3% of children in that country. In contrast, in 2000 ITNs were used by 4% of children in Rwanda; in 2007–08 ITNs were used by 56% of Rwandan children. Even

FIGURE 3.7

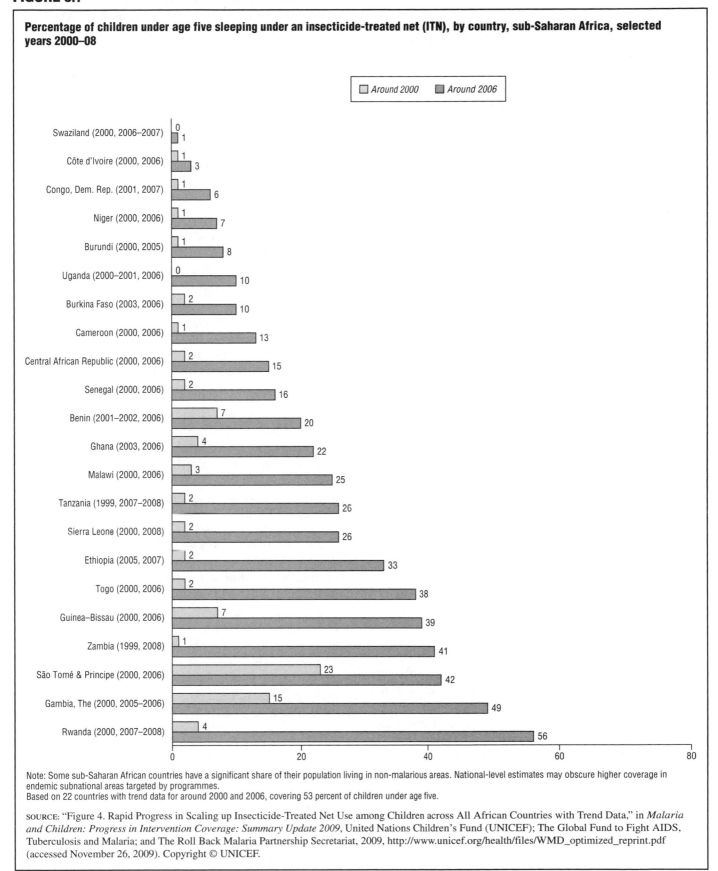

Percentage of children under age five sleeping under an insecticide-treated net (ITN), by country, sub-Saharan Africa, selected years 2000–08

Note: Some sub-Saharan African countries have a significant share of their population living in non-malarious areas. National-level estimates may obscure higher coverage in endemic subnational areas targeted by programmes.
Based on 22 countries with trend data for around 2000 and 2006, covering 53 percent of children under age five.

SOURCE: "Figure 4. Rapid Progress in Scaling up Insecticide-Treated Net Use among Children across All African Countries with Trend Data," in *Malaria and Children: Progress in Intervention Coverage: Summary Update 2009*, United Nations Children's Fund (UNICEF); The Global Fund to Fight AIDS, Tuberculosis and Malaria; and The Roll Back Malaria Partnership Secretariat, 2009, http://www.unicef.org/health/files/WMD_optimized_reprint.pdf (accessed November 26, 2009). Copyright © UNICEF.

though progress still needs to be made, UNICEF notes that "19 of 22 African countries with trend data at least tripled coverage during this time, with 17 of them experiencing at least a fivefold increase."

FIGURE 3.8

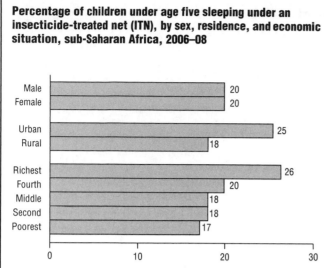

Percentage of children under age five sleeping under an insecticide-treated net (ITN), by sex, residence, and economic situation, sub-Saharan Africa, 2006–08

SOURCE: "Figure 5. Use of Insecticide-Treated Nets is Lowest among African Children in Rural Areas and the Poorest Households," in *Malaria and Children: Progress in Intervention Coverage: Summary Update 2009*, United Nations Children's Fund (UNICEF); The Global Fund to Fight AIDS, Tuberculosis and Malaria; and The Roll Back Malaria Partnership Secretariat, 2009, http://www.unicef.org/health/files/WMD_optimized_reprint.pdf (accessed November 26, 2009). Copyright © UNICEF.

UNICEF also points out that the use of ITNs is lowest among African children living in rural areas and in the poorest households. Figure 3.8 shows that in 2006–08 ITNs were used by 25% of children under the age of five living in urban areas of sub-Saharan Africa, but by only 18% of under-five children living in the region's rural areas. Additionally, ITN use correlated positively with wealth; that is, ITNs were used by 26% of children who lived in sub-Saharan Africa's richest households and by only 17% of children who lived in the poorest households.

SANITATION AND CLEAN WATER. Clean water for drinking, food preparation, and bathing and effective sanitation of wastewater is essential in disease control. Clean water is free of disease-causing organisms. Effective sanitation keeps fecal waste separate from water supplies and treats wastewater to kill pathogens (disease-causing microbes). Even though urine is virtually free of microbes, fecal waste contains a variety of species of microbes, many of which are capable of causing disease. Food prepared with contaminated water can transmit disease as well. Moreover, bathing with contaminated water can result in infections of the skin, mucous membranes, ears, nose, and throat. Diseases that are commonly transmitted by contaminated water include those that cause severe diarrhea. In 2000 diarrheal diseases were the fourth-most common cause of death in sub-Saharan Africa. (See Table 3.3.)

According to UNICEF, in *Soap, Toilets, and Taps: A Foundation for Healthy Children* (February 2009, http://www.unicef.org/wash/files/26351FINALLayoutEn1(1).pdf), from 1990 to 2006 progress was made in sanitation in sub-Saharan Africa, most specifically in reductions in the practice of open defecation (expelling feces without using a toilet). In a rural environment this practice may occur simply on the land, such as in a field; in an urban environment open defecation may mean relieving oneself in a gutter, onto a newspaper, or into a plastic bag. Oftentimes, this fecal material ends up in the water sources that people use for drinking, food preparation, and bathing. Furthermore, in many cultures women are not allowed to be seen uncovered, so they often have to wait until dark to relieve themselves. As a result, they not only develop health issues from delayed defecation and possibly urination but also risk bodily harm as they travel in the darkness alone. Improved sanitation (the use of toilets) rids women of these health and safety problems, restores some level of dignity to both genders, dramatically reduces disease, and reduces childhood deaths. UNICEF notes that in spite of the recent progress made in improved sanitation, 1.2 billion people worldwide have no sanitation facilities and defecate in the open.

Figure 3.9 shows changes in the use of sanitation facilities from 1990 to 2006 for various regions of the world. Globally, open defecation decreased 6% during this period, from 24% to 18%. In developing countries, open defecation decreased 8%, from 31% to 23%, and in sub-Saharan Africa the practice decreased 8% as well, from 36% to 28%.

In spite of this progress in sanitation, sub-Saharan Africa still lags behind other regions of the world in the use of improved drinking water sources that supply clean water. Being without clean water means living more than 0.6 of a mile (1 km) from the nearest safe water source. People without a source of clean water nearby usually collect water from unsafe sources, such as drains, ditches, and streams. These sources are often shared with animals and are likely to be contaminated with disease-causing organisms, such as bacteria and viruses, which may cause severe illness and death.

Figure 3.10 shows the progress that was made in access to clean water from 1990 to 2006 in various regions of the world. The percentage of people in sub-Saharan Africa who had drinking water piped into their home remained stagnant at 16% from 1990 to 2006. However, the presence of other improved sources of clean water, such as nearby protected wells and streams or a public standpipe (communal water tap), rose from 33% in 1990 to 42% in 2006. Consequently, the percentage of the population in sub-Saharan Africa without an improved water source dropped from 51% in 1990 to 42% in 2006. Even greater progress was made in developing countries in

FIGURE 3.9

Global changes in the use of sanitation facilities, by region, 1990–2006

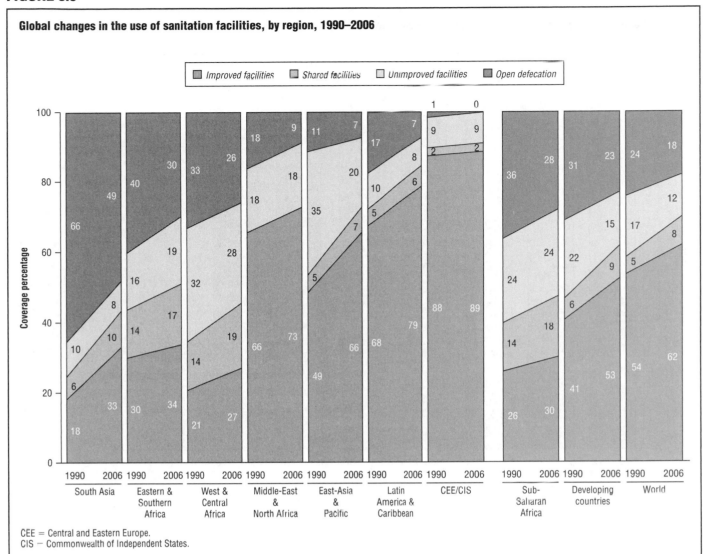

CEE = Central and Eastern Europe.
CIS – Commonwealth of Independent States.

SOURCE. "Open Defecation Is Decreasing," in *Soap, Toilets, and Taps—A Foundation for Healthy Children: How UNICEF Supports Water, Sanitation and Hygiene*, United Nation's Children's Fund (UNICEF), February 2009, http://www.unicef.org/wash/files/26351FINALLayoutEn1(1).pdf (accessed December 5, 2009). Copyright © UNICEF.

general from 1990 to 2006: having piped drinking water in the home increased from 36% to 46% of the population of developing countries, having other improved water sources increased from 35% to 38%, and having unimproved sources fell from 29% to 16%.

Education and Literacy

Table 3.4 shows that 74% of all children of primary school age in sub-Saharan Africa were enrolled in primary school in 2008. Even though the percentage of children enrolled in primary school may seem low, great progress has been made in recent years. In 2000, 58% of all children of primary school age were enrolled in primary school, and by 2005 this number increased to 69%. Thus, in just eight years the number of children enrolled in primary school in sub-Saharan Africa rose 16 percentage points. Strides have also been made in primary

school completion rates in sub-Saharan Africa. In 2000 only 50% of all children of primary school age completed primary school. By 2005, 59% completed primary school and by 2008, 63% completed this course of study.

The UN finds in *Millennium Development Goals Report, 2009* (2009, http://www.un.org/millenniumgoals/pdf/MDG_Report_2009_ENG.pdf) that primary school enrollment in developed nations was 96% in 2007. By contrast, sub-Saharan Africa had an extremely low rate of primary school enrollment, at 74%. Along with poverty and a lack of resources in the region, the two other major reasons for this low rate are the high prevalence of disease and military conflict.

The prevalence of disease—particularly HIV/AIDS and malaria—takes an especially heavy toll on school-aged children in sub-Saharan Africa. Besides the many

FIGURE 3.10

Global changes in the use of improved drinking water sources, by region, 1990–2006

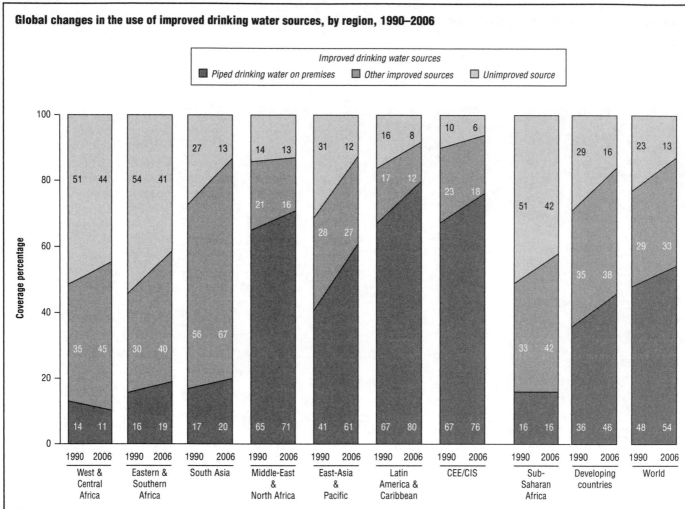

CEE = Central and Eastern Europe.
CIS = Commonwealth of Independent States.

SOURCE: "Africa Lags behind in Use of Improved Drinking Water Sources," in *Soap, Toilets, and Taps—A Foundation for Healthy Children: How UNICEF Supports Water, Sanitation and Hygiene*, United Nation's Children's Fund (UNICEF), February 2009, http://www.unicef.org/wash/files/26351FINALLayoutEn1(1).pdf (accessed December 5, 2009). Copyright © UNICEF.

children who must leave school because they suffer from diseases such as HIV and malaria, many others are affected in another way: by the loss of their teachers. The National Academy of Public Administration states in *Mitigating HIV/AIDS' Impacts on Teachers and Administrators in Sub-Saharan Africa* (December 2005, http://www.napawash.org/Pubs/africa.pdf) that "some 200,000 of Sub-Saharan Africa's 650,000 teachers are projected to die from AIDS." Figure 3.11 shows the effects of HIV/AIDS on education and vice versa. The high prevalence of HIV/AIDS in sub-Saharan Africa not only reduces the quality of education and expands illiteracy but also feeds the growth of the prevalence of HIV infection.

Persistent military conflicts in many African countries also make it nearly impossible for many children, particularly those living in rural areas, to attend school, even if schools still exist. Decades of political, economic, and social turmoil have decimated the educational sector

on the continent. Schools have been destroyed, students and teachers have been killed, and teaching materials and supplies are virtually nonexistent. Merely walking to school can be deadly due to the existence of land mines.

Low rates of primary schooling result in low rates of literacy. According to the UN Educational, Scientific, and Cultural Organization (UNESCO), in *Education for All Global Monitoring Report 2009: Overcoming Inequality—Why Governance Matters* (2008, http://unesdoc.unesco.org/images/0017/001776/177683e.pdf), the rate of adult literacy in sub-Saharan Africa was 53% in 1985–94, compared with a 99% rate of adult literacy in developed countries. Approximately 133 million adults in sub-Saharan Africa were illiterate during this period. In 2000–06 the rate of adult literacy in this region increased to 62%. The number of adult illiterates rose as well, to about 161.1 million. However, UNESCO projects that by 2015 the adult literacy rate will rise to 72% in sub-Saharan Africa and that

TABLE 3.4

Sub-Saharan Africa's progress in reaching Millennium Development Goals (MDGs), selected years, 1990–2008

	1990	1995	2000	2005	2000
Goal 1: Eradicate extreme poverty and hunger					
Employment to population ratio, 15 I, total (%)	64	64	64	64	64
Employment to population ratio, ages 15–24, total (%)	50	50	49	49	49
GDP per person employed (annual % growth)	−5	2	1	4	—
Income share held by lowest 20%	—	—	—	—	—
Malnutrition prevalence, weight for age (% of children under 5)	—	—	—	26.5	26.5
Poverty gap at $1.25 a day (PPP) (%)	—	—	—	—	—
Poverty headcount ratio at $1.25 a day (PPP) (% of population)	58	59	58	51	—
Prevalence of undernourishment (% of population)	32	32	—	29	—
Vulnerable employment, total (% of total employment)	—	—	—	—	—
Goal 2: Achieve universal primary education					
Literacy rate, youth female (% of females ages 15–24)	59	—	65	67	67
Literacy rate, youth male (% of males ages 15–24)	71	—	76	77	77
Persistence to last grade of primary, total (% of cohort)	—	—	—	—	—
Primary completion rate, total (% of relevant age group)	51	—	50	59	63
Total enrollment, primary (% net)	—	—	58	69	74
Goal 3: Promote gender equality and empower women					
Proportion of seats held by women in national parliaments (%)	—	10	12	16	18
Ratio of female to male enrollments in tertiary education	—	—	63	68	67
Ratio of female to male primary enrollment	83	—	85	88	90
Ratio of female to male secondary enrollment	76	—	81	80	79
Share of women employed in the nonagricultural sector (% of total nonagricultural employment)	—	—	—	—	—
Goal 4: Reduce child mortality					
Immunization, measles (% of children ages 12–23 months)	57	54	55	69	73
Mortality rate, infant (per 1,000 live births)	108	105	98	91	89
Mortality rate, under-5 (per 1,000)	183	178	164	151	146
Goal 5: Improve maternal health					
Adolescent fertility rate (births per 1,000 women ages 15–19)	—	134	130	122	118
Births attended by skilled health staff (% of total)	—	—	—	45	45
Contraceptive prevalence (% of women ages 15–49)	15	—	—	22	22
Maternal mortality ratio (modeled estimate, per 100,000 live births)	920	—	—	900	—
Pregnant women receiving prenatal care (%)	—	—	—	72	72
Unmet need for contraception (% of married women ages 15–49)	—	—	—	24	24
Goal 6: Combat HIV/AIDS, malaria, and other diseases					
Children with fever receiving antimalarial drugs (& of children under age 5 with fever)	—	—	—	35	35
Condom use, population ages 15–24, female (% of females ages 15–24)	—	—	—	15	15
Condom use, population ages 15–24, male (% of males ages 15–24)	—	—	—	36	36
Incidence of tuberculosis (per 100,000 people)	176	237	325	384	369
Prevalence of HIV, female (% ages 15–24)	—	—	—	3.3	3.3
Prevalence of HIV, male (% ages 15–24)	—	—	—		
Prevalence of HIV, total (% of population ages 15–49)	2.1	4.4	5.5	5.1	5.0
Tuberculosis cases detected under DOTS (%)	—	33	40	45	47
Goal 7: Ensure environmental sustainability					
CO_2 emissions (kg per PPP $ of GDP)	0.8	0.7	0.6	0.5	—
CO_2 emissions (metric tons per capita)	0.9	0.8	0.8	0.9	—
Forest area (% of land area)	30	28	27	26	—
Improved sanitation facilities (% of population with access)	26	27	29	31	31
Improved water source (% of population with access)	49	51	55	58	58
Marine protected areas, (% of surface area)	—	—	—	—	—
Nationally protected areas (% of total land area)	—	—	—	11.3	11.3
Goal 8: Develop a global partnership for development					
Aid per capita (current US$)	35	32	20	43	44
Debt service (PPG and IMF only, % of exports, excluding workers' remittances)	—	10	9	8	4
Internet users (per 100 people)	0.0	0.1	0.5	2.2	4.5
Mobile cellular subscriptions (per 100 people)	0	0	2	12	32
Telephone lines (per 100 people)	1	1	1	1	1

the number of adult illiterates will fall to approximately 147.7 million despite the educational obstacles facing the people of this region. One major reason for this positive projection is that the youth in sub-Saharan Africa are making gains in the rates of primary school enrollment and literacy. Youth literacy rates (for those aged 15 to 24) in sub-Saharan Africa are higher than adult literacy rates (for those aged 15 years and older). Females aged 15 to 24 years had a literacy rate of 67% in both 2005 and 2008, and males in the same age group for the same years had a literacy rate of 77%, compared with the adult literacy rate of 62% during 2000–06. (See Table 3.4.)

Economic Well-Being

In *World Development Report 2006: Equity and Development* (2005, http://www-wds.worldbank.org/), the World

TABLE 3.4

Sub-Saharan Africa's progress in reaching Millennium Development Goals (MDGs), selected years, 1990–2008 [CONTINUED]

Other	1990	1995	2000	2005	2008
Fertility rate, total (births per woman)	6.3	5.9	5.6	5.2	5.1
GNI per capita, Atlas method (current US$)	555	529	486	757	1,082
GNI, Atlas method (current US$) (billions)	284.3	310.5	326.1	575.5	885.3
Gross capital formation (% of GDP)	17.9	18.4	17.3	19.1	22.6
Life expectancy at birth, total (years)	50	50	50	51	52
Literacy rate, adult total (% of people ages 15 and above)	54	—	59	62	62
Population, total (millions)	512.1	587.1	670.8	760.3	818.0
Trade (% of GDP)					

PPP = Purchasing Power Parity. GDP = Gross Domestic Product. PPG = Public and Publicly Guaranteed. DOTS = Development Outcome Tracking System.

SOURCE: "Sub-Saharan Africa Millennium Development Goals," The World Bank, World Development Indicators Database, http://ddp-ext.worldbank.org/ext/ddpreports/ViewSharedReport?&CF=1&REPORT_ID=1336&REQUEST_TYPE=VIEWADVANCED&HF=N (accessed December 5, 2009). Copyright © International Bank for Reconstruction and Development/The World Bank 2008.

FIGURE 3.11

The effect of HIV/AIDS on education

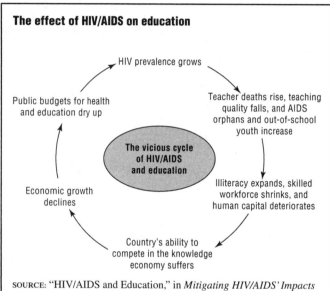

SOURCE: "HIV/AIDS and Education," in *Mitigating HIV/AIDS' Impacts on Teachers and Administrators in Sub-Saharan Africa*, National Academy of Public Administration, 2006, http://www.napawash.org/Pubs/africa.pdf (accessed December 5, 2009). Data adapted from The World Bank, www.developmentgoals.org, 2004.

Bank states, "An individual's consumption, his or her income, or his or her wealth have all been used as indicators of the command of an individual over goods and services that can be purchased in the market and that contribute directly to well-being. It is clear too, that individuals' economic status can determine and shape in many ways the opportunities they face to improve their situations. Economic well-being can also contribute to improved education outcomes and better health care. In turn, good health and good education are typically important determinants of economic status."

The interconnectedness of health, education, and economic status is true in all countries. Circumstances in Africa, including armed conflicts, under- and malnutrition, little access to clean water and improved sanitation, and the

HIV/AIDS and malaria epidemics, have led to a long history of extreme poverty. Table 3.4 shows that the percentage of people living on less than $1.25 per day (in 2005 U.S. dollars) in sub-Saharan Africa decreased from 59% in 1995 to 51% in 2005. In spite of this progress, the UN explains in *Millennium Development Goals Report, 2009* that the global economic crisis that began in 2007 derailed the progress being made in reducing poverty in this region and in others around the world. The UN notes that "in sub-Saharan Africa and Southern Asia, both the number of poor and the poverty rate are expected to increase further in some of the more vulnerable and low-growth economies." Thus, it will be difficult and almost impossible for sub-Saharan Africa to reach its Millennium Development Goal (MDG) of 28.5% by 2015, and even if this goal were to be reached, it would mean that more than one out of every four people in the region would still be living in extreme poverty.

ASIA: THE LARGEST AND MOST POPULOUS CONTINENT

In terms of both number of people and land mass, Asia is the largest continent, with 4 billion people (about two-thirds of the world's population) in approximately 55 countries covering over 17 million square miles (44 million sq km), including parts of Siberia (North Asia); China, Japan, Taiwan, and the Korea Peninsula (East Asia, or the Far East); the Middle East, including the Arabian Peninsula, the Persian Gulf countries, Armenia, Georgia, Azerbaijan, the Near East countries of Israel, Jordan, Syria, Lebanon, and Iraq, and parts of North Africa (West Asia); India, Pakistan, Nepal, Bhutan, Bangladesh, Sri Lanka, and the Maldives (South Asia, or the Indian subcontinent); Indonesia, Malaysia, the Philippines, Vietnam, Thailand, Laos, and Cambodia (Southeast Asia); and Afghanistan and the republics of Kazakhstan, Kyrgyzstan, Tajikistan, Turkmenistan, and Uzbekistan (central Asia). Because the borders around Asia have never been permanently defined, experts disagree on the total number of countries on the continent, and even the distinctions outlined here are in dispute. For example, sometimes East and Southeast Asia are discussed together as East Asia and the Pacific.

Asia is a region of geographic, ethnic, and cultural diversity as well as of immense economic differences. The region houses—at the same time—some of the wealthiest people in the world and some of the most startlingly poor, many of whom reside in the 14 LDCs of Asia and the Pacific.

THE LEAST DEVELOPED COUNTRIES OF ASIA AND THE PACIFIC

The UN Office of the High Representative for the Least Developed Countries, Landlocked Developing Countries, and Small Island Developing States (2009, http://www.unohrlls.org/en/ldc/related/62/) lists 49 LDCs in the world: 33 are in Africa and 15 are in Asia and the Pacific (the remaining LDC is Haiti). (See Table 3.1.) The UNDP and the UN Economic and Social Commission (UNESCAP) discuss the LDCs in *Voices of the Least Developed Countries of Asia and the Pacific: Achieving the Millennium Development Goals through a Global Partnership* (2005, http://www.unescap.org/unis/Library/pub_pdf/LDCMDG-Voices.pdf). This publication is unique because it deals with the LDCs of Asia and the Pacific as a unit and their progress in reaching the Millennium Development Goals (MDGs). Other publications divide Asia and the Pacific into the following regions: southern, western, eastern, and southeastern. The LDCs of Asia and the Pacific are found in both the southern and southeastern portions of Asia and the Pacific.

As of February 2010, *Voices of the Least Developed Countries of Asia and the Pacific* was the most up-to-date publication focusing on the LDCs of only Asia and the Pacific and these countries' poverty and progress toward the MDGs. The UNDP and UNESCAP state that the LDCs of Asia and the Pacific together account for 37% of the total population of all LDCs. These countries range in size from Bangladesh, which has 130 million people, to Tuvalu with 11,000 people. The LDCs of Asia and the Pacific are Afghanistan, Bangladesh, Bhutan, Cambodia, Kiribati, Lao People's Democratic Republic (Laos), Maldives, Myanmar, Nepal, Samoa, Solomon Islands, Timor-Leste, Tuvalu, Vanuatu, and Yemen.

The UNDP and UNESCAP examine in *Voices of the Least Developed Countries of Asia and the Pacific* the status and progress of the LDCs in Asia and the Pacific in reducing poverty. In 1990, 55% of the population of the LDCs in Asia and the Pacific were living below their countries' national poverty lines. By 2000 that proportion had decreased to 46.8%, but the reduction was not enough to be on track to reach the 2015 target of 27.5%. At the current trajectory, 37.9% of the population of the LDCs in Asia and the Pacific will be impoverished in 2015.

Even though Asia as a whole has experienced much growth, and the large Asian economies of China and India have expanded in the early 21st century and reduced their rates of overall poverty to a greater degree than the LDCs of the Asian and Pacific region, 22% of the population of developing countries in Asia lived on less than $1 per day (now referred to as $1.25 per day) in 2004, whereas 38% of the population of the Asian and Pacific LDCs lived on less than $1 per day in that same year.

Afghanistan

Afghanistan is considered the second least developed country in the world and had the lowest poverty index (HPI-1) in 2009. (See Table 1.2 in Chapter 1.) More than two decades of near-constant war and natural disasters left Afghanistan with an HDI ranking of 181 out of 182 countries in 2009. (Africa's Niger was ranked 182.) By comparison, Norway had the world's highest HDI ranking and the United States ranked 13th in 2009. (See Table 1.3 in Chapter 1.) According to Jeni Klugman of the UNDP, in *Human Development Report 2009—Overcoming Barriers: Human Mobility and Development* (2009, http://hdr.undp.org/en/media/HDR_2009_EN_Complete.pdf), Afghanistan's Gender-related Development Index (GDI; examines the basic quality of life but is adjusted for inequalities between men and women) had a GDI ranking of 154 out of 155 countries and a GDI value of 0.31 in 2007. Australia ranked first in the world, with a GDI value of 0.966, Norway was second at 0.961, and the United States was 19th at 0.942. Niger ranked last with a GDI value of 0.308.

Individual poverty indicators are equally low. In *Afghanistan Human Development Report 2007: Bridging Modernity and Tradition—Rule of Law and the Search for Justice* (2007, http://hdr.undp.org/en/reports/national reports/asiathepacific/afghanistan/nhdr2007.pdf), the UNDP indicates that Afghanistan's GDP per capita was $683 in 2002 but rose to $964 in 2005. According to the Central Intelligence Agency (CIA), in *World Factbook: Afghanistan* (February 4, 2010, https://www.cia.gov/library/publications/the-world-factbook/geos/af.html), Afghanistan's GDP per capita in 2009 was $800 (all in purchasing power parity [PPP] terms; see Chapter 1). As a comparison, Klugman indicates that the GDP per capita average in PPP terms for low human development countries was $862 in 2007, whereas the average for medium human development countries was $3,963. The average GDP per capita worldwide was $9,972 and the average GDP per capita for the United States was $45,592.

HEALTH AND MORTALITY IN AFGHANISTAN. The UNDP notes in *Afghanistan Human Development Report 2007* that life expectancy at birth in Afghanistan fell from 44.5 years in 2003 to 43.1 years in 2005. According to Klugman, by 2007 life expectancy at birth in Afghanistan rose slightly to 43.6

TABLE 3.5

Afghanistan's progress in reaching Millennium Development Goals (MDGs), 2005

MDG	Indicator	Kuchi*	Rural	Urban	National average
1 Eradicate extreme poverty and hunger	Proportion of population below minimum level of dietary energy consumption (%)	24	30	31	30
2 Achieve universal primary education	Net enrollment rate in primary education	9	36	53	37
	Literacy rate of 15–24 year-olds (%)	5	25	63	31
3 Promote gender equality and empower women	Ratio of girls to boys in primary education	0.5	0.6	0.9	0.7
	Ratio of literate women to men, 15–24 years old	0.9	0.3	0.8	0.5
4 Reduce child mortality	Proportion of 1-year-old children immunized against measles (%)	35	51	63	53
5 Improve maternal health	Proportion of births attended by skilled health personnel (%)	7	9	52	53
6 Combat HIV/AIDS, malaria and other diseases	Use of condoms (%)	17	8	9	8
7 Ensure environmental sustainability	Proportion of population using solid fuels (%)	98	98	75	94
	Proportion of population with sustainable access to an improved water source, urban and rural (%)	16	26	63	31
	Proportion of population with access to improved sanitation, urban and rural (%)	0	3	28	7
	Prop. households with secure housing tenure (%)	28	44	83	49
8 Develop a global partnership for development	Telephone lines and cellular subscribers per 100 population	0.1	0.3	8.3	1.5
	Personal computers in use per 100 people	0.00	0.01	0.52	0.09
	Internet users per 100 people	0	0.01	0.18	0.03

*Nomad population.

SOURCE: "Table 1.4. Some Indicators of Progress of AMDGs," in *Afghanistan Human Development Report 2007—Bridging Modernity and Tradition: Rule of Law and the Search for Justice*, United Nations Development Programme and Kabul University, Center for Policy and Human Development, 2007, http://hdr.undp.org/en/reports/nationalreports/asiathepacific/afghanistan/nhdr2007.pdf (accessed December 11, 2009).

years. The UNDP explains that even though the incidence of malaria and tuberculosis has dropped, the health indicators for both women and children remain low, with widespread violence against women a serious threat to health and life. In addition, the mortality rates of infants, children, and mothers are some of the highest in the world. Only 11 of the country's 31 provinces have obstetric care available, and Afghan women report that the care they do receive is inadequate. Table 3.5 shows that nationally only 53% of births were attended by skilled health personnel in 2005. Only 7% of Kuchi (nomadic) women and 9% of women who lived in rural areas were attended by skilled health personnel while giving birth.

UNICEF notes in *State of the World's Children 2008: Child Survival* (December 2007, http://www.unicef.org/sowc08/docs/sowc08.pdf) that Afghanistan is one of 11 countries in which 20% or more of the children die before they reach their fifth birthday. An estimated 257 per 1,000 children in Afghanistan died before reaching the age of five in 2006, which ranked Afghanistan the third highest in the rate of under-five mortality. The two countries in which the rate of under-five mortality was higher in 2006 were Sierra Leone (270) and Angola (260).

Besides the many children dying before the age of five in Afghanistan, the UNDP notes in *Afghanistan Human Development Report 2007* that an estimated 54% of children under the age of five suffered from chronic malnutrition

resulting in moderate to severe stunting of growth in 2006. The government of Afghanistan and the UNDP state in the joint report *Millennium Development Goals Islamic Republic of Afghanistan—Vision 2020: Annual Progress Report 2008* (September 2008, http://www.undp.org.af/Publications/KeyDocuments/2008_MDGAnnualProgressR.pdf) that the 2015 target for reducing the prevalence of underweight children under five years of age is 15%. Table 3.5 shows that nearly one-third (30%) of the population of Afghanistan lived below the minimum level of dietary energy consumption in 2005, whereas the *Vision 2020* report for 2005–07 places this figure at 39%.

In *Afghanistan Human Development Report 2007*, the UNDP notes that the annual number of malaria cases in Afghanistan has fallen by about half in recent years. In 2002 there were 626,839 documented cases of malaria, whereas in 2006 there were 329,754 cases. The UNDP explains that "the expansion of the BPHS [the Basic Package of Health Services instituted by the Afghan government in 2003] has facilitated the detection and treatment of malaria cases in vast areas of the country."

The BPHS initiative may be effective in decreasing the prevalence of malaria, but it has been less successful in lowering the incidence of tuberculosis (TB). The incidence of TB in Afghanistan is one of the highest in the world. According to the UNDP, of the 22 countries that had high incidences of this disease in 2005, Afghanistan ranked 17th. The prevalence of TB in Afghanistan was estimated at about 228 cases per 100,000 in 2005. Approximately 12,000 people die from TB in Afghanistan each year, and women of reproductive age have the highest incidence of TB.

Diseases such as measles and polio—which have been largely eradicated in developed countries—continue to afflict Afghan children. Table 3.5 shows that the national average for immunization of one-year-old children against measles was only 53% in 2005. The *Vision 2020* report for 2005–07 places this figure at 68%. Table 3.5 shows that those in urban areas had the highest percentage (63%) of immunization, whereas the Kuchi population had the lowest (35%). According to the UNDP, the 2005 rates for immunization of one-year-olds against TB and polio were somewhat higher: 73% of one-year-olds were immunized against TB and 76% against polio. Afghanistan is one of only six countries where polio still exists.

EDUCATION AND LITERACY. As a result of the country's long-standing military engagements, many of Afghanistan's schools have been seriously damaged or destroyed. So even though the 1964 Afghan constitution guarantees free and compulsory (required) education for all citizens, in 2005 only 37% of children aged six to 13 were enrolled in primary school, and less than one-third (31%) of the 15- to 24-year-old populace were literate. (See Table 3.5.) Those living in urban areas fared better. In 2005 more than half (53%) of urban children were enrolled in primary school and 63% of urban-dwellers were literate. By contrast, 36% of children living in rural areas were enrolled in primary school and 25% of 15- to 24-year-olds were literate, and only 9% of Kuchi children were enrolled in primary school and 5% of the 15- to 24-year-old Kuchi population were literate in 2005.

Access to education is limited and schools remain substandard in Afghanistan. Most classes are held in tents or in the open air, with few materials available. In more remote areas schools are often located inside mosques, where girls and women are not allowed. In areas where gender segregation is enforced, schools must either hold separate sessions for girls and boys, or there must be separate schools altogether. Some parents continue to resist sending their daughters to school due to cultural beliefs and a lack of value for female education. Nonetheless, the gender gap in schooling in Afghanistan is narrowing, especially for those living in cities. In *Afghanistan Human Development Report 2007*, the UNDP indicates that in 2005 in urban areas 55% of males and 51% of females were enrolled in primary schools. In rural areas 44% of males and 27% of females were enrolled, and in Kuchi populations 11% of males and 6% of females were enrolled.

ACCESS TO NATURAL RESOURCES. The ongoing military conflict in Afghanistan is another example of a cyclical situation that is both a cause and a consequence of poverty. On the one hand, it has caused environmental destruction that prevents many Afghans from earning a good living. On the other hand, because they cannot earn a living wage, Afghans continue to join militias and fight, thus causing more damage to natural resources and preventing other Afghans from getting out of poverty. Besides the environmental effects of war, Afghanistan has suffered from natural soil erosion and drought, which make agricultural work extremely difficult. A rapidly diminishing water table due to drought and infrastructure mismanagement has made safe water and sanitation rare in Afghanistan.

The scarcity and poor quality of water is a tremendous threat to human development in Afghanistan. Wetlands in the country have disappeared, along with the wildlife they housed and the agriculture they supported. According to the UNDP, in *Afghanistan Human Development Report 2007*, 73% of Afghan households had sanitation facilities within their compounds, and only 31% had access to safe drinking water in 2005. Moreover, Klugman indicates that in 2006 only 22% of Afghan households had sustainable access to safe water.

Access to arable (farmable) land is also linked to the health and livelihood of impoverished Afghans. The UNDP indicates in *Afghanistan Annual Report 2006* (August 2007, http://www.undp.org.af/Publications/KeyDocuments/UNDP%20AF%20ANNUAL%20REPORT%202006.pdf) that Afghanistan is one of the most heavily mined countries in the world and that removing land mines is important in helping provide more arable land. According to the CIA, in *World Factbook: Afghanistan*, just 12.1% of Afghanistan's land can be used as farmland. As a result, competition among rural farmers over land and water often leads to outbreaks of violence, and families can become displaced (forced to move to urban areas to survive) when they lose valuable land on which to farm or let their livestock graze, leaving them even more vulnerable to malnutrition and disease.

Timor-Leste

Afghanistan is the world's least developed country in terms of social and human development indicators, but Timor-Leste (formerly known as East Timor) is commonly cited as among the world's poorest in terms of income poverty. Table 1.2 in Chapter 1 shows that in 2009 Timor-Leste was ranked 122 out of 135 countries on the Human Poverty Index and that 77.5% of its people lived on less than US $2 per day. As with many extremely poor countries, Timor-Leste has experienced violent conflict throughout much of its history that has contributed to reducing its potential for economic development and keeping much of the population in poverty.

Timor-Leste makes up about half of the island of Timor in Southeast Asia and is surrounded by the Banda Sea to the north and the Timor Sea to the south. This island country experienced 24 years of control by Indonesia (which controls the other half of the island) and three years of UN administration. The people of Timor-Leste voted for independence from Indonesia in 1999, but violence ensued, carried out by militia groups, resulting in the displacement of three-quarters of the population and the destruction of about 75% of the country's infrastructure. In May 2002 Timor-Leste officially became an independent republic, and since then it has been struggling to rebuild its infrastructure, stabilize its economy, and develop its government. In 2006 the country had a setback in trying to achieve these goals when nearly half of its army went on strike. The government subsequently fired the striking soldiers, and, once again, violence took over the country. With the assistance of international forces, order was eventually restored and Prime Minister Mari Alkatiri (1949–) resigned. In May 2007 José Ramos-Horta (1949–), the winner of a Nobel Peace Prize, was elected president of the country. He survived an assassination attempt in February 2008 and was the president as of February 2010.

ECONOMIC CONDITIONS. In spite of Timor-Leste's status of being extremely poor, it has substantial oil and natural gas reserves. After gaining independence in 2002, Timor-Leste signed a treaty with Australia that governs petroleum exploration and development in the part of the Timor Sea to which both countries claim jurisdiction. The treaty describes the method of joint administration by Australia and Timor-Leste of petroleum exploration and development in the Timor Sea.

In *Democratic Republic of Timor-Leste: Selected Issues* (July 2009, http://www.imf.org/external/pubs/ft/scr/2009/cr09220.pdf), Tobias Rasmussen indicates that income from oil and natural gas has raised the gross national income (GNI; the total value produced within a country plus income from other countries minus payments made to other countries) per capita from over $350 in 2002 to over $1,600 in 2007. Clearly, Timor-Leste is developing its petroleum resources to its economic advantage. However, according to Rasmussen, poverty is still pervasive within Timor-Leste and the standard of living in the country is one of the lowest in the world.

How can a small country such as Timor-Leste be rich in oil revenues yet have most of its citizens living in poverty? Where does the money go? Rasmussen explains that the oil revenues are deposited into the Petroleum Fund, which was established in 2005. The money in the fund is invested abroad with an eye to long-term sustainability. Withdrawals are made only to fund shortfalls in the country's budget. Rasmussen states, "This helps ensure that all revenue is properly accounted for, that the government budget remains the primary vehicle for public policy, and that wealth is preserved for future generations."

One factor that helps reduce poverty is high employment, but high employment is not a benefit of Timor-Leste's petroleum reserves. Rasmussen explains that the petroleum industry provides few jobs for the people of Timor-Leste because this natural resource is piped to Australia and processed there. Meanwhile, the non–oil economy of Timor-Leste has remained stagnant. According to the CIA, in *World Factbook: Timor-Leste* (January 15, 2010, https://www.cia.gov/library/publications/the-world-factbook/geos/tt.html), 90% of those employed in Timor-Leste in 2009 worked in agriculture, and the unemployment rate was high, at 20%. The challenge for Timor-Leste is to determine how best to use its petroleum revenues in the short term to help the non–oil economy and reduce poverty while sustaining the Petroleum Fund assets for the long term. Rasmussen states that "the overarching economic challenge remains to translate the petroleum wealth into a broad-based and sustainable increase in living standards."

HEALTH. According to the World Bank and the Asian Development Bank (ADB), in *Economic and Social Development Brief* (August 2007, http://www.adb.org/Documents/Books/ESDB-Timor-Leste/ESDB-Timor-Leste.pdf), the Timorese rate of maternal mortality is one of the highest in the region, at 800 deaths per 100,000 live births in 2001–02. In that same year, only 24% of births were attended by skilled practitioners. The rate of infant mortality was also high, at 88 deaths per 1,000 live births. In *Improving Maternal, Newborn, and Child Health in the South East Asia Region: Timor-Leste* (April 2005, http://www.searo.who.int/LinkFiles/Improving_maternal_newborn_and_child_health_timor-leste.pdf), the WHO reports that the mortality rate of children under the age of five decreased from 160 deaths per 1,000 children in the 1989–93 period to slightly over 80 deaths per 1,000 children in the 1999–2003 period.

The World Bank and the ADB state that in 2007 Timor-Leste had 1 national hospital, 5 regional hospitals, 66 community health centers, and 155 health posts to service a population of nearly a million people. The country has had a serious shortage of doctors since the violence of 1999, when many health care professionals fled to Indonesia. In 2007 there were only 17 Timorese doctors; however, over 300 Cuban doctors were in the country to help reduce the doctor shortage. The health care system also had 763 nurses and 255 midwives. The numbers of health care workers are beginning to reach an acceptable ratio of workers to residents, but these workers are unevenly distributed throughout the country, so that some segments of the population have a more difficult time accessing health care practitioners than do others. The lack of technical services, clean water, reliable electricity, and communications systems adds to the problems experienced by the Timorese medical system.

Common childhood diseases in Timor-Leste include acute respiratory and diarrheal diseases, malaria, and dengue fever. Additionally, many Timorese children suffer from intestinal parasites, which can lead to severe malnutrition. From 2000 to 2006 nearly half (46%) of all children under the age of five were underweight. (See Table 1.2 in Chapter 1.) Other serious diseases prevalent in Timor-Leste include malaria, leprosy, lymphatic filariasis (an infection of the lymph system by parasitic worms), Japanese encephalitis (inflammation of the brain), yaws (a bacterial infection of the skin), typhoid fever, and TB.

The Timorese childhood immunization program was revived in 2000, and immunization rates have improved in recent years. According to the World Bank and the ADB, in *Economic and Social Development Brief*, 56% of children were immunized against diphtheria, tetanus, and pertussis (whooping cough; collectively these three diseases are called DTP in Timor-Leste and DPT in the United States) in 2001–02, and this percentage rose to 63% in 2006. The WHO (2009, http://www.who.int/ immunization_monitoring/en/globalsummary/timeseries/ tscoveragedtp1.htm) indicates that 85% of Timorese children received their first dose of DTP vaccine in 2008. In 2001–02, 47% of children were immunized against measles; by 2006 this percentage rose to 61% and— according to WHO (2009, http://www.who.int/immuni zation_monitoring/en/globalsummary/timeseries/tscover agemcv.htm)—to 73% in 2008.

ACCESS TO ESSENTIAL SERVICES. The lack of access to essential services such as water and sanitation is a strong indicator of poverty, especially among those living in rural areas. The World Bank and the ADB note in *Economic and Social Development Brief* that 51% of the rural population of Timor-Leste had access to drinkable water and only 10% had access to sanitation in 2001–02. Table 1.2 in Chapter 1 shows that 62% of the total population had access to clean water by 2006. According to the CIA, in *World Factbook: Timor-Leste*, in 2008 the country had only basic telephone service, which was limited to urban areas. There were 21 radio stations and 1 television station in Timor-Leste, and only 1,800 people were using the Internet in 2008. This poor communications system makes communication across even short distances almost nonexistent in Timor-Leste.

EDUCATION. During the Timorese fight for independence and during the more recent unrest in 2006, many of the country's schools were destroyed. Regardless, UNICEF indicates in "At a Glance: Timor-Leste" (2009, http:// www.unicef.org/infobycountry/Timorleste_statistics .html) that the majority of children in Timor-Leste attended primary school from 2000 to 2007: 76% of males and 74% of females. Secondary school attendance percentages were much lower, with only 53% of males and 54% of females attending.

CHAPTER 4
EMERGING AND TRANSITION ECONOMIES: WIDENING THE POVERTY GAP

An *emerging economy* is one that is moving from developing to developed (or industrial); a *transition economy* is one evolving from a planned economy (meaning one controlled by the government, as in the former Soviet bloc countries) to a free market economy such as those in North America and Europe. A country may be both emerging and transitional. Countries undergoing these economic shifts experience varying degrees of progress regarding their impoverished citizens. Generally, a large number of people are able to enter the middle class during such a transition due to increased business opportunities. At the same time, the incidence of poverty and extreme poverty can increase as the very poor have little or no access to such opportunities—the rich get richer and the poor get poorer. A similar phenomenon can also occur with public infrastructure. Those with economic means generally have access to electricity, sanitation, and clean water, whereas those who are poor generally do not.

Researchers who study poverty use a measurement called the Gini coefficient to discuss income equality—that is, the poverty gap. Developed by the Italian statistician Corrado Gini (1884–1965) in 1912, the Gini coefficient is a number between 0 and 1, with 0 representing perfect (absolute) equality and 1 representing perfect (absolute) inequality. Scholars often use the Gini coefficient to express how wide the gap is between the very poor and those with higher incomes. The more income-unequal countries of the world tend to have Gini coefficients close to 0.5, whereas the more income-equal countries tend have Gini coefficients closer to 0.3.

ASIA

At the turn of the 21st century several Asian countries that had suffered long-term extreme poverty began to experience unprecedented economic growth. The reasons for this growth include rapidly expanding economies and increasing acceptance into the global marketplace; the burgeoning fields of technology and science in both East Asia and the Indian subcontinent that have allowed for greater educational and employment opportunities; the outsourcing of jobs from developed countries to the developing world; and the relative loss in value of the U.S. dollar, which has in general increased the values of foreign currencies.

Developing Asia

Table 4.1 shows the Asian Development Bank's (ADB) list of developing Asian countries, which are found throughout the various regions of Asia. In *Asian Development Outlook 2009: Rebalancing Asia's Growth* (2009, http://www.adb.org/Documents/Books/ADO/2009/ado2009.pdf), the ADB indicates that developing Asia has had remarkable economic growth in recent years and was weathering quite well the global economic storm that began in 2007. Growth in developing Asia continued through 2007, with a 9.7% increase in the gross domestic product (GDP; the total value of all goods and services produced by a country in a year). GDP growth continued at a slowed 6.3% in 2008. By comparison, the Central Intelligence Agency (CIA) indicates in *World Factbook: United States* (February 4, 2010, https://www.cia.gov/library/publications/the-world-factbook/geos/us.html) that the United States' GDP grew an estimated 0.4% in 2008, which was down from 2.1% in 2007.

According to the ADB, in *Key Indicators for Asia and the Pacific 2009* (August 2009, http://www.adb.org/documents/books/key_indicators/2009/pdf/Key-Indicators-2009.pdf), the percentage of the population in poverty according to national measures in developing Asian countries ranged from a high of 44.4% in 2003 in the country of Tajikistan to a low of 1% in 2007 in Chinese Taipei (Taipei is the capital city of the country Republic of China, commonly called Taiwan or Chinese Taipei).

TABLE 4.1

Asian Development Bank's developing member countries, 2009

East Asia	Central and West Asia
China, People's Rep. of	Afghanistan
Hong Kong, China	Armenia
Korea, Rep. of	Azerbaijan
Mongolia	Georgia
Taipei, China	Kazakhstan
Southeast Asia	Kyrgyz Republic
Cambodia	Pakistan
Indonesia	Tajikistan
Lao People's Democratic Republic	Turkmenistan
Malaysia	Uzbekistan
Myanmar	**Pacific**
Philippines	Cook Islands
Singapore	Fiji Islands
Thailand	Kiribati
Vietnam	Marshall Islands
South Asia	Micronesia, Fed. States of
Bangladesh	Nauru
Bhutan	Palau
India	Papua New Guinea
Maldives	Samoa
Nepal	Solomon Islands
Sri Lanka	Timor-Leste
	Tonga
	Tuvalu
	Vanuatu

SOURCE: Created by Sandra Alters for Gale, 2009.

The rate of poverty as measured by the international standard of US $1.25 per day was 21.5% in 2004 in Tajikistan. The rate for Chinese Taipei was not available.

The Gini coefficients listed by the ADB for the developing countries of Asia range from a low (more equality) of 0.168 in 2005 in Azerbaijan to a high (less equality) of 0.473 in 2003 in Nepal. Chinese Taipei, with a Gini coefficient of 0.339 in 2003, had the lowest percentage of poverty among the developing Asian countries in 2007, but it did not have the lowest Gini index figure. However, its Gini coefficient shows that it is a somewhat income-equal country. The developing countries of Asia that had high Gini coefficients were Nepal, 0.473 (2003); Bhutan, 0.468 (2003); the Philippines, 0.44 (2006); Samoa, 0.43 (2002); Thailand, 0.425 (2004); Tonga, 0.42 (2001); People's Republic of China (mainland China, commonly referred to as China), 0.415 (2005); Sri Lanka, 0.411 (2002); Georgia, 0.408 (2005); and Cambodia, 0.407 (2007). The developing countries of Asia that had low Gini coefficients were Pakistan, 0.312 (2004); Lao People's Democratic Republic (Laos), 0.326 (2002); Kyrgyzstan, 0.329 (2004); and Mongolia, 0.33 (2005).

Central Asia

Some of the developing countries of central Asia (Armenia, Azerbaijan, Georgia, Kazakhstan, Kyrgyzstan, Tajikistan, Turkmenistan, and Uzbekistan) have abundant oil supplies that make them a major region of net oil exports. According to IndexMundi's country comparison of oil production (January 1, 2009, http://www.indexmundi.com/g/r.aspx?c=am&v=88), Kazakhstan, Azerbaijan, Turkmeni-

stan, and Uzbekistan are the big oil producers of the central Asian region. Georgia, Kyrgyzstan, and Tajikistan produce some oil, and Armenia produces virtually none. Because of high oil prices, the GDP of this region was developing at a double-digit pace. In 2006 the GDP of this region grew 13.3%, and in 2007 it grew at a rate of 12%. (See Table 4.2.) However, the economic world crisis that began in 2007 had an effect on the growth rate of the GDP in this region, slowing it to 5.7% in 2008. Nonetheless, this growth rate was exceptional in a year in which the world economy slowed dramatically. The ADB projected that the slowdown of central Asia's GDP will continue in 2009 with a GDP growth rate of only 0.5%, but that by 2010 growth will begin to recover and increase to 3.6%.

Prior to the economic downturn, Armenia, Azerbaijan, Kazakhstan, and Turkmenistan in particular had rapidly expanding economies and were experiencing growth in industries such as tourism, communications, and oil and natural gas (with the exception of Armenia). Furthermore, government investment in modern infrastructure had increased employment and exports in other industries. With the onset of the economic crisis, however, the ADB expects that the GDP growth rates in the non- and low oil producing countries of central Asia will fall with that of their main trade and financial partner, the Russian Federation.

The ADB notes in *Key Indicators for Asia and the Pacific 2009* that even with their strong economic growth, Armenia, Kazakhstan, and Turkmenistan continued to experience somewhat high rates of poverty, with the following percentages of their populations living on less than US $2 per day: Armenia, 43.5% (2003); Kazakhstan, 17.2% (2003); and Turkmenistan, 49.7% (1998). By 2005 Azerbaijan had brought its rate down to 0.3%. Table 4.3 shows the proportion of the population in these countries that live on less than $1.25 per day: Armenia, 10.6% (2003); Kazakhstan, 3.1% (2003); and Turkmenistan, 24.8% (1998). The region of central Asia will be discussed further in Chapter 5.

East Asia

In developing East Asia (which includes Hong Kong, Mongolia, the People's Republic of China, the Republic of Korea [South Korea], and Chinese Taipei) GDP growth was strong in 2006 at 9.4% and in 2007 at 10.5%, but slowed in 2008 to 6.5%. (See Table 4.2.) The ADB projects further slowing in 2009 to a 4.4% GDP growth rate but an upturn in 2010 to 7.1%. The acceptance of China into the World Trade Organization (WTO) in 2001 added to the economic expansion of East Asia, which was led largely by Chinese exports. Relaxed government policies in China have allowed entrepreneurs to compete—many for the first time—in the global marketplace. Besides the success of exported products such as steel and manufactured goods, real estate in China has also seen rapid growth.

TABLE 4.2

Percent growth of gross domestic product (GDP) for Central Asia, East Asia, and South Asia, 2006–10

Subregion/economy	2006	2007	2008	2009 projected	2010 projected
Central Asia	13.3	12.0	5.7	0.5	3.6
Armenia	13.2	13.8	6.8	−9.9	0.9
Azerbaijan	34.5	25.4	10.8	3.0	4.5
Georgia	9.4	12.3	2.1	−4.0	2.5
Kazakhstan	10.7	8.9	3.3	−1.0	2.5
Kyrgyz Republic	3.1	8.5	7.6	1.0	2.0
Tajikistan	7.0	7.8	7.9	0.5	2.0
Turkmenistan	11.4	11.6	9.8	8.0	10.0
Uzbekistan	7.2	9.5	9.0	7.0	6.5
East Asia	9.4	10.5	6.5	4.4	7.1
China, People's Rep. of	11.6	13.0	9.0	8.2	8.9
Hong Kong, China	7.0	6.4	2.4	−4.0	3.0
Korea, Rep. of	5.2	5.1	2.2	−2.0	4.0
Mongolia	8.6	10.2	8.9	2.8	4.3
Taipei, China	4.8	5.7	0.1	−4.9	2.4
South Asia	9.0	8.6	6.3	5.6	6.4
Afghanistan	8.2	12.1	3.4	15.7	8.5
Bangladesh	6.6	6.4	6.2	5.9	5.2
Bhutan	6.4	14.1	11.5	6.0	6.5
India	9.7	9.0	6.7	6.0	7.0
Maldives	18.0	7.2	5.8	−3.5	3.5
Nepal	4.1	2.7	5.3	3.8	4.0
Pakistan	5.8	6.8	4.1	2.0	3.0
Sri Lanka	7.7	6.8	6.0	4.0	6.0

SOURCE: Adapted from "Table A1. Growth Rate of GDP (% per Year)," in *Asian Development Outlook 2009 Update: Broadening Openness for a Resilient Asia*, Asian Development Bank (ADB), September 2009, http://www.adb.org/Documents/Books/ADO/2009/Update/statistical.pdf (accessed December 7, 2009)

Table 4.3 shows the percentage of people living on less than $1.25 per day in three developing countries of East Asia. The People's Republic of China has made extraordinary progress in slashing the proportion of people living on less than $1.25 per day. In 1990, 60.2% of people were living below this poverty line, but by 2005, 15.9% did. Conversely, Mongolia has lost ground in the fight to lessen the proportion of people living on less than $1.25 per day. In 1995, 18.8% of the people of Mongolia lived below this poverty line, but by 2005, 22.4% did. Less than 2% of the people in the Republic of Korea in urban areas lived on less than $1.25 per day in 1998, but no recent data were available to see if the country maintained this low percentage. In addition, no rural data were available.

Table 4.4 shows the net enrollment ratios in primary education in the developing countries of Asia and the Pacific. These ratios are the percentage of the number of children of primary school age that are enrolled in primary school. A percentage of 100%, for example, means that all children of primary school age in an area were enrolled in primary school, and a percentage of 50% means that only half were enrolled. The developing countries of East Asia have high net enrollment ratios, all of which are close to or over 95%.

Thus, most of the children of primary school age of the developing countries of East Asia enroll in primary school, and most students in East Asian countries stay in school and complete this portion of their education. There are variations among countries, however. Table 4.5 shows the percent of students who started Grade 1 and who reached the last grade of primary school in three developing countries of East Asia. In 2002 the primary school completion rate in Hong Kong was 99.3% and it remained the same in 2004. A slightly higher percentage of girls (100% in both years) than boys (98.7% and 98.6%, respectively) completed primary school in this country.

By contrast, the Republic of Korea (South Korea) and Mongolia have both slipped slightly in their primary school completion rates. In 1999, 99.5% of children who began primary school in the Republic of Korea completed their primary schooling, but by 2006 this rate had dropped to 97.4%. In this country, the rates of completion for girls and boys were extremely close.

The primary school completion rates in Mongolia are lower than in Hong Kong and the Republic of Korea (South Korea). In 1999, 87.2% of children completed their primary school education, but by 2006 this rate fell to 84.1%. The rate of primary school completion for girls dropped during this period, from 89.7% to 82.6%, but it rose for boys, from 84.7% to 85.5%. Thus, in 1999 a greater proportion of girls than boys completed their primary schooling in Mongolia, but by 2006 a greater proportion of boys completed this portion of their education.

South Asia

The developing countries of South Asia (Afghanistan, Bangladesh, Bhutan, India, Maldives, Nepal, Pakistan, and

TABLE 4.3

Percent of people living on less than $1.25 per day, Asia and the Pacific, by region and country, selected years 1990–2006

Developing member countries	$1.25 (PPP) a day			
	Earliest year		Latest year	
Central and West Asia				
Afghanistan	—		—	
Armenia	17.5	(1996)	10.6	(2003)
Azerbaijan	15.6	(1995)	<2.0	(2005)
Georgia	4.5	(1996)	13.4	(2005)
Kazakhstan	4.2	(1993)	3.1	(2003)
Kyrgyz Republic	18.6	(1993)	21.8	(2004)
Pakistan	64.7	(1991)	22.6	(2005)
Tajikistan	44.5	(1999)	21.5	(2004)
Turkmenistan	63.5	(1993)	24.8	(1998)
Uzbekistan	32.1	(1998)	46.3	(2003)
East Asia				
China, People's Rep. of	60.2[a]	(1990)	15.9[a]	(2005)
Hong Kong, China	—		—	
Korea, Rep. of	—		<2.0[b]	(1998)
Mongolia	18.8	(1995)	22.4	(2005)
Taipei, China	—		—	
South Asia				
Bangladesh	66.8[c]	(1992)	49.6[c]	(2005)
Bhutan	—		26.2	(2003)
India	49.4[a]	(1994)	41.6[a]	(2005)
Maldives	—		—	
Nepal	68.4	(1996)	55.1	(2004)
Sri Lanka	15.0	(1991)	14.0	(2002)
Southeast Asia				
Brunei Darussalam[d]	—		—	
Cambodia	48.6	(1994)	40.2	(2004)
Indonesia	—		—	
Lao PDR	55.7	(1992)	44.0	(2002)
Malaysia	<2.0	(1992)	<2.0	(2004)
Myanmar	—		—	
Philippines	30.7	(1991)	22.6	(2006)
Singapore	—		—	
Thailand	5.5	(1992)	<2.0	(2004)
Viet Nam	63.7	(1993)	21.5	(2006)
The Pacific				
Cook Islands	—		—	
Fiji Islands	—		—	
Kiribati	—		—	
Marshall Islands	—		—	
Micronesia, Fed. States of	—		—	
Nauru	—		—	
Palau	—		—	
Papua New Guinea	—		35.8	(1996)
Samoa	—		—	
Solomon Islands	—		—	
Timor-Leste	—		—	
Tonga	—		—	
Tuvalu	—		—	
Vanuatu	—		—	

TABLE 4.3

Percent of people living on less than $1.25 per day, Asia and the Pacific, by region and country, selected years 1990–2006 [CONTINUED]

Developed member countries	$1.25 (PPP) a day	
	Earliest year	Latest year
Australia	—	—
Japan	—	—
New Zealand	—	—

—Data not available at cut-off date.
PPP = Purchasing Power Parity.
[a]Weighted average of urban and rural estimates.
[b]Refers to urban areas only.
[c]Estimate is adjusted by spatial consumer price index information.
[d]Brunei Darussalam is a regional member of the Asian Development Bank (ADB), but it is not classified as a developing member country.

SOURCE: Adapted from "Table 1.1.—1.1. Proportion of Population below the Poverty Line (Percent)," in *Key Indicators for Asia and the Pacific 2009*, 40th ed., Asian Development Bank (ADB), August 2009, http://www.adb.org/Documents/Books/Key_Indicators/2009/pdf/Key-Indicators-2009.pdf (accessed December 6, 2009). Data from the Millennium Indicators Database Online (UNSD 2009), Pacific Regional Information System (SPC), and country sources.

achieved GDP growth of 12.1% in 2007, but that slowed to 3.4% in 2008 with the global recession. The ADB projected that Afghanistan's GDP growth will see a rebound in 2009 with a 15.7% rate and a lesser 8.5% rate in 2010, provided that donor funding continues to flow into the country and that drought or other factors do not negatively affect licit agricultural production. (Note that direct revenues from opium cultivation are not included in the country's GDP.)

Table 4.3 shows the under-$1.25-per-day poverty rate for five developing South Asian countries. Four shown in this list have made progress in reducing their poverty rates. Bangladesh reduced the percentage of its people living on less than $1.25 per day from 66.8% in 1992 to 49.6% in 2005. India reduced its poverty rate from 49.4% in 1994 to 41.6% in 2005. Nepal's percentages went from 68.4% in 1996 to 55.1% in 2004. Sri Lanka, already at a comparatively low rate of under-$1.25-per-day poverty, went from 15% in 1991 to 14% in 2002. Bhutan's rate of under-$1.25-per-day poverty was 26.2% in 2003.

Table 4.4 shows the net enrollment ratios in primary education in the developing countries of South Asia, which do not have, in general, the high enrollment ratios of developing countries of East Asia. In the most recent year available, the net enrollment ratios ranged from 76.5% in Nepal to 96.7% in Sri Lanka. In Bangladesh the net enrollment ratios were higher for girls (93%) than for boys (86.3%). In India and Nepal the net enrollment ratios were higher for boys (96.1% and 78.3%, respectively) than for girls (92.2% and 74.6% respectively). In Bhutan and Maldives the net enrollment ratios for girls and boys were about equal, with 80.1% of girls and 79.7% of boys enrolled in primary education in Bhutan, and 97.6% of girls and 96.5% of boys enrolled in primary education in Maldives.

Sri Lanka) have also experienced strong rates of growth, allowing many people in the region to attain relative prosperity in the early years of the 21st century. (See Table 4.2.) GDP growth in many of these countries is fueled by development in industry and agriculture as well as by high consumer spending, which results as economic conditions improve. Bhutan's economic growth is focused primarily on its expanding hydropower capabilities, and war-torn Afghanistan is externally funded development. (This country also has a huge illicit economy driven by opium, supplying about 90% of the world's opium.) Afghanistan—which is among the world's least developed countries—

TABLE 4.4

Percent primary enrollment, Asia and the Pacific, by region and country, selected years 1991–2007

Developing member countries	Total 1991		Total 2007		Girls 1991	Girls 2007	Boys 1991	Boys 2007
Central and West Asia								
Afghanistan	—		—		—	—	—	—
Armenia	92.8	(2001)	93.9		93.6	95.5	92.0	92.5
Azerbaijan	88.8		95.4		—	94.7	—	96.1
Georgia	97.1		94.5		—	93.1	—	95.8
Kazakhstan	86.7		99.0		—	99.4	—	98.6
Kyrgyz Republic	92.3		92.4		—	92.4	—	92.5
Pakistan	57.2	(2001)	65.6	(2006)	46.0	57.3	67.8	73.5
Tajikistan	76.7		97.5		—	95.7	—	99.3
Turkmenistan	—		—		—	—	—	—
Uzbekistan	78.2		93.6		—	92.3	—	94.8
East Asia								
China, People's Rep. of	98.3		—		—	—	—	—
Hong Kong, China	97.5	(2001)	94.9	(2005)	95.5	92.8	99.5	96.9
Korea, Rep. of	99.7		98.5	(2006)	—	—	—	—
Mongolia	95.7		97.6		—	99.0	—	96.2
Taipei, China	98.7		99.3		—	—	—	—
South Asia								
Bangladesh	89.5	(2005)	89.6	(2006)	92.5	93.0	86.7	86.3
Bhutan	56.4	(1999)	79.9	(2006)	53.0	80.1	59.8	79.7
India	84.9	(2000)	94.3	(2006)	77.1	92.2	92.0	96.1
Maldives	98.0	(1999)	97.0		98.3	97.6	97.7	96.5
Nepal	67.0	(1999)	76.5		58.7	74.6	74.7	78.3
Sri Lanka	99.1	(2001)	96.7	(2004)	99.4	—	98.9	—
Southeast Asia								
Brunei Darussalam*	92.7		96.5		—	96.9	—	96.2
Cambodia	75.1		89.4		—	87.4	—	91.3
Indonesia	96.7		98.0		—	—	—	—
Lao PDR	61.9		86.3		—	84.1	—	88.5
Malaysia	97.7	(1999)	97.5	(2006)	96.7	97.3	98.7	97.6
Myanmar	98.6		—		—	—	—	—
Philippines	96.3		91.7		—	92.7	—	90.6
Singapore	—		—		—	—	—	—
Thailand	87.7		—		—	—	—	—
Viet Nam	90.5		94.0	(2001)	—	91.2	—	96.6
The Pacific								
Cook Islands	86.3	(1999)	68.8		84.5	67.4	87.9	70.0
Fiji Islands	99.4		94.2	(2006)	—	94.4	—	94.1
Kiribati	99.2	(1999)	99.7	(2002)	—	—	—	—
Marshall Islands	88.1	(2001)	66.5		88.4	66.3	87.8	66.8
Micronesia, Fed. States of	—		—		—	—	—	—
Nauru	—		72.3		—	72.7	—	71.9
Palau	96.8	(1999)	96.4	(2000)	93.9	94.5	99.4	98.3
Papua New Guinea	—		—		—	—	—	—
Samoa	94.2	(1999)	99.1	(2004)	93.9	—	94.5	—
Solomon Islands	63.3	(2003)	61.8	(2005)	62.3	61.5	64.2	62.1
Timor-Leste	68.1	(2005)	63.0		66.6	61.9	69.6	64.1
Tonga	88.2	(1999)	98.5	(2005)	86.2	—	90.1	—
Tuvalu	—		—		—	—	—	—
Vanuatu	91.9	(1999)	87.7		91.4	87.1	92.3	88.2
Developed member countries								
Australia	99.8		97.2		—	97.6	—	96.9
Japan	99.7		99.8		—	—	—	—
New Zealand	98.8		99.3		—	99.6	—	98.9

—Data not available at cut-off date.
*Brunei Darussalam is a regional member of the Asian Development Bank, but it is not classified as a developing member country.

SOURCE: Adapted from "Table 2.1.—2.1. Total Net Enrollment Ratio in Primary Education (Percent)," in *Key Indicators for Asia and the Pacific 2009*, 40th ed., Asian Development Bank (ADB), August 2009, http://www.adb.org/Documents/Books/Key_Indicators/2009/pdf/Key-Indicators-2009.pdf (accessed December 6, 2009). Data from the Millennium Indicators Database Online (UNSD 2009); for Taipei, China: economy sources.

Unlike the developing countries of East Asia, a large percentage of students in developing South Asian countries drop out before completing this portion of their education. In the most recent year available, the proportion of students starting Grade 1 who reach the last grade of primary education ranged from 54.8% in Bangladesh

TABLE 4.5

Percent of students of relevant age group completing primary school, Asia and the Pacific, by region, country, and sex, selected years 1999–07

Developing member countries	Total 1999		Total 2006		Girls[a] 1999	Girls[a] 2006	Boys[a] 1999	Boys[a] 2006
Central and West Asia								
Afghanistan	—		—		—	—	—	—
Armenia	79.3	(2001)	97.7		80.4	97.4	78.2	98.0
Azerbaijan	96.6		98.7		97.7	100.0	95.6	97.6
Georgia	99.4		100.0		100.0	—	98.8	—
Kazakhstan	95.9	(2000)	99.5	(2007)	93.3	100.0	98.4	99.1
Kyrgyz Republic	94.5		96.5		93.9	97.0	95.1	96.0
Pakistan	—		69.7	(2004)	—	72.4	—	67.8
Tajikistan	96.7		99.4		93.6	97.3	99.7	—
Turkmenistan	—		—		—	—	—	—
Uzbekistan	99.5		99.2		99.4	99.2	99.7	99.3
East Asia								
China, People's Rep. of	—		—		—	—	—	—
Hong Kong, China	99.3	(2002)	99.3	(2004)	100.0	100.0	98.7	98.6
Korea, Rep. of	99.5		97.4		99.3	97.3	99.6	97.5
Mongolia	87.2		84.1		89.7	82.6	84.7	85.5
Taipei, China	—		—		—	—	—	—
South Asia								
Bangladesh	—		54.8	(2005)	—	57.6	—	52.2
Bhutan	81.3		84.4	(2005)	85.7	87.8	77.8	81.2
India	62.0		65.8	(2005)	60.4	65.3	63.3	66.2
Maldives	—		—		—	—	—	—
Nepal	58.0		61.6	(2007)	61.4	63.6	55.7	59.7
Sri Lanka	—		93.4	(2005)	—	93.6	—	93.2
Southeast Asia								
Brunei Darussalam[b]	98.0	(2003)	98.2		96.0	99.3	100.0	97.2
Cambodia	48.6		54.5		45.0	55.8	51.9	53.3
Indonesia	85.9	(2001)	94.7		88.7	81.4	83.3	—
Lao PDR	54.3		61.5		53.6	61.1	54.9	61.7
Malaysia	97.7	(2002)	89.3	(2005)	97.3	89.6	98.0	89.1
Myanmar	55.2	(2000)	72.7		55.2	—	55.3	—
Philippines	75.3	(2001)	73.2		79.8	78.4	71.1	68.6
Singapore	—		—		—	—	—	—
Thailand	—		—		—	—	—	—
Viet Nam	82.8		92.1	(2005)	86.2	—	79.9	—
The Pacific								
Cook Islands	—		—		—	—	—	—
Fiji Islands	82.1		75.6		82.0	—	82.2	—
Kiribati	69.7	(2001)	81.4	(2003)	67.4	88.8	72.0	75.0
Marshall Islands	—		—		—	—	—	—
Micronesia, Fed. States of	—		—		—	—	—	—
Nauru	—		25.4	(2001)	—	30.1	—	21.5
Palau	—		—		—	—	—	—
Papua New Guinea	—		—		—	—	—	—
Samoa	92.4		95.9	(2000)	94.1	—	90.9	—
Solomon Islands	—		—		—	—	—	—
Timor-Leste	—		—		—	—	—	—
Tonga	94.6	(2000)	90.9	(2005)	—	91.9	—	89.9
Tuvalu	72.7	(2000)	62.6	(2001)	—	—	—	—
Vanuatu	68.9		—		71.0	—	67.0	—
Developed member countries								
Australia	—		—		—	—	—	—
Japan	—		—		—	—	—	—
New Zealand	—		—		—	—	—	—

—Data not available at cut-off date.

[a]Figures refer to the same year as indicated in the column for "total."

[b]Brunei Darussalam is a regional member of ADB, but it is not classified as a developing member country.

SOURCE: Adapted from "Table 2.1.—2.2. Proportion of Pupils Starting Grade 1 Who Reach Last Grade of Primary (Percent)," in *Key Indicators for Asia and the Pacific 2009*, 40th ed., Asian Development Bank (ADB), August 2009, http://www.adb.org/Documents/Books/Key_Indicators/2009/pdf/Key-Indicators-2009 .pdf (accessed December 6, 2009). Data from the Millennium Indicators Database Online (UNSD 2009); for Taipei, China: economy sources.

to 93.4% in Sri Lanka. (See Table 4.5.) Among the developing countries of South Asian, Sri Lanka had both the highest net enrollment ratio and the highest proportion of students who finish their primary education. In addition, the percentage of girls and boys who enroll in and complete their primary education was nearly equal.

THE PEOPLE'S REPUBLIC OF CHINA: AN EMERGING AND TRANSITIONAL ECONOMY

According to the CIA, in *World Factbook: China* (February 4, 2010, https://www.cia.gov/library/publications/the-world-factbook/geos/ch.html), the People's Republic of China is the most populous country in the world, with 1.3 billion people and a variety of different ethnic groups. The primary ethnic group is the Han Chinese, which made up 91.5% of the population in 2009. (Han refers to the Han dynasty in Chinese history; this group is sometimes referred to as "traditional" Chinese.) The CIA estimates that China had a GDP (purchasing power parity) of $8.8 trillion in 2009.

The United Nations Development Programme (UNDP) reports in *Human Development Report China 2007/08* (November 2008, http://www.undp.org.cn/downloads/nhdr2008/NHDR2008_en.pdf) that China ranked 81st globally on the United Nations (UN) Human Development Index (HDI) in 2007 (using 2005 data). The UNDP notes that "the scale of China's economic transition and social transformation is evident in its spectacular economic growth rates, averaging nearly 10 percent per annum for the last 30 years. Its HDI score has increased from 0.53 in 1975, just barely above the low-human development floor, to 0.781 in 2006, very close to high human development." However, poverty is high in rural China. China's rural poverty—as well as its contemporary status as an emerging and transitional economic power—has many causes that are forged in large part by its complex political history.

From Dynasties to Communism to a Free(er) Market Economy

China is one of the oldest ongoing civilizations in the world, with organized city-states having been developed about 5,000 years ago. Early human beings are believed to have inhabited the region 65,000 years ago, and agriculture is known to have developed about 8,000 years ago. Approximately 2,000 years ago the region was unified for the first time under a single system of government, although over the centuries China experienced periods of political upheaval followed by reunification.

Until the early 20th century China was governed by a series of dynasties—that is, unified governments controlled by a single leader, with leadership passed down to successive generations. This system of political elitism depended heavily on a massive rural peasant class that provided food and other necessities to all of China. This social and political organization is known as feudalism and still exists in China.

Over the centuries conflict between the ruling elite class and the poverty-stricken peasants often erupted into rebellions. The Republican Revolution of 1911 brought an end to the dynastic system. For the next several decades, China was nominally unified at best. Various regions were controlled by warlords, who vacillated between supporting and not supporting a national government.

Among the groups vying for power were the communists. The Chinese Communist Party (CCP) was formed in 1920 and quickly grew in strength. It benefited from the anger many Chinese felt toward Western nations, which were supporting Japanese control over the Chinese region of Shandong. Mao Zedong (1893–1976) was one of the early members of the CCP, and by 1931 he rose to become its leader. By this time the CCP was one of the two most powerful factions in China, the other being the Nationalist Party.

When Japan invaded China in 1937, both the Communists and the Nationalists fought back, while remaining at odds with each other. Fighting with Japan continued throughout World War II (1939–1945) and was marked by brutal atrocities by the Japanese. Under Mao's direction, the Communist's Red Army succeeded in waging guerrilla warfare against the Japanese, gaining further support for the CCP. When Japan surrendered in 1945, China became free from occupation, but the country was soon plunged into civil war between the Communists and the Nationalists. The Red Army conquered most of China by 1949, largely due to Mao's successful recruiting of peasants, and the formation of the People's Republic of China was declared. The Nationalists remained in control of the island of Taiwan.

Mao created what was called a democratic dictatorship, meaning that all the classes of Chinese society were represented by the centralized government; however, detractors from Mao's system were sent to prison camps or simply executed. It is not known exactly how many people were killed under Mao's democratic dictatorship. He admitted to having approximately 800,000 people executed, but the number is believed to be in the millions.

Despite Mao's stated commitment to empowering the peasantry, many of contemporary China's problems with rural poverty can be traced to his economic policies. As a communist country, the government strictly controlled most aspects of the economy, and Mao directed much of its resources toward collectivization, industrialization, and modernization, regardless of the cost to the average Chinese. The purges of the Cultural Revolution (1966–1976) nearly bankrupted the country intellectually and economically by ridding China of anyone accused of holding so-called counterrevolutionary ideas.

After years of isolation, China was drawn back into the international community when U.S. president Richard M. Nixon (1913–1994) visited the country in 1972 and reestablished relations. Following Mao's death in 1976, a series of reforms loosened state controls somewhat and boosted productivity. However, calls for democratic reform were suppressed, including the massacre that ended the Tiananmen Square protests in 1989.

In 1998 the Chinese government began a program to privatize some of the economy. That same year diplomatic relations with the United States improved after a summit was held with U.S. president Bill Clinton (1946–). By November 1999 the United States and China had reached a trade agreement that loosened trade barriers and made way for China's acceptance into the WTO; China officially earned WTO membership in December 2001. Since then, China has experienced unprecedented economic growth. In 2006 its GDP grew 11.6%, and in 2007 it grew 13%. (See Table 4.2.) Even with the economic global crisis that began in 2007, China's GDP grew at a rate of 9% in 2008. Furthermore, it was projected to continue at a rate of 8.2% in 2009 and 8.9% in 2010. China has become one of the world's largest and most important manufacturing centers, much of it for export but also for its expanding domestic market.

China's Growing Middle Class

A large part of the success of China's economy since the late 1990s has been the expansive building and business boom in its cities, which has fueled the urban economy by increasing employment opportunities. With so many people finding work in China's large cities, and massive government investment in fueling this urbanization, the urban middle class has swelled. This new middle class is both a result and a cause of China's evolution from an agrarian economy to an industrial one. As the middle class continues to expand in the urban setting, the more it needs items such as automobiles. These needs affect not only the way people shop and do business but also the likelihood that they will pay for goods and services they would not have purchased before, thus increasing overall consumerism.

The Chinese government reports in the press release "China Auto Production, Sales Hit Record 8.8 mln Units in 2007" (January 13, 2008, http://english.gov.cn/2008-01/13/content_856987.htm) that private ownership of vehicles—which had been anathema to CCP leaders throughout much of the 20th century—is on the rise. In 2007 China's auto manufacturers produced 8.9 million new vehicles, up 22% from 2006. Sales totaled 8.8 million vehicles in 2007, up 21.8% from 2006 and twice the number of sales as in 2003. China was the second-largest car market after the United States in 2007. In the press release "China's Retail Sales up 16.9% in 2009" (January 21, 2010, http://english.gov.cn/2010-01/21/content_1516849.htm), the Chinese government states that it became the world's largest car market in 2009, when auto sales climbed 46.2% over sales in 2008.

To accommodate the growing number of vehicles, China has been updating and expanding its highway infrastructure. According to the Chinese government, in the press release "China FactFile: Highways" (February 16, 2006, http://english.gov.cn/2006-02/08/content_182515.htm), in 2003 the country embarked on a National Expressway Network Plan and by 2008 it planned on having five north-south and seven east-west national highways completed, totaling 22,000 miles (35,000 km).

In "China's Retail Sales up 16.9% in 2009," the Chinese government also reports that in 2009 retail sales in general had increased 16.9% from 2008. In addition, Edward Cody notes in "Chinese Lawmakers Approve Measure to Protect Private Property Rights" (*Washington Post*, March 17, 2007) that the Chinese legislature passed a law in March 2007 to protect private property rights of individuals, which legal experts consider "a milestone on the path toward a market economy."

Income Distribution

Inevitably, as a large segment of a country's population moves up in social and economic status, the divide between the rich and the poor becomes wider and deeper. In countries that have a planned economy, in which the centralized government controls prices and wages, income is distributed to ensure a certain level of equality and market competition is discouraged. In China, however, the rural communal farm system was never really equitable. Urban factories were owned by the central government, with workers receiving a low but dependable level of health care and compulsory education, whereas the farm communes in the countryside were operated by provincial landlords. To guarantee the health of the urban economy so that China could compete in the world market, investment was concentrated in eastern manufacturing centers along the coast, while the prices of crops produced in the interior were suppressed. This guaranteed that more money would be available for the country to pursue industry, but it also created inequalities of income and living standards between those who lived in urban centers and those who lived in rural areas.

According to the UNDP, in *Human Development Report China 2007/08*, the urban per capita (per person) income in 1978 was 2.6 times that of the rural provinces, and in 2007 it was 3.3 times that of the rural provinces. Economic growth has occurred for both groups, however, and China has worked hard to reduce both urban and rural poverty even though the per capita income gap has grown.

Poverty Decreases

Great advancements have been made in the country's human development indicators since government reforms began in the late 1970s. The UNDP lists China as a developing country with a medium level of human development. (See Table 1.2 in Chapter 1.) In 2009 China had an HDI rank of 92, and a Human Poverty Index (HPI-1) rank of 36 out of 135 developing countries and areas. Approximately 2.8% of the population lived below the national poverty line from 2000 to 2006, which the Chinese government calls the absolute poverty population. Those living above the official poverty line but below the $1.25-per-day line are called the low income population by the Chinese government. From 2000 to 2007, 15.9% of China's population earned less than $1.25 per day. Even though the percentage of those living below the $1.25-per-day line was higher in China than in some developing countries with medium human development, such as Armenia (10.6%), Paraguay (6.5%), the Dominican Republic (5%), and Thailand (less than 2%), it was lower than in some developing countries with medium human development, such as the Philippines (22.6%), Ghana (30%), India (41.6%), and Madagascar (67.8%).

Other Human Development Indicators

Other human development indicators include the prevalence of maternal mortality (death as a result of pregnancy or childbirth), the under-five mortality rate (U5MR), underweight children under the age of five, access to clean water, access to basic sanitation, and primary enrollment in school.

Table 4.6 presents the rates of maternal mortality in Asia and the Pacific. The maternal mortality rate for China was 45 maternal deaths per 100,000 live births in 2005. Compared with the other countries and regions shown, China had a low maternal mortality rate in 2005. Countries with a low maternal mortality rate have a high proportion of births attended by skilled health personnel. China raised its proportion between 1995 and 2006. In 1995, 89% of births in the People's Republic of China were attended by a skilled health professional, and in 2006, 98% of births were attended by a health professional. (See Table 4.7.)

Table 4.8 shows the mortality rate for children under the age of five and the infant mortality rate for 1990, 2000, and 2007. China's U5MR was 22 deaths per 1,000 children under the age of five in 2007, down from 37 per 1,000 in 2000 and 45 per 1,000 in 1990. In addition, China cut its infant mortality rate in half, from a rate of 36 deaths per 1,000 live births in 1990 to a rate of 19 deaths per 1,000 in 2007. The 2015 Millennium Development Goal (MDG; http://www.undp.org/mdg/basics.shtml) targets in these areas of child health is to cut the U5MR and infant mortality rate by two-thirds from 1990 to 2015. China has made a great deal of progress toward these goals.

A related indicator to the U5MR is the prevalence of underweight children who are younger than five years old. Table 4.9 shows that 7% of Chinese children under the age of five were underweight in 2005. As it did with the U5MR, China has more than halved the percentage of underweight children in this age group, thereby achieving

TABLE 4.6

Maternal mortality rate, Asia and the Pacific, by region and country, 2005 and 2007

[per 100,000 live births]

Developing member countries	2005	
Central and West Asia		
Afghanistan	1800	
Armenia	76	
Azerbaijan	82	
Georgia	66	
Kazakhstan	140	
Kyrgyz Republic	150	
Pakistan	320	
Tajikistan	170	
Turkmenistan	130	
Uzbekistan	24	
East Asia		
China, People's Rep. of	45	
Hong Kong, China	1	(2007)
Korea, Rep. of	14	
Mongolia	46	
Taipei, China	7	(2007)
South Asia		
Bangladesh	570	
Bhutan	440	
India	450	
Maldives	120	
Nepal	830	
Sri Lanka	58	
Southeast Asia		
Brunei Darussalam*	13	
Cambodia	540	
Indonesia	420	
Lao PDR	660	
Malaysia	62	
Myanmar	380	
Philippines	230	
Singapore	14	
Thailand	110	
Viet Nam	150	
The Pacific		
Cook Islands	—	
Fiji Islands	210	
Kiribati	—	
Marshall Islands	—	
Micronesia, Fed. States of	—	
Nauru	—	
Palau	—	
Papua New Guinea	470	
Samoa	—	
Solomon Islands	220	
Timor-Leste	380	
Tonga	—	
Tuvalu	—	
Vanuatu	—	
Developed member countries		
Australia	4	
Japan	6	
New Zealand	9	

—Data not available at cut-off date.
*Brunei Darussalam is a regional member of the Asian Development Bank, but it is not classified as a developing member country.

SOURCE: Adapted from "Table 5.1.—5.1. Maternal Mortality Ratio (per 100,000 Live Births)," in Key Indicators for Asia and the Pacific 2009, 40th ed., Asian Development Bank (ADB), August 2009, http://www.adb.org/Documents/Books/Key_Indicators/2009/pdf/Key-Indicators-2009.pdf (accessed December 6, 2009). Data from the Millennium Indicators Database Online (UNSD 2009); for Hong Kong, China and Taipei, China: economy sources.

TABLE 4.7

Percent of births attended by a skilled health professional, Asia and the Pacific, by region and country, selected years 1991–2007

Developing member countries	1995		2006	
Central and West Asia				
Afghanistan	12	(2000)	14	(2003)
Armenia	96	(1997)	98	(2005)
Azerbaijan	100	(1998)	88	
Georgia	96	(1998)	98	(2005)
Kazakhstan	100		100	
Kyrgyz Republic	98	(1997)	98	
Pakistan	19	(1991)	39	(2007)
Tajikistan	79	(1996)	83	(2005)
Turkmenistan	96	(1996)	100	
Uzbekistan	98	(1996)	100	
East Asia				
China, People's Rep. of	89		98	
Hong Kong, China	—		—	
Korea, Rep. of	—		—	
Mongolia	94	(1998)	99	
Taipei, China	—		—	
South Asia				
Bangladesh	10	(1994)	18	(2007)
Bhutan	15	(1994)	56	(2003)
India	34	(1993)	47	
Maldives	90	(1994)	84	(2004)
Nepal	9	(1996)	19	
Sri Lanka	94	(1993)	99	(2007)
Southeast Asia				
Brunei Darussalam*	98	(1994)	99	(1999)
Cambodia	34	(1998)	44	(2005)
Indonesia	50		73	(2007)
Lao PDR	19	(2001)	20	
Malaysia	96		98	(2005)
Myanmar	56	(1997)	57	(2001)
Philippines	56	(1998)	60	(2003)
Singapore	100	(1998)	—	
Thailand	99	(2000)	97	
Viet Nam	77	(1997)	88	
The Pacific				
Cook Islands	100	(1998)	98	(2001)
Fiji Islands	100	(1998)	99	(2000)
Kiribati	72	(1994)	85	(1998)
Marshall Islands	95	(1998)	—	
Micronesia, Fed. States of	93	(1999)	88	(2001)
Nauru	—		—	
Palau	100	(1998)	100	(2002)
Papua New Guinea	53	(1996)	41	(2000)
Samoa	100	(1998)	—	
Solomon Islands	85	(1994)	85	(1999)
Timor-Leste	26	(1997)	18	(2003)
Tonga	92	(1991)	95	(2000)
Tuvalu	99	(1997)	100	(2002)
Vanuatu	89		88	(1999)
Developed member countries				
Australia	100	(1999)	—	
Japan	100	(1996)	—	
New Zealand	100		—	

—Data not available at cut-off date.

*Brunei Darussalam is a regional member of the Asian Development Bank, but it is not classified as a developing member country.

SOURCE: Adapted from "Table 5.1.—5.2. Proportion of Births Attended by Skilled Health Personnel (Percent)," in *Key Indicators for Asia and the Pacific 2009*, 40th ed., Asian Development Bank (ADB), August 2009, http://www.adb.org/Documents/Books/Key_Indicators/2009/pdf/Key-Indicators-2009.pdf (accessed December 6, 2009). Data from the Millennium Indicators Database Online (UNSD 2009); for Hong Kong, China and Taipei, China: economy sources.

the 2015 MDG target. Compared with the other regions and countries shown, the prevalence of underweight children under the age of five in China was low in the most recent years shown. In a related human development factor, China made progress in lowering the proportion of the population below the minimum level of dietary energy consumption, from 15% of the population in 1990–92 to 9% in 2003–05. (See Table 4.10.) The MDG target is to halve the proportion of the population below the minimum level of dietary energy consumption between 1990 and 2015. China did not reach this target but was on track to achieve it.

Access to improved (clean) water sources is related to under-five mortality and underweight children because unclean water contains disease-causing microbes that can make children sick and even kill them. Table 4.11 provides data for access to improved water sources in both rural and urban locations. China was succeeding with both of these indicators in 2006—81% of rural inhabitants and 98% of urban inhabitants had access to clean water, up from 55% and 97%, respectively, in 1999. China reached its 2015 MDG target by cutting in half the proportion of people without access to clean water. In 1990, 33% of the population did not have access to clean water, and by 2006, 12% did not.

Sanitation and clean water are linked, for without appropriate sanitation facilities, groundwater is often polluted with excrement and the microbes present in that excrement. Table 4.12 shows that only 43% of China's rural population had access to basic sanitation in 1990, but by 2006, 59% did. In 1990 only 61% of China's urban population had access to basic sanitation, but by 2006, 74% did. The country did not reach its MDG target of cutting in half the percentage of the population not using an improved sanitation facility, but it was making progress toward that goal. In 1990, 52% of the population did not have access to improved sanitation, and by 2006, 35% did not. China's goal is to lower the percentage of the population not having access to improved sanitation to 26%.

Even though China still has progress to make in the area of basic sanitation, the country is doing well regarding the percentage of children enrolled in primary school out of the total number of children of primary school age. Table 4.4 does not have a recent figure available for the primary school net enrollment ratio, but it does show that the net enrollment ratio was 98.3% in 1991. The UN Children's Fund (UNICEF) notes in "China" (2009, http://www.unicef.org/infobycountry/china_statistics.html) that the net enrollment ratio for primary school was 99% from 2000 to 2007.

INDIA: AN EMERGING AND TRANSITIONAL ECONOMY

India has one of the oldest civilizations in the world, with evidence of permanent human settlements dating back 9,000 years. It is also the world's largest democracy

TABLE 4.8

Under-five and infant mortality rates, Asia and the Pacific, by region and country, 1990, 2000, and 2007

[per 1,000 live births]

Developing member countries	Under-five mortality rate			Infant mortality rate		
	1990	2000	2007	1990	2000	2007
Central and West Asia[a]	130	119	107	98	89	80
Afghanistan	260	257	257	168	165	165
Armenia	56	36	24	48	32	22
Azerbaijan	98	69	39	78	58	34
Georgia	47	35	30	41	31	27
Kazakhstan	60	44	32	51	38	28
Kyrgyz Republic	74	50	38	62	43	34
Pakistan	132	106	90	102	84	73
Tajikistan	117	94	67	91	75	57
Turkmenistan	99	71	50	81	59	45
Uzbekistan	74	62	41	61	53	36
East Asia[a]	44	36	22	35	29	19
China, People's Rep. of	45	37	22	36	30	19
Hong Kong, China	—	—	—	6	3	2
Korea, Rep. of	9	5	5	8	5	4
Mongolia	98	63	43	71	49	35
Taipei, China	—	—	—	5	6	5
South Asia[a]	121	90	70	85	66	53
Bangladesh	151	91	61	105	66	47
Bhutan	148	106	84	91	68	56
India	117	91	72	83	67	54
Maldives	111	55	30	79	43	26
Nepal	142	85	55	99	63	43
Sri Lanka	32	23	21	26	18	17
Southeast Asia[a]	77	47	34	53	35	27
Brunei Darussalam[b]	11	9	9	10	8	8
Cambodia	119	107	91	87	80	70
Indonesia	91	48	31	60	36	25
Lao PDR	163	101	70	120	77	56
Malaysia	22	14	11	16	11	10
Myanmar	130	110	103	91	78	74
Philippines	62	37	28	43	29	23
Singapore	8	4	3	6	3	2
Thailand	31	13	7	26	11	6
Viet Nam	56	30	15	40	23	13
The Pacific[a]	98	77	65	73	59	51
Cook Islands	32	24	18	26	20	16
Fiji Islands	22	18	18	19	16	16
Kiribati	88	70	63	65	52	46
Marshall Islands	92	68	54	63	55	49
Micronesia, Fed. States of	58	47	40	45	38	33
Nauru	—	30	30	—	25	25
Palau	21	14	10	18	13	9
Papua New Guinea	94	76	65	69	57	50
Samoa	50	34	27	40	28	22
Solomon Islands	121	88	70	86	65	53
Timor-Leste	184	129	97	138	100	77
Tonga	32	26	23	26	22	19
Tuvalu	53	42	37	42	35	30
Vanuatu	62	48	34	48	38	28
Developed member countries[a]	7	5	4	6	3	3
Australia	9	6	6	8	5	5
Japan	6	5	4	5	3	3
New Zealand	11	7	6	9	6	5

—Data not available at cut-off date.
[a]Estimated using data on births provided by the United Nations Children's Fund as weights.
[b]Brunei Darussalam is a regional member of the Asian Development Bank, but it is not classified as a developing member country.

SOURCE: Adapted from "Table 4.1.—4.1. Under-Five Mortality Rate (per 1,000 Live Births)" and "Table 4.1.—4.2 Infant Mortality Rate (per 1,000 Live Births)," in *Key Indicators for Asia and the Pacific 2009*, 40th ed., Asian Development Bank (ADB), August 2009, http://www.adb.org/Documents/Books/Key_Indicators/2009/pdf/Key-Indicators-2009.pdf (accessed December 6, 2009). Data from the Millennium Indicators Database Online (UNSD 2009); for Hong Kong, China: Census and Statistics Department and Centre for Health Protection, Department of Health; for Taipei, China: Directorate-General of Budget, Accounting and Statistics; ADB staff estimates.

TABLE 4.9

Percent of underweight children under age five, Asia and the Pacific, by region, country, and sex, selected years, 1990–2007

Developing member countries	Earliest year Total		Latest year Total	Girls	Boys	
Central and West Asia						
Afghanistan	48	(1997)	39[a]	40	38	(2003–2004)
Armenia	4	(1998)	4	6	2	(2005)
Azerbaijan	10	(1996)	10	10	9	(2006)
Georgia	3	(1999)	2	2	2	(2005)
Kazakhstan	8	(1995)	4	4	4	(2006)
Kyrgyz Republic	11	(1997)	3	3	4	(2006)
Pakistan	40	(1991)	38	36	38	(2001–2002)
Tajikistan	—		17	17	18	(2005)
Turkmenistan	12	(2000)	11	10	12	(2005)
Uzbekistan	19	(1996)	5	5	5	(2006)
East Asia						
China, People's Rep. of	19	(1990)	7	—	—	(2005)
Hong Kong, China	—		—	—	—	
Korea, Rep. of	—		—	—	—	
Mongolia	12	(1992)	6	7	6	(2005)
Taipei, China	—		—	—	—	
South Asia						
Bangladesh	67	(1992)	48	49	46	(2004)
Bhutan	—		19[a]	17	20	(1999)
India	53	(1993)	48	49	46	(2005–2006)
Maldives	39	(1994)	30	30	31	(2001)
Nepal	49	(1995)	39	40	38	(2006)
Sri Lanka	38	(1993)	29[b]	30	29	(2000)
Southeast Asia						
Brunei Darussalam[c]	—		—	—	—	
Cambodia	40	(1993)	36	36	35	(2005)
Indonesia	34	(1995)	28	—	—	(2003)
Lao PDR	44	(1993)	37	38	37	(2006)
Malaysia	23	(1993)	8	—	—	(2005)
Myanmar	32	(1990)	32	32	31	(2003)
Philippines	34	(1990)	28	—	—	(2003)
Singapore	—		3	3	4	(2000)
Thailand	19	(1993)	9	10	9	(2005)
Viet Nam	45	(1994)	20	19	21	(2006)
The Pacific						
Cook Islands	—		—	—	—	
Fiji Islands	—		—	—	—	
Kiribati	—		—	—	—	
Marshall Islands	—		—	—	—	
Micronesia, Fed. States of	—		—	—	—	
Nauru	—		—	—	—	
Palau	—		—	—	—	
Papua New Guinea	—		—	—	—	
Samoa	—		—	—	—	
Solomon Islands	—		—	—	—	
Timor-Leste	43	(2002)	49	45	53	(2007)
Tonga	—		—	—	—	
Tuvalu	—		—	—	—	
Vanuatu	—		—	—	—	
Developed member countries						
Australia	—		—	—	—	
Japan	—		—	—	—	
New Zealand	—		—	—	—	

—Data not available at cut-off date.
[a]For children aged 6–59 months.
[b]For children aged 3–59 months.
[c]Brunei Darussalam is a regional member of the Asian Development Bank, but it is not classified as a developing member country.

SOURCE: Adapted from "Table 1.3.—1.8. Prevalence of Underweight Children under Five Years of Age (Percent)," in *Key Indicators for Asia and the Pacific 2009*, 40th ed., Asian Development Bank (ADB), August 2009, http://www.adb.org/Documents/Books/Key_Indicators/2009/pdf/Key-Indicators-2009.pdf (accessed December 6, 2009). Data from the Millennium Indicators Database Online (UNSD 2009) and Monitoring the Situation of Children and Women Online (UNICEF 2009).

and is home to the greatest concentration of poor people. The CIA notes in *World Factbook: India* (February 18, 2010, https://www.cia.gov/library/publications/the-world-factbook/geos/in.html) that out of 1.2 billion people living on 1.3 million square miles (3.3 million sq km) of land, 25% lived below the country's poverty line in 2007.

TABLE 4.10

Percent undernourished, Asia and the Pacific, by region and country, 1990–92, 1995–97, and 2003–05

Developing member countries	1990–1992	1995–1997	2003–2005
Central and West Asia			
Afghanistan	—	—	—
Armenia	46	34	21
Azerbaijan	27	27	12
Georgia	47	24	13
Kazakhstan	<5	<5	<5
Kyrgyz Republic	17	13	<5
Pakistan	22	18	23
Tajikistan	34	42	34
Turkmenistan	9	9	6
Uzbekistan	5	5	14
East Asia			
China, People's Rep. of	15[a]	12[a]	9[a]
Hong Kong, China	—	—	—
Korea, Rep. of	<5	<5	<5
Mongolia	30	40	29
Taipei, China	—	—	—
South Asia			
Bangladesh	36	40	27
Bhutan	—	—	—
India	24	21	21
Maldives	9	9	7
Nepal	21	24	15
Sri Lanka	27	24	21
Southeast Asia			
Brunei Darussalam[b]	<5	<5	<5
Cambodia	38	41	26
Indonesia	19	13	17
Lao PDR	27	26	19
Malaysia	<5	<5	<5
Myanmar	44	34	19
Philippines	21	18	16
Singapore	—	—	—
Thailand	29	21	17
Viet Nam	28	21	14
The Pacific			
Cook Islands	—	—	—
Fiji Islands	8	5	<5
Kiribati	8	5	5
Marshall Islands	—	—	—
Micronesia, Fed. States of	—	—	—
Nauru	—	—	—
Palau	—	—	—
Papua New Guinea	—	—	—
Samoa	9	10	<5
Solomon Islands	25	13	9
Timor-Leste	18	13	22
Tonga	—	—	—
Tuvalu	—	—	—
Vanuatu	10	10	7
Developed member countries			
Australia	<5	<5	<5
Japan	<5	<5	<5
New Zealand	<5	<5	<5

—Data not available at cut-off date.

[a]Includes Hong Kong, China; Macao, China; and Taipei, China.

[b]Brunei Darussalam is a regional member of the Asian Development Bank, but it is not classified as a developing member country.

SOURCE: Adapted from "Table 1.3.—1.9. Proportion of Population below Minimum Level of Dietary Energy Consumption (Percent)," in *Key Indicators for Asia and the Pacific 2009*, 40th ed., Asian Development Bank (ADB), August 2009, http://www.adb.org/Documents/Books/Key_Indicators/2009/pdf/Key-Indicators-2009.pdf (accessed December 6, 2009). Data from the Millennium Indicators Database Online (UNSD 2009) and Monitoring the Situation of Children and Women Online (UNICEF 2009).

Two historic factors have caused much of India's poverty. First, like Africa, India was colonized by outsiders from the 16th century until it achieved independence from British rule in 1947. Second, like China, it has had a class system that keeps many people in extreme poverty and uses them to perform labor that benefits wealthier citizens. Since 1991 India has experienced economic expansion similar to China's, which has left its population even more divided between the so-called haves and have-nots.

Colonialism and the Caste System in India

Four major world religions originated in India: Buddhism, Hinduism, Jainism, and Sikhism. This has made the country rich with cultural and philosophical traditions, but it has also led to violent disputes that made India vulnerable to colonial takeover, to wars with neighboring countries, and to the creation of Hinduism's caste (class or birth-ranking) system that continues to keep many Indians in poverty, in part because of the legal entrenchment of castes during the period of British colonialism from 1757 to 1947.

According to the CIA, in *World Factbook: India*, Hinduism is India's dominant religion, with 80.5% of Indians counted as followers in 2001. One tenet of Hinduism that has strongly influenced secular Indian society is that of castes—that is, the categories into which different kinds of occupations are placed based on the labor or social class into which a person is born. As in early China, the early Indian government was based on a series of dynasties, which further aggravated tensions between the rich and the poor.

THE INDIAN APARTHEID. The result of centuries of adherence to the caste system is a social structure that still closely resembles that of South Africa's apartheid (a legal and social policy of racial segregation). The people who were formerly called Untouchables are now called Dalits, but they are nonetheless at the bottom of the Indian social hierarchy, especially in the rural states and villages. According to Bob Clifford, in "'Dalit Rights Are Human Rights': Caste Discrimination, International Activism, and the Construction of a New Human Rights Issue" (*Human Rights Quarterly*, vol. 29, no. 1, February 2007), there are approximately 240 million Dalits in India, even though the concept and practice of "untouchability" was outlawed by the Indian constitution in 1950. The Dalits are routinely discriminated against: they typically cannot own or access land, they must work in the most undesirable occupations (dealing with corpses and waste), they are abused by local police and denied rights, their living quarters and public spaces are strictly segregated, and their children do not receive equal education. Dalit children are also the ones most commonly sold into debt bondage and forced labor. Dalit workers commonly earn just $0.38 to $0.88 per day. Dalit women suffer perhaps the most: they are routinely

TABLE 4.11

Percent using improved water sources, Asia and The Pacific, by region, country, and rural/urban location, selected years 1990–2007

Developing member countries	1990						2006					
	Total		Urban		Rural		Total		Urban		Rural	
Central and West Asia												
Afghanistan	21	(1995)	37	(1995)	17	(1995)	22		37		17	
Armenia	91	(1995)	99	(1995)	75	(1995)	98		99		96	
Azerbaijan	68		82		51		78		95		59	
Georgia	76		91		58		99		100		97	
Kazakhstan	96		99		91		96		99		91	
Kyrgyz Republic	77	(1995)	97	(1995)	65	(1995)	89		99		83	
Pakistan	86		96		81		90		95		87	
Tajikistan	56	(1995)	91	(1995)	42	(1995)	67		93		58	
Turkmenistan	—		—		—		—		—		—	
Uzbekistan	90		97		85		88		98		82	
East Asia												
China, People's Rep. of	67		97		55		88		98		81	
Hong Kong, China	—		—		—		—		—		—	
Korea, Rep. of	91	(1995)	97	(1995)	71	(1995)	92	(2000)	97	(2000)	71	(2000)
Mongolia	64		97		21		72		90		48	
Taipei, China	84		—		—		92	(2007)	—		—	
South Asia												
Bangladesh	78		88		76		80		85		78	
Bhutan	81	(2000)	98	(2000)	79	(2000)	81		98		79	
India	71		90		65		89		96		86	
Maldives	96		100		95		83		98		76	
Nepal	72		97		70		89		94		88	
Sri Lanka	67		91		62		82		98		79	
Southeast Asia												
Brunei Darussalam*	—		—		—		—		—		—	
Cambodia	19	(1995)	47	(1995)	14	(1995)	65		80		61	
Indonesia	72		92		63		80		89		71	
Lao PDR	41	(1995)	73	(1995)	34	(1995)	60		86		53	
Malaysia	98		100		96		99		100		96	
Myanmar	57		86		47		80		80		80	
Philippines	83		92		75		93		96		88	
Singapore	100		100		na		100		100		na	
Thailand	95		98		94		98		99		97	
Viet Nam	52		87		43		92		98		90	
The Pacific												
Cook Islands	94		99		87		95		98		88	
Fiji Islands	48		43		51		47		43		51	
Kiribati	48		76		33		65		77		53	
Marshall Islands	96		95		97		88	(2000)	83	(2000)	96	(2000)
Micronesia, Fed. States of	88		93		86		94		95		94	
Nauru	—		—		—		—		—		—	
Palau	90		73		98		89		79		94	
Papua New Guinea	39		88		32		40		88		32	
Samoa	91		99		89		88		90		87	
Solomon Islands	69		94		65		70		94		65	
Timor-Leste	61	(2000)	77	(2000)	56	(2000)	62		77		56	
Tonga	100		100		100		100		100		100	
Tuvalu	90		92		89		93		94		92	
Vanuatu	61		93		53		59	(2000)	86	(2000)	52	(2000)
Developed member countries												
Australia	100		100		100		100		100		100	
Japan	100		100		100		100		100		100	
New Zealand	97		100		82		97	(1995)	100	(1995)	82	(1995)

—Data not available at cut-off date.
*Brunei Darussalam is a regional member of the Asian Development Bank, but it is not classified as a developing member country.

SOURCE: Adapted from "Table 7.3.—7.8. Population Using Improved Water Sources (Percent)," in *Key Indicators for Asia and the Pacific 2009*, 40th ed., Asian Development Bank (ADB), August 2009, http://www.adb.org/Documents/Books/Key_Indicators/2009/pdf/Key-Indicators-2009.pdf (accessed December 6, 2009). Data from the Millennium Indicators Database Online (UNSD 2009); for Taipei, China: economy sources.

raped as punishment for any offenses their family members commit, and their numbers are increasing in the commercial sex trade due to poverty and the lack of other financial opportunities.

Economics of Contemporary India

India is an example of a country that is both emerging and transitional: even though it has been a democracy since its independence in 1947, certain elements of its

TABLE 4.12

Percent using improved sanitation, Asia and the Pacific, by region, country, and rural/urban location, selected years 1990–2006

Developing member countries	1990			2006		
	Total	Urban	Rural	Total	Urban	Rural
Central and West Asia						
Afghanistan	32 (1995)	42 (1995)	29 (1995)	30	45	25
Armenia	89 (1995)	94 (1995)	78 (1995)	91	96	81
Azerbaijan	80 (1995)	90 (1995)	70 (1995)	80	90	70
Georgia	94	96	91	93	94	92
Kazakhstan	97	97	96	97	97	98
Kyrgyz Republic	92 (1995)	93 (1995)	92 (1995)	93	94	93
Pakistan	33	76	14	58	90	40
Tajikistan	83 (1995)	88 (1995)	81 (1995)	92	95	91
Turkmenistan	—	—	—	—	—	—
Uzbekistan	93	97	91	96	97	95
East Asia						
China, People's Rep. of	48	61	43	65	74	59
Hong Kong, China	—	—	—	—	—	—
Korea, Rep. of	—	—	—	—	—	—
Mongolia	47 (1995)	66 (1995)	23 (1995)	50	64	31
Taipei, China	—	—	—	—	—	—
South Asia						
Bangladesh	26	56	18	36	48	32
Bhutan	52 (2000)	71 (2000)	50 (2000)	52	71	50
India	14	44	4	28	52	18
Maldives	57 (1995)	100 (1995)	42 (1995)	59	100	42
Nepal	9	36	6	27	45	24
Sri Lanka	71	85	68	86	89	86
Southeast Asia						
Brunei Darussalam*	—	—	—	—	—	—
Cambodia	8 (1995)	43 (1995)	2 (1995)	28	62	19
Indonesia	51	73	42	52	67	37
Lao PDR	13 (1995)	48 (1995)	6 (1995)	48	87	38
Malaysia	94 (2000)	95 (2000)	93 (2000)	94	95	93
Myanmar	23	47	15	82	85	81
Philippines	58	71	46	78	81	72
Singapore	100	100	na	100	100	na
Thailand	78	92	72	96	95	96
Viet Nam	29	62	21	65	88	56
The Pacific						
Cook Islands	96	100	91	100	100	100
Fiji Islands	68	87	55	71	87	55
Kiribati	22	26	20	33	46	20
Marshall Islands	75	88	51	81 (2000)	93 (2000)	57 (2000)
Micronesia, Fed. States of	29	54	20	25	61	14
Nauru	—	—	—	—	—	—
Palau	61	76	54	67	96	52
Papua New Guinea	44	67	41	45	67	41
Samoa	98	100	98	100	100	100
Solomon Islands	29	98	18	32	98	18
Timor-Leste	40 (2000)	64 (2000)	32 (2000)	41	64	32
Tonga	96	98	96	96	98	96
Tuvalu	78	83	74	89	93	84
Vanuatu	49 (1995)	78 (1995)	42 (1995)	50 (2000)	78 (2000)	42 (2000)
Developed member countries						
Australia	100	100	100	100	100	100
Japan	100	100	100	100	100	100
New Zealand	—	—	88	—	—	88 (1995)

—Data not available at cut-off date.
*Brunei Darussalam is a regional member of the Asian Development Bank, but it is not classified as a developing member country.

SOURCE: Adapted from "Table 7.3.—7.9. Population Using Improved Sanitation Facilities (Percent)," in *Key Indicators for Asia and the Pacific 2009*, 40th ed., Asian Development Bank (ADB), August 2009, http://www.adb.org/Documents/Books/Key_Indicators/2009/pdf/Key-Indicators-2009.pdf (accessed December 6, 2009). Data from the Millennium Indicators Database Online (UNSD 2009); for Taipei, China: economy sources.

economy have been planned to encourage social equality. To make up for centuries of discrimination against the lower-caste Indians by those in upper castes and by British rulers, the post-independence Indian government developed a mixed economy, with a certain amount of market freedom in the private sector (independent, privately owned businesses) and socialist-style control of the public sector (services such as the railroad and postal systems). With India failing to keep up with the huge growth of other Asian economies in the 1980s, in 1991 the Indian government began to open up the country's markets—including parts of the public sector—to private ownership, foreign investment, and increased trade in an effort to stimulate the economy.

Table 4.2 shows that the Indian economy grew at a rate of 9.7% in 2006, 9% in 2007, and 6.7% in 2008. It was projected to continue at a rate of 6% in 2009 and 7% in 2010. The main reason for India's high rate of growth—outside of the loosening of the country's markets—is its abundance of well-educated, English-speaking workers who are willing to accept relatively low wages for steady jobs. Western countries have responded by outsourcing jobs and setting up operations in India, especially in information technology, to save money and to take advantage of the talented labor force. In general, the economy of India weathered the global economic crisis that began in 2007 and extended into 2010 relatively well. However, the ADB notes in *Asian Development Outlook 2009* that the slowdown in India's rate of growth of its GDP in 2008 and projected slowdown in 2009 was due to not only investors limiting their exposure to emerging markets, such as India, during the economic crisis, but also to reduced earnings from a slump in worldwide information technology business.

Comparing Income Inequality in India and China

In *Key Indicators for Asia and the Pacific 2009*, the ADB lists the Gini coefficient for India in 1993 as 0.329 and shows that India's income inequality worsened by 2005, when its Gini coefficient stood at 0.368. However, China had worse conditions of income inequality than India in both years, with a Gini coefficient of 0.407 in 1993 and of 0.415 in 2005.

COMPARING OTHER HUMAN DEVELOPMENT INDICATORS. Table 4.6 shows that the maternal mortality rate for India was 450 maternal deaths per 100,000 live births in 2005, which was ten times higher than China's 45 maternal deaths per 100,000 live births. The proportion of births attended by skilled health personnel differed dramatically as might be expected from the maternal mortality data. In India only 47% of births were attended by skilled health personnel in 2006, whereas in China 98% of births were attended by skilled health professionals. (See Table 4.7.) Both countries have made strides in this area. In 1993 only 34% of births in India were attended by skilled health professionals, 13 percentage points less than in 2006. In 1995, 89% of births in China were attended by skilled health professionals, 9 percentage points less than in 2006.

In 2007 India's U5MR was 72 deaths per 1,000 children under the age of five. (See Table 4.8.) India's U5MR was much higher than China's rate of 22 deaths per 1,000 children under the age of five. Both India and China have made progress toward their MDG targets in this area of cutting their 1990 rates by two-thirds. India's U5MR target by 2015 was 39 and China's was 15. The differences in each country's infant mortality rate was equally dramatic. In 2007 India's infant mortality rate was 54 deaths per 1,000 live births, whereas China's was 19 deaths per 1,000 live births.

Table 4.9 shows that the prevalence of underweight children under the age of five in India was about 48% in 2005–06, compared with China's 7% in 2005. The 2015 MDG target in this area of child health is to cut the prevalence of underweight children by half from 1990 to 2015. India was not on target to meet its MDG of 26.5% in 2015, but China already achieved and surpassed its 2015 MDG target of 9.5%.

One human development indicator in which India surpassed China was access to clean water in rural areas. Table 4.11 shows that in 2006, 86% of rural inhabitants in India had access to clean water, whereas 81% of rural inhabitants in China did. In urban communities the proportions were nearly the same. In 2006, 96% of urban inhabitants in India had access to clean water, whereas 98% of urban inhabitants of China did. Overall, India met its MDG target for this indicator, reducing the percentage of people not having access to clean water by more than half, from 29% in 1990 to 11% in 2006. China also met its MDG target for this indicator, reducing the percentage of people not having access to clean water by more than half, from 33% in 1990 to 12% in 2006.

Regarding access to basic sanitation, China has far surpassed India in access. Table 4.12 shows that only 18% of India's rural population had access to basic sanitation in 2006, whereas 59% of China's rural population did. Greater proportions of both countries' populations used improved sanitation facilities in urban areas, but urban Chinese had better access than urban Indians. In 2006, 52% of India's urban population had access to basic sanitation, whereas 74% of China's urban population did.

Concerning the percentage of children enrolled in primary school out of the total number of children of primary school age, India lagged behind China. In 2006 India had a 94.3% primary enrollment rate. (See Table 4.4.) As mentioned previously, Table 4.4 does not have a recent figure available for the primary school net enrollment ratio for China, but UNICEF indicates in "China" that the net enrollment ratio for primary school in China was 99% from 2000 to 2007.

CHAPTER 5
POVERTY IN THE DEVELOPING WORLD

Developing countries are those with incomes (in terms of gross domestic product, or GDP—the total value of all goods and services produced by a country in a year) that fall between the least developed countries and the industrialized nations. Most countries in the world can be described as developing: neither desperately poor nor excessively rich. These countries have segments of deep, absolute poverty and instances of great wealth in their populations, but their overall economies fall below even that of a middle-income country such as Russia. At the same time, however, in terms of government and general standards of living, progress can be seen over time. Industry and technology in developing nations show progress as well—often aided by an abundance of natural resources—but they may be hampered by militarism, violent unrest between classes and ethnic groups, political instability, and persistent poverty. Nevertheless, many developing countries have experienced impressive economic growth due to their increasingly important role in the global market as they open their economies to international trade and learn to leverage their natural resources for greater returns.

LATIN AMERICA AND THE CARIBBEAN
Poverty Reduction and Economic Growth

In *Poverty Reduction and Growth: Virtuous and Vicious Circles* (February 2006, http://siteresources.world bank.org/EXTLACOFFICEOFCE/Resources/870892-1139 877599088/virtuous_circles1_complete.pdf), Guillermo E. Perry et al. cite Latin America's high US $2-or-less-per-day poverty rate as one of the major causes and consequences of its overall low growth rate. This overall low growth rate is discussed by the U.S. Agency for International Development's Bureau for Latin America and the Caribbean in *Latin America and the Caribbean: Selected Economic and Social Data, 2009* (September 2009, http://pdf.usaid.gov/pdf_docs/PNADQ200.pdf). From 1998 to 2005 the GDP growth rate for this region

ranged annually from less than 1% in 1999, 2001, and 2002, to a high of 6% in 2004. The percentage of the population living below $2 per day in Latin America and the Caribbean (LAC) ranged from a low of 4.5% in 2005 in Uruguay to a high of 72.1% in 2001 in Haiti, but most LAC countries had double-digit percentages of their populations living on less than $2 per day. (See Table 5.1.)

Each country within the LAC region has its own standard for measuring poverty, which typically differs significantly from the other countries. This lack of consistency makes comparing rates of poverty in different LAC countries difficult. Thus, Table 5.1 compares poverty in LAC countries using both the national poverty line as determined by each country and the standard under-US-$1.25-per-day and the under-$2-per-day poverty line.

Comparing the $2-per-day poverty line against the poverty lines of individual countries yields a somewhat confusing picture. For example, in Honduras 50.7% of the population lived below the country's poverty line in 2004, whereas 34.8% lived on less than $2 per day in 2005 and 29.7% in 2006. (See Table 5.1.) In contrast, 18.7% of people in Jamaica lived below the country's poverty line in 2000, whereas 8.7% made less than $2 per day in 2002 and 5.8% in 2004. In no countries were the two numbers nearly the same.

Table 5.1 also shows the differences in urban and rural poverty rates using the national poverty measure. Of the 24 countries listed, only Trinidad and Tobago had a higher percentage of poverty in its urban areas as opposed to its rural areas. For all other countries listed, and as is usually the case in developing countries, poverty is much more prevalent in rural areas than in urban areas.

As noted earlier, Perry et al. suggest that widespread poverty hampers the rate of growth of the GDP. Conversely, the World Bank notes in *World Development Report 2006: Equity and Development*

TABLE 5.1

Percent living in poverty, Latin America and the Caribbean, by region, country, and rural/urban location, selected years 1989–2007

	Survey year	Rural %	Urban %	National %	Survey year	Population below $1.25/day	Population below $2/day
Caribbean							
Dominican Republic	2000	45.3	18.2	27.7	2003	6.1	16.3
	2004	55.7	34.7	42.2	2005	5.0	15.1
Guyana	1993	—	—	43.2	1993	5.8	15.0
	1998			35.0	1998	7.7	16.8
Haiti	1987	—	—	65.0	2001	54.9	72.1
	1995	66.0	—	—	—	—	—
Jamaica	1995	37.0	18.7	27.5	2002	<2.0	8.7
	2000	25.1	12.8	18.7	2004	<2.0	5.8
St. Lucia	—	—	—	—	1995	20.9	40.6
Suriname	—	—	—	—	1999	15.5	27.2
Trinidad and Tobago	1992	20.0	24.0	21.0	1988	<2.0	8.6
	—	—	—	—	1992	4.2	13.5
Central America							
Costa Rica	1992	25.5	19.2	22.0	2003	5.6	11.5
	2004	28.3	20.8	23.9	2005	2.4	8.6
El Salvador	1995	64.8	38.9	50.6	2003	14.3	25.3
	2002	49.8	28.5	37.2	2005	11.0	20.5
Guatemala	1989	71.9	33.7	57.9	2002	16.9	29.8
	2000	74.5	27.1	56.2	2006	11.7	24.3
Honduras	1999	71.2	28.6	52.5	2005	22.2	34.8
	2004	70.4	29.5	50.7	2006	18.2	29.7
Nicaragua	1993	76.1	31.9	50.3	2001	19.4	37.5
	1998	68.5	30.5	47.9	2005	15.8	31.8
Panama	1997	64.9	15.3	37.3	2004	9.2	18.0
	—	—	—	—	2006	9.5	17.8
South America							
Argentina	1995	—	28.4	—	2002	9.9	19.7
	1998	—	29.9	—	2005	4.5	11.3
Bolivia	1999	81.7	50.6	62.7	2002	22.8	34.2
	2002	83.5	53.9	65.2	2005	19.6	30.3
Brazil	1998	51.4	14.7	22.0	2005	7.8	18.3
	2003	41.0	17.5	21.5	2007	5.2	12.7
Chile	1996	—	—	19.9	2003	<2.0	5.3
	1998	—	—	17.0	2006	<2.0	2.4
Colombia	1995	79.0	48.0	60.0	2003	15.4	26.3
	1999	79.0	55.0	64.0	2006	16.0	27.9
Ecuador	1995	56.0	19.0	34.0	2005	9.8	20.4
	1998	69.0	30.0	46.0	2007	4.7	12.8
Paraguay	1990	28.5	19.7	20.5	2005	9.3	18.4
	—	—	—	—	2007	6.5	14.2
Peru	2001	77.1	42.0	54.3	2005	8.2	19.4
	2004	72.1	42.9	53.1	2006	7.9	18.5
Uruguay	1994	—	20.2	—	2005	<2.0	4.5
	1998	—	24.7	—	2006	<2.0	4.2
Venezuela	1989	—	—	31.3	2005	10.0	19.8
	—	—	—	—	2006	3.5	10.2
LAC							
Mexico	2002	34.8	11.4	20.3	2004	2.8	7.0
	2004	27.9	11.3	17.6	2006	<2.0	4.8

SOURCE: Adapted from "2.1. Incidence of Poverty Percentage," in *Latin America and the Caribbean: Selected Economic and Social Data, 2009*, United States Agency for International Development (USAID), Bureau for Latin American and the Caribbean, September 2009, http://pdf.usaid.gov/pdf_docs/PNADQ200 .pdf (accessed December 6, 2009). Data from The World Bank, World Development Indicators (online version) as of May, 2009.

(2005, http://www-wds.worldbank.org/) that economic growth is necessary for sustained poverty reduction. In LAC countries, widespread poverty and slow economic growth are a vicious cycle.

Great income disparity within a region or country makes both poverty reduction and economic growth more difficult. As in other countries with a wide income gap—even in developed ones—the challenge is to provide equal opportunities to all people, not only to promote fairness and provide a decent life for all but also to foster economic opportunity and growth in all sectors of society and the economy. The World Bank states these ideas this way: "Institutions and policies that promote a level playing field—where all members of society have similar chances to become socially active, politically influential, and economically productive—contribute to sustainable growth and development."

Income Inequality

Income inequality in LAC countries is among the highest in the world. For example, Jeni Klugman of the United Nations Development Programme (UNDP) indicates in *Human Development Report 2009—Overcoming Barriers: Human Mobility and Development* (2009, http://hdr.undp.org/en/media/HDR_2009_EN_Complete.pdf) that in 2007 Venezuela's Gini coefficient was 43.4, Peru's was 49.6, Brazil's was 55, and Colombia's was 58.5. The Gini coefficient is a number between 0 and 100, with 0 representing perfect equality and 100 representing perfect inequality. The more income-unequal countries of the world tend to have Gini coefficients close to 50, whereas the more income-equal countries tend to have Gini coefficients closer to 30. (Sometimes a scale of 0 to 1 is used, so that the coefficient is expressed as, for example, 0.5 instead of 50.)

COLONIZATION AND INEQUALITY IN LATIN AMERICA. Latin American economic, political, and social inequality dates back to the late 15th century, when the region was first colonized by Spanish and Portuguese explorers. The indigenous peoples of what are now the Caribbean, Mexico, Central America, and South America had lived there for thousands of years. However, when the Europeans arrived, they brought with them infectious diseases against which the native inhabitants had no natural immunity. Historians estimate that by the 1530s approximately 90% of the indigenous population had died— some in battle against the Europeans and others as a result of the brutal working conditions imposed on them by the conquerors, but most because of diseases such as smallpox, typhoid fever, influenza, and measles. To make up for the loss in potential workers, the European colonizers began importing slaves from Africa. The Europeans, Africans, and natives occasionally intermarried. However, instead of creating a society of equals, intermarriage actually resulted in a group of permanent underclasses; children of mixed unions, as well as descendants of natives, continue to be socially and economically oppressed even into the 21st century.

Besides this social and economic inequality, the LAC countries have a history of unequal land distribution and of denying native peoples land rights. Native land claims were first officially addressed when the LAC countries adopted the International Labour Office's C107 Indigenous and Tribal Populations Convention in 1957, which recommended methods for protecting and assimilating native peoples while recognizing their individual rights and cultures. Since the 1970s native land rights have become a central issue in Latin American legal and social reform.

Other Human Development Indicators

Human development indicators include not only poverty, economic growth, and income inequality but also the rate of infant mortality, hunger and undernutrition, and the completion of primary school.

Table 5.2 shows the rates of infant mortality in the LAC countries annually, from 2005 to 2009. This table reveals the great diversity in poverty levels in Latin America, measured here through infant mortality rates. Whereas some countries have infant mortality rates as low as the wealthiest countries in the world, others have rates as high as the world's poorest regions. As a comparison, the Central Intelligence Agency (CIA) indicates in *World Factbook: United States* (February 4, 2010, https://www.cia.gov/library/publications/the-world-factbook/geos/us.html) that the United States had an infant mortality rate of 6.2 deaths per 1,000 live births in 2009. The LAC countries with equally low rates or lower in 2009 were Bermuda (2.5 deaths per 1,000 live births), Anguilla (3.5), the Cayman Islands (6.9), the Virgin Islands (7.6), and Chile (7.7). As is the case with Chile, countries on the coastline generally (but not always) have a less severe hunger problem than inland countries and have a lower infant mortality rate. Chile is a narrow South American country with an extensive coastline. The other countries in the list are small islands.

The LAC countries with the highest infant mortality rates in 2009 were Haiti (59.7 deaths per 1,000 live births) and Bolivia (44.7). Even though Haiti is a half-island (sharing the island with the Dominican Republic), it is one of the poorest countries in the world and has an extremely high infant mortality rate. By contrast, Bolivia is landlocked and has a high elevation. The high elevations of Bolivia's mountainous west provide cold and windy plateaus, which present difficult growing conditions for the subsistence farmers who live there.

Low consumption of calories is correlated to undernutrition and death in children. The U.S. Department of Health and Human Services and the U.S. Department of Agriculture (USDA) estimate in *Dietary Guidelines for Americans, 2005* (January 2005, http://www.health.gov/dietaryguidelines/dga2005/document/pdf/DGA2005.pdf), the most recent publication as of February 2010, the number of calories needed to maintain health. Moderately active females aged 19 to 30 require 2,000 to 2,200 calories per day, whereas moderately active males of the same age require 2,600 to 2,800 calories per day. Older people and small children do not require as many calories. People who do not eat as many calories as they require to maintain health on a regular basis are undernourished.

Figure 5.1 shows the percent of the population in the LAC region that is undernourished. The highest prevalence of undernourishment is in Central America. However, undernourishment in this region has declined in recent years, from nearly 20% of the population in 1992 to about 14% of the population in 2005. In 1992 the prevalence of undernourishment was slightly higher in South America

TABLE 5.2

Infant mortality rate, Latin America and the Caribbean, by region, country, and sex, 2005–09

[per 1,000 live births]

	Both sexes					Female					Male				
	2005	2006	2007	2008	2009	2005	2006	2007	2008	2009	2005	2006	2007	2008	2009
Caribbean	**19.1**	**18.4**	**17.8**	**17.3**	**16.8**	**17.1**	**16.4**	**15.9**	**15.4**	**14.9**	**21.0**	**20.3**	**19.7**	**19.1**	**18.6**
Anguilla	3.6	3.6	3.6	3.5	3.5	3.1	3.1	3.1	3.1	3.0	4.1	4.1	4.0	4.0	4.0
Antigua and Barbuda	21.8	20.2	18.8	17.5	16.2	18.1	16.9	15.7	14.6	13.6	25.3	23.5	21.8	20.2	18.8
Aruba	15.8	15.3	14.8	14.3	13.8	10.4	10.1	9.8	9.5	9.2	21.0	20.3	19.6	18.9	18.3
Bahamas	25.2	24.7	24.2	23.7	23.2	19.3	19.0	18.6	18.3	18.0	31.0	30.3	29.6	28.9	28.2
Barbados	14.1	13.7	13.2	12.7	12.3	12.5	12.1	11.6	11.1	10.7	15.6	15.2	14.8	14.3	13.9
Belize	25.5	24.9	24.2	23.6	23.1	22.2	21.8	21.2	20.8	20.0	28.7	27.8	27.2	26.4	26.0
Bermuda	2.4	2.5	2.5	2.5	2.5	2.3	2.3	2.4	2.4	2.4	2.5	2.5	2.6	2.6	2.6
British Virgin Islands	17.0	16.4	15.8	15.2	14.7	14.6	14.1	13.6	13.1	12.6	19.2	18.5	17.9	17.2	16.6
Cayman Islands	7.6	7.5	7.3	7.1	6.9	6.5	6.3	6.2	6.0	5.9	8.8	8.6	8.4	8.2	8.0
Dominica	15.6	15.1	14.6	14.1	13.7	9.9	9.6	9.3	9.0	8.7	21.1	20.4	19.7	19.0	18.3
Dominican Republic	30.1	29.0	27.9	26.9	26.0	27.9	26.8	25.8	24.8	23.8	32.3	31.1	30.1	29.0	28.0
Grenada	14.7	14.3	13.9	13.6	13.2	15.1	14.7	14.3	13.9	13.5	14.2	13.9	13.6	13.2	12.9
Guyana	33.3	32.2	31.4	30.4	29.6	29.4	28.4	27.6	26.8	26.1	36.9	35.8	34.9	33.9	33.0
Haiti	66.7	64.9	63.1	61.4	59.7	59.3	57.7	56.1	54.5	53.0	73.8	71.8	69.9	68.0	66.2
Jamaica	16.5	16.2	15.9	15.6	15.2	15.8	15.5	15.2	14.9	14.6	17.1	16.8	16.5	16.2	15.8
Montserrat	20.1	17.4	16.8	16.5	16.1	25.8	22.2	21.5	20.9	20.4	14.6	12.7	12.4	12.2	12.0
Netherlands Antilles	10.2	9.9	9.6	9.4	9.1	9.4	9.2	8.9	8.6	8.4	10.9	10.6	10.3	10.0	9.8
Puerto Rico	9.3	8.6	8.5	8.5	8.4	8.9	7.2	7.1	7.1	7.1	9.7	9.9	9.8	9.8	9.7
St. Kitts and Nevis	15.6	15.2	14.7	14.3	13.9	13.6	13.2	12.8	12.5	12.1	17.4	17.0	16.5	16.1	15.7
St. Lucia	15.0	14.6	14.2	13.8	13.4	16.4	15.8	15.4	14.9	14.4	13.7	13.3	13.1	12.8	12.5
St. Vincent and Grenadines	17.1	16.6	16.1	15.6	15.1	15.5	15.1	14.6	14.2	13.8	18.6	18.0	17.5	17.0	16.5
Suriname	21.5	20.8	20.1	19.4	18.8	17.4	16.8	16.2	15.7	15.2	25.4	24.5	23.7	23.0	22.2
Trinidad and Tobago	34.8	33.5	32.2	31.1	29.9	33.7	32.3	31.1	29.8	28.7	35.8	34.7	33.4	32.2	31.1
Turks and Caicos Islands	15.8	15.3	14.8	14.3	13.9	13.3	12.9	12.4	12.0	11.6	18.3	17.7	17.1	16.6	16.0
Virgin Islands (U.S.)	8.2	8.0	7.9	7.7	7.6	7.5	7.3	7.1	7.0	6.8	8.9	8.7	8.6	8.4	8.3
Central America	**22.8**	**22.1**	**21.4**	**20.7**	**20.0**	**20.3**	**19.6**	**19.0**	**18.3**	**17.7**	**25.2**	**24.4**	**23.7**	**22.9**	**22.2**
Costa Rica	9.8	9.5	9.2	9.0	8.8	8.7	8.5	8.3	8.1	7.8	10.7	10.4	10.2	9.9	9.7
El Salvador	24.3	23.6	22.9	22.2	21.5	21.3	20.6	19.9	19.2	18.5	27.2	26.5	25.8	25.1	24.4
Guatemala	31.8	30.8	29.8	28.8	27.8	29.1	28.1	27.2	26.2	25.4	34.5	33.3	32.3	31.2	30.2
Honduras	26.5	25.8	25.2	24.6	24.0	23.0	22.5	21.9	21.4	20.9	29.7	29.0	28.3	27.6	27.0
Nicaragua	28.8	27.8	26.8	25.9	25.0	25.2	24.3	23.4	22.6	21.8	32.2	31.1	30.1	29.1	28.1
Panama	15.7	15.0	14.2	13.4	12.7	14.4	13.8	13.1	12.4	11.8	16.9	16.1	15.2	14.3	13.5
South America	**23.9**	**23.2**	**22.5**	**21.9**	**21.2**	**20.8**	**20.1**	**19.5**	**18.9**	**18.3**	**26.9**	**26.2**	**25.5**	**24.7**	**24.1**
Argentina	12.9	12.5	12.1	11.8	11.4	11.4	11.0	10.7	10.4	10.1	14.3	13.9	13.5	13.1	12.8
Bolivia	50.0	48.6	47.3	46.0	44.7	45.7	44.4	43.1	41.8	40.6	54.1	52.7	51.3	49.9	48.6
Brazil	25.7	24.9	24.1	23.3	22.6	21.8	21.0	20.2	19.5	18.8	29.4	28.6	27.8	26.9	26.2
Chile	8.5	8.3	8.1	7.9	7.7	7.6	7.4	7.2	7.1	6.9	9.4	9.1	8.9	8.7	8.5
Colombia	21.4	20.8	20.1	19.5	18.9	17.5	16.9	16.3	15.7	15.1	25.3	24.6	23.9	23.2	22.5
Ecuador	23.7	22.9	22.2	21.6	20.9	19.8	19.1	18.5	17.8	17.2	27.4	26.6	25.9	25.1	24.4
Paraguay	28.4	27.4	26.4	25.6	24.7	23.7	22.8	22.0	21.2	20.4	32.8	31.8	30.7	29.7	28.8
Peru	32.4	31.4	30.5	29.5	28.6	29.7	28.8	27.8	26.9	26.1	35.0	34.0	33.0	32.0	31.1
Uruguay	12.8	12.4	12.0	11.7	11.3	11.2	10.8	10.5	10.2	9.9	14.3	13.9	13.5	13.1	12.7
Venezuela	23.5	23.0	22.5	22.0	21.5	19.7	19.2	18.7	18.3	17.8	27.2	26.7	26.1	25.6	25.1
LAC	**20.8**	**20.1**	**19.5**	**18.9**	**18.3**	**18.5**	**17.8**	**17.2**	**16.7**	**16.2**	**23.1**	**22.3**	**21.7**	**21.0**	**20.4**
Mexico	20.9	20.3	19.6	19.0	18.4	18.9	18.2	17.6	17.0	16.4	22.9	22.2	21.5	20.9	20.3

SOURCE: "3.1. Infant Mortality Rate per 1,000 Live Births," in *Latin America and the Caribbean: Selected Economic and Social Data, 2009*, United States Agency for International Development (USAID), Bureau for Latin American and the Caribbean, September 2009, http://pdf.usaid.gov/pdf_docs/PNADQ200 .pdf (accessed December 6, 2009)

(15%) than in the Caribbean (slightly under 15%), but South America has made greater strides in reducing the percentage of the undernourished population than has the Caribbean. In 2005 just over 10% of the population in South America was undernourished, whereas 13% of the population in the Caribbean was undernourished.

In *Food Security Assessment, 2008–09* (June 2009, http://www.ers.usda.gov/Publications/GFA20/GFA20.pdf), Shahla Shapouri et al. of the USDA's Economic Research Service (ERS) define food-insecure people as those consuming less than 2,100 calories per day. The number of

food-insecure people in the LAC region decreased in 2000 and 2001 from 1999, but then rose to near 1999 levels in 2002. (See Figure 5.2.) The percentage decreased again through 2005 and then somewhat stabilized. The LAC region has enough agricultural resources to feed its population, but equitable food distribution is a problem in the region. In addition, the low-income countries, which cannot afford to import much of their food, are therefore the countries most affected by hunger when severe weather events (e.g., hurricanes and droughts) strike and threaten a season's harvest.

The United Nations Children's Fund (UNICEF) describes in *Progress for Children: A Report Card on Nutrition* (May 2006, http://www.unicef.org/media/files/PFC_Nutrition.pdf) the correlation between poverty and underweight in children in the LAC region. In the LAC region, children living in the poorest households were 3.6 times more likely to be underweight than children living in the richest households in 2004. Among the countries listed, Paraguay's poor children found themselves in the worst situation, because they were 7.3 times more likely

to be underweight than children living in the richest Paraguayan households. By contrast, Trinidad and Tobago's poor children were 2.4 times more likely to be underweight than children living in the richest Trinidadian and Tobagonian households.

The rate of completion of primary school is a human development factor on which the LAC region is progressing well. The World Bank states in *World Development Indicators 2006* (April 2006, http://devdata.worldbank.org/wdi2006/contents/cover.htm) that "education is the foundation of all societies and globally competitive economies. It is the basis for reducing poverty and inequality, improving health, enabling the use of new technologies, and creating and spreading knowledge. In an increasingly complex, knowledge-dependent world, primary education, as the gateway to higher levels of education, must be the first priority." Most LAC countries are close to or on track to achieving the Millennium Development Goal (MDG; http://www.undp.org/mdg/basics.shtml) of universal primary education—that is, having all primary school–aged children complete their primary education.

Table 5.3 shows the net and gross enrollment ratios for both primary and secondary education in the LAC region. Net enrollment ratios are the percentage of students enrolled in primary or secondary education that are of primary or secondary school age. Gross enrollment ratios are the percentage of students enrolled in primary or secondary education regardless of age. Thus, gross enrollment ratios (percentages) can be over 100% because they include students outside of the age group appropriate for the particular level of schooling.

FIGURE 5.1

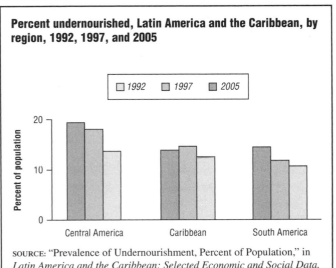

Percent undernourished, Latin America and the Caribbean, by region, 1992, 1997, and 2005

SOURCE: "Prevalence of Undernourishment, Percent of Population," in *Latin America and the Caribbean: Selected Economic and Social Data, 2009*, United States Agency for International Development (USAID), Bureau for Latin American and the Caribbean, September 2009, http://pdf.usaid.gov/pdf_docs/PNADQ200.pdf (accessed December 6, 2009). Data from The World Bank, World Development Indicators (online) as of May, 2009.

FIGURE 5.2

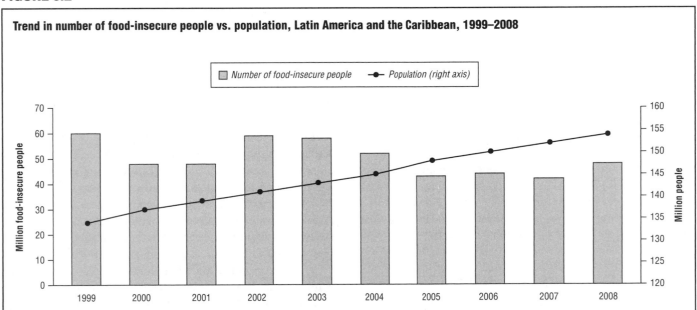

Trend in number of food-insecure people vs. population, Latin America and the Caribbean, 1999–2008

SOURCE: Shahla Shapouri et al., "LAC: Trend in Number of Food-Insecure People vs. Population," in *Food Security Assessment, 2008–09*, U.S. Department of Agriculture (USDA), Economic Research Service (ERS), June 2009, http://www.ers.usda.gov/Publications/GFA20/GFA20.pdf (accessed November 25, 2009)

TABLE 5.3

Percent school enrollment by level, Latin America and the Caribbean, by region and country, 2005 and 2007

	Pre-primary (gross)		Primary (gross)		Secondary (gross)		Tertiary (gross)		Primary (net)		Secondary (net)	
	2005	2007	2005	2007	2005	2007	2005	2007	2005	2007	2005	2007
Caribbean												
Antigua and Barbuda	—	72	—	102	—	105	—	—	—	74	—	—
Aruba	93	96	114	114	98	105	33	33	99	100	76	82
Bahamas	—	—	100	103	90	94	—	—	90	91	84	86
Barbados	89	91	100	105	103	103	—	53	94	97	88	90
Belize	31	35	122	123	84	79	—	—	95	97	71	67
Bermuda	—	—	102	—	89	—	19	—	98	—	—	—
Cayman Islands	93	—	90	—	102	—	—	—	81	—	96	—
Dominica	77	—	91	—	107	—	—	—	83	—	91	—
Dominican Republic	30	32	104	107	71	79	—	—	80	82	53	61
Grenada	81	80	93	81	100	99	—	—	84	76	79	—
Guyana	99	87	124	112	104	107	11	12	—	—	—	—
Jamaica	92	—	95	—	87	—	—	—	90	—	78	—
St. Kitts and Nevis	102	120	99	94	94	105	—	—	93	87	86	84
St. Lucia	74	68	113	109	83	93	13	9	97	99	73	—
St. Vincent and Grenadines	88	—	111	102	75	—	—	—	90	91	64	—
Suriname	88	85	120	119	74	80	—	—	94	94	68	—
Trinidad and Tobago	85	—	95	—	76	—	11	—	85	—	65	—
Central America												
Costa Rica	69	61	110	110	79	87	25	—	—	—	—	64
El Salvador	52	49	116	118	65	64	20	22	94	92	55	54
Guatemala	28	29	113	113	51	56	—	18	94	95	35	—
Honduras	34	36	113	117	76	61	—	—	92	96	—	—
Nicaragua	39	—	112	—	66	—	—	—	87	—	43	—
Panama	62	70	111	113	70	70	44	—	98	98	64	—
South America												
Argentina	66	—	112	—	84	—	64	—	99	—	78	—
Bolivia	50	—	—	—	—	—	—	—	—	—	—	—
Brazil	69	—	137	—	105	—	25	—	94	—	79	—
Chile	55	—	104	—	91	—	48	—	—	—	—	—
Colombia	41	41	116	116	79	85	29	32	90	87	61	67
Ecuador	80	100	117	118	65	70	—	—	97	97	55	59
Paraguay	34	—	111	—	66	—	26	—	94	—	57	—
Peru	66	—	116	—	92	—	34	—	96	—	70	—
Uruguay	76	—	114	—	101	—	45	—	97	—	—	—
Venezuela	58	62	104	106	74	79	—	—	91	92	63	68
LAC												
Mexico	96	—	112	—	85	—	25	—	98	—	69	—

SOURCE: "4.3. Gross and Net Enrollment Ratios Percent of Relevant Age Group," in *Latin America and the Caribbean: Selected Economic and Social Data, 2009*, United States Agency for International Development (USAID), Bureau for Latin American and the Caribbean, September 2009, http://pdf.usaid.gov/pdf_docs/PNADQ200.pdf (accessed December 6, 2009). Data from The World Bank, World Development Indicators (online) as of May, 2009.

In 2007 Aruba had achieved a net rate of primary enrollment of 100%, thus achieving its MDG target in this area. (See Table 5.3.) St. Lucia had a net rate of primary enrollment of 99%, and Panama had a net rate of primary enrollment of 98%. Barbados, Belize, and Ecuador had all achieved a 97% net rate of primary enrollment. The countries that still needed to make significant progress in this area in 2007 were Antigua and Barbuda, with a 74% net primary enrollment rate, Grenada with a 76% rate, the Dominican Republic with an 82% rate, and St. Kitts and Nevis and Colombia, with 87% rates.

THE CENTRAL ASIAN REPUBLICS

The central Asian republics (Kazakhstan, Kyrgyzstan, Tajikistan, Turkmenistan, and Uzbekistan) were all republics of the Soviet Union until they achieved independence in 1991. Officially, they are now a part of the Commonwealth of Independent States (CIS). However, the central Asian republics, while having a 20th-century history rooted in the Soviet bloc and still being politically tied to Russia, are fundamentally different ethnically, religiously, and economically. In one sense, the central Asian republics are transition economies. They all had planned economies during the Soviet era and have gradually opened to the international market since the 1990s. However, their general adherence to authoritarianism and their high rates of extreme poverty make them far less developed than other former Soviet countries. The central Asian republics have abundant natural resources and growing economies, but their human development indicators are seriously lacking because overall poverty has increased and human security has decreased since independence. For example, these countries have experienced a decline in life expectancy at birth in the years since the dissolution of the Soviet Union.

FIGURE 5.3

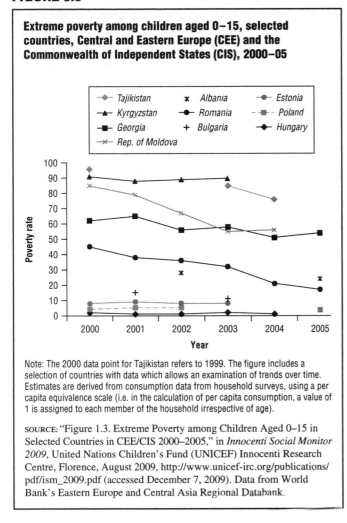

Extreme poverty among children aged 0–15, selected countries, Central and Eastern Europe (CEE) and the Commonwealth of Independent States (CIS), 2000–05

Note: The 2000 data point for Tajikistan refers to 1999. The figure includes a selection of countries with data which allows an examination of trends over time. Estimates are derived from consumption data from household surveys, using a per capita equivalence scale (i.e. in the calculation of per capita consumption, a value of 1 is assigned to each member of the household irrespective of age).

SOURCE: "Figure 1.3. Extreme Poverty among Children Aged 0–15 in Selected Countries in CEE/CIS 2000–2005," in *Innocenti Social Monitor 2009*, United Nations Children's Fund (UNICEF) Innocenti Research Centre, Florence, August 2009, http://www.unicef-irc.org/publications/pdf/ism_2009.pdf (accessed December 7, 2009). Data from World Bank's Eastern Europe and Central Asia Regional Databank.

FIGURE 5.4

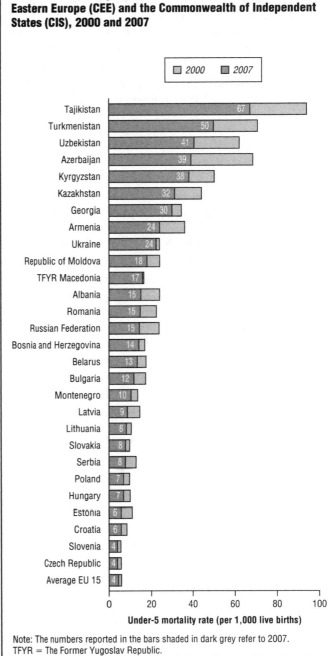

Under-five mortality rates, selected countries, Central and Eastern Europe (CEE) and the Commonwealth of Independent States (CIS), 2000 and 2007

Note: The numbers reported in the bars shaded in dark grey refer to 2007. TFYR = The Former Yugoslav Republic.
EU 15 = Austria, Belgium, Denmark, Finland, France, Germany, Greece, Ireland, Italy, Luxembourg, the Netherlands, Portugal, Spain, Sweden and the United Kingdom

SOURCE: "Figure 1.7. Under-Five Mortality Rates, 2000 and 2007," in *Innocenti Social Monitor 2009*, United Nations Children's Fund (UNICEF) Innocenti Research Centre, Florence, August 2009, http://www.unicef-irc.org/publications/pdf/ism_2009.pdf (accessed December 7, 2009). Data from www.childinfo.org.

The World Bank maintains a regional databank on 29 east European and central Asian countries, including Albania, Armenia, Azerbaijan, Belarus, Bosnia and Herzegovina, Bulgaria, Poland, Lithuania, the Russian Federation, Hungary, Turkey, Tajikistan, Turkmenistan, and Uzbekistan. In Figure 5.3, UNICEF's Innocenti Research Centre uses these World Bank regional data to show the rates of extreme poverty among children aged 15 years and younger in selected countries in central and eastern Europe and the CIS. For some of the countries shown, such as Tajikistan, the Republic of Moldova, Georgia, and Romania, extreme poverty among children declined in the first few years in the first decade of the 21st century. In other countries, such as Kyrgyzstan, Estonia, Poland, and Hungary, extreme poverty rates among children stayed about the same during those years. Countries with high rates of extreme childhood poverty include the Democratic Republic of Georgia, Kyrgyzstan, the Republic of Moldova, and Tajikistan. Countries with low rates of extreme childhood poverty include Estonia, Hungary, and Poland.

Figure 5.4 shows under-five mortality rates (U5MRs) for this region in 2000 and 2007. The rates dropped in all the countries shown, particularly in countries with high U5MRs, such as Tajikistan (97 to 67 deaths per 1,000 children under the age of five), Turkmenistan (70 to 50), Uzbekistan (60 to 41), Azerbaijan (68 to 39), Kyrgyzstan (50 to 38), and Kazakhstan (45 to 32). The Czech Republic and Slovenia had among the lowest U5MRs in the world at 4 deaths per 1,000 children under the age of five. Croatia (6), Estonia (6), Hungary (7) and Poland (7) all had U5MRs lower than the United States' rate of 8 deaths per 1,000 children under the age of five in 2005 as reported by the World Health Organization (WHO; November 2006, http://www.who.int/whosis/mort/profiles/mort_amro_usa_unitedstatesofamerica.pdf). Serbia, Slovakia, and Lithuania all had U5MRs on par with the United States, at 8 deaths per 1,000 children under the age of five.

Figure 5.5 shows U5MRs by level of GDP per capita and makes clear the negative correlation between poverty and the U5MR. Countries that had the lowest GDP per capita, such as Tajikistan, Kyrgyzstan, Uzbekistan, Turkmenistan, and Azerbaijan, had the highest U5MR. As the GDP per capita increases, the U5MR decreases.

One human development area in which the CIS has been making substantial progress is in reducing the number of food-insecure people in the region. Figure 5.6 shows that approximately 14 million people in this region were food-insecure in 2000. This number decreased every year through 2007 but increased suddenly in 2008 to approximately 6 million people. Shapouri et al. report that this increase was due not only to higher food and fuel prices but also to a sharp decline in food production caused by poor weather.

Access to clean water is another important area of development. Figure 5.7 reveals that access to piped water in the home was primarily a problem in rural areas in the region during 2005–06. In Serbia, Montenegro, Armenia, and Macedonia, less than 10% of the urban population

did not have water piped into the home from a public water network. Of the countries listed in Figure 5.7, the Republic of Moldova had the highest proportion of urban residents not having safe water piped into the home, at 27%. Concerning the rural populations in the central Asian republics, large percentages of the

FIGURE 5.5

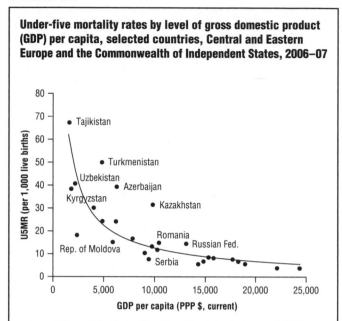

Under-five mortality rates by level of gross domestic product (GDP) per capita, selected countries, Central and Eastern Europe and the Commonwealth of Independent States, 2006–07

SOURCE: "Figure 1.1. Under-Five Mortality Rates by Level of GDP per Capita, 2006–2007," in *Innocenti Social Monitor 2009*, United Nations Children's Fund (UNICEF) Innocenti Research Centre, Florence, August 2009, http://www.unicef-irc.org/publications/pdf/ism_2009.pdf (accessed December 7, 2009). Data from www.childinfo.org and World Development Indicators 2008.

FIGURE 5.6

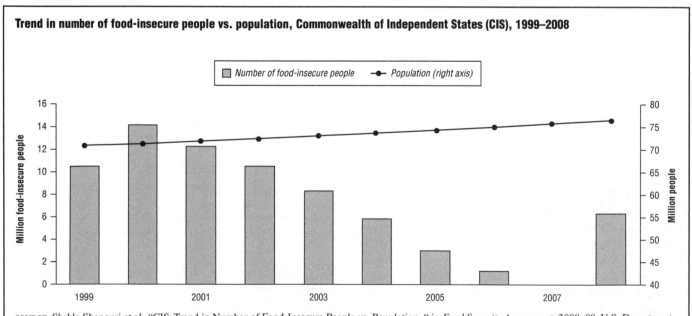

Trend in number of food-insecure people vs. population, Commonwealth of Independent States (CIS), 1999–2008

SOURCE: Shahla Shapouri et al., "CIS: Trend in Number of Food-Insecure People vs. Population," in *Food Security Assessment, 2008–09*, U.S. Department of Agriculture (USDA), Economic Research Service (ERS), June 2009, http://www.ers.usda.gov/Publications/GFA20/GFA20.pdf (accessed November 25, 2009)

FIGURE 5.7

Percent living in dwellings not connected to the public water supply, selected countries, Central and Eastern Europe and the Commonwealth of Independent States, 2005–06

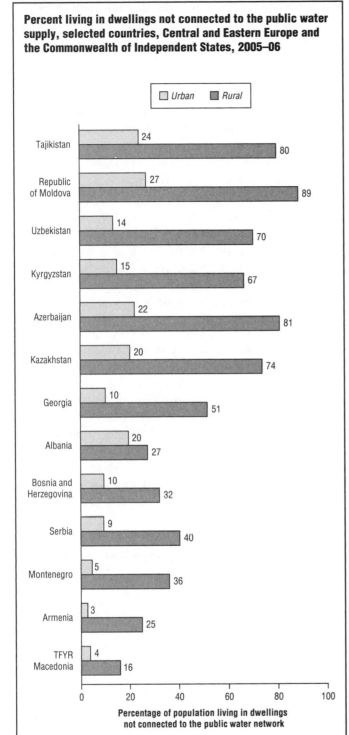

Note: The household connection only takes into account piped water that is distributed in the house or just outside (yard) and that can be considered as used privately. Countries are ordered by decreasing levels of the national average of household water connections.
TFYR = The Former Yugoslav Republic.

SOURCE: "Figure 1.13. Urban/Rural Population Living in Dwellings Not Connected to the Public Water Network, 2005–2006," in *Innocenti Social Monitor 2009*, United Nations Children's Fund (UNICEF) Innocenti Research Centre, Florence, August 2009, http://www.unicef-irc.org/publications/pdf/ism_2009.pdf (accessed December 7, 2009)

population did not have access to safe water piped into the home. In Kazakhstan, for example, three-quarters (74%) of the rural population did not have water piped into the home.

Kazakhstan

The UNDP reports in *The Great Generation of Kazakhstan: Insight into the Future* (2005, http://hdr.undp.org/en/reports/nationalreports/europethecis/kazakhstan/kazakhstan_2005_en.pdf) that Kazakhstan saw a dramatic decline in its human development indicators immediately after independence from the Soviet Union in 1991, dropping in rank from 54th to 93rd on the United Nations' (UN) Human Development Index (HDI) of 177 countries. However, from 1995 to 2003 it rose to the 80th place. The UNDP notes that the other CIS countries experienced a similar pattern of decline and then recovery.

The HDI measures poverty using a combination of life expectancy, literacy, and amount of education, along with the domestic purchasing power of the GDP (how much citizens of a country are able to buy based on the country's GDP). The HDI was devised by the UNDP, and its purpose is to measure how well a country is progressing toward development. A low HDI ranges from 0.3 to 0.499, a medium HDI from 0.5 to 0.799, and a high HDI from 0.8 to 1. The UNDP reports that in 1990 Kazakhstan's HDI value was 0.776 and fell to 0.726 in 1995. In 2004 its HDI had risen to 0.782. In the fact sheet "Human Development Report 2009: Kazakhstan" (2009, http://hdrstats.undp.org/en/countries/country_fact_sheets/cty_fs_KAZ.html), the UNDP indicates that by 2007 Kazakhstan had become a high human development country with an HDI value of 0.804.

The UNDP explains in *Great Generation of Kazakhstan* that the total poverty rate in Kazakhstan was 12.2% in 2004, down from 34.5% in 1999. This indicates that Kazakhstan exceeded the first MDG target of reducing by half the proportion of people with an income below the national subsistence minimum. Table 1.2 in Chapter 1 shows that from 2000 to 2006, 15.4% of the population lived below the Kazakhstan national poverty line. Nevertheless, in Kazakhstan, as in many countries, poverty is more prevalent in rural than in urban areas. According to the UNDP, in 2001 the poverty rate in rural regions was 38.5% and in urban areas it was 20%. However, in 2003 poverty had declined to 30.9% in rural regions and to 10.8% in urban areas. In *Millennium Development Goals in Kazakhstan, 2007* (2007, http://www.un.kz/assets/docs/MDGs_2007.pdf), the UN notes that by 2006 the rural poverty rate had dropped further to 24.4% and the urban poverty rate rose to 13.6%.

A large gap also exists between urban and rural households in the availability of in-house utilities. The UN reports in *Millennium Development Goals in*

Kazakhstan, 2005 (2005, http://www.un.kz/assets/docs/ MDGs_2005.pdf) that even though 81% of urban households had piped water in 2004, only 8.3% of rural households did, with just 0.8% of rural houses having a hot water supply versus 56.1% of urban houses. By 2007, 95.2% of urban residents and 57.2% of rural residents had access to piped water, according to the UN, in *Millennium Development Goals in Kazakhstan, 2007*.

Even though nearly 100% of both rural and urban households had electricity in 2004, according to the UN, in *Millennium Development Goals, 2005*, just 1.9% of rural homes had central heating, compared with 68.6% of urban homes. Concerning sanitation, only 4.3% of rural households in 2004 were using improved sanitation, such as toilets or pit latrines, whereas 73.7% of urban households had such access. However, the World Bank notes in *World Bank Group Data Profile: Kazakhstan* (September 2009, http://ddp-ext.worldbank.org/ext/ddpreports/View SharedReport?&CF=&REPORT_ID=9147&REQUEST _TYPE=VIEWADVANCED) that in 2000, 97% of the urban population in Kazakhstan had access to improved sanitation facilities. It was unclear whether the urban sanitation situation had worsened by 2004 or whether the data differed because of data collection differences among the reporting organizations.

EDUCATION AND LITERACY. According to the UNDP, in *National Human Development Report 2008: Climate Change and Its Impact on Kazakhstan's Human Development* (February 2009, http://hdr.undp.org/en/reports/national reports/europethecis/kazakhstan/Kazakhstan_nhdr_2008

.pdf), not only do many of the poor people of Kazakhstan live in rural areas but also these rural residents often live in isolated groups without proper medical, cultural, transportation, or educational services. Concerning education, the country has a high inequality ratio, especially in secondary education, because of the great differences between rural and urban areas. In *Millennium Development Goals in Kazakhstan, 2005*, the UN notes that 47% of school-aged children lived in rural areas in 2004. Hundreds of Kazakhstan's rural communities have no schools, and even in the areas where schools are present, children may have to travel long distances to attend them. As a result, rural children find it increasingly difficult to attain the skills they need to succeed. Furthermore, because Kazakh and Russian are the dominant languages used in school, the smallest of Kazakhstan's 100 or more ethnic groups have problems in school. The quality of teacher training is also an issue in Kazakhstan, with 18% of urban teachers and 42% of rural teachers rated as unqualified.

Table 5.4 shows that rate of completion of primary school is high in Kazakhstan. The primary completion rate is the percentage of students completing the last year of primary school out of the total number of children of official graduation age. The number can be higher than 100% because some students may be older than the official graduation age. The rate rose from 94% in 2000 to over 100% between 2005 and 2008. Girls and boys complete primary school in nearly equal numbers, as shown by ratios between 2000 and 2008 that are very close to 100%.

TABLE 5.4

Selected world development indicators, Kazakhstan, 2000, 2005, 2007, 2008

	2000	2005	2007	2008
World view				
Population, total (millions)	14.88	15.15	15.48	15.67
Population growth (annual %)	−0.3	0.9	1.1	1.2
Surface area (sq. km) (thousands)	2,724.9	2,724.9	2,724.9	2,724.9
GNI per capita, PPP (current international $)	4,460	7,830	9,510	9,690
People				
Life expectancy at birth, total (years)	66	66	66	—
Fertility rate, total (births per woman)	1.8	2.2	2.4	—
Adolescent fertility rate (births per 1,000 women ages 15–19)	33	30	31	—
Contraceptive prevalence (% of women ages 15–49)	—	—	—	—
Births attended by skilled health staff (% of total)	—	99	—	—
Mortality rate, under-5 (per 1,000)	44	35	32	—
Malnutrition prevalence, weight for age (% of children under 5)	—	—	—	—
Primary completion rate, total (% of relevant age group)	94	107	101	104
Ratio of girls to boys in primary and secondary education (%)	102	99	99	99
Prevalence of HIV, total (% of population ages 15–49)	0.1	0.1	0.1	—
Economy				
GDP (current US$) (billions)	18.29	57.12	104.85	132.23
GDP growth (annual %)	9.8	9.7	8.9	3.2

GNI = Gross National Income. PPP = Purchasing Power Parity. GDP = Gross Domestic Product. US$ = United States dollars.

SOURCE: Adapted from "Kazakhstan," in *The World Bank Group Data Profile*, The World Bank, April 2009, http://ddpext.worldbank.org/ext/ddpreports/ ViewSharedReport?&CF=&REPORT_ID=9147&REQUEST_ TYPE=VIEWADVANCED (accessed December 10, 2009). Copyright © International Bank for Reconstruction and Development/The World Bank 2009.

As expected with such a high primary completion rate, adult illiteracy is nearly nonexistent at 0.4% from 1999 to 2007. (See Table 1.2 in Chapter 1.)

HEALTH AND MORTALITY. According to the WHO, in "Kazakhstan" (2010, http://www.who.int/countries/kaz/en/), life expectancy for Kazakhstani males was 59 years and 70 years for females in 2006. Healthy life expectancy (includes an adjustment for time spent in poor health) at birth in 2003 was 53 years for males and 59 years for females. Table 5.4 shows the overall life expectancy in 2000, 2005, and 2007 to be 66 years.

As noted previously in this chapter, Kazakhstan has a high U5MR compared with other countries having a high level of human development. However, the U5MR in Kazakhstan has declined in recent years. Table 5.4 shows that in 2000 the U5MR was 44 deaths per 1,000 children under the age of five. This rate declined to 35 deaths per 1,000 children under the age of five in 2005 and to 32 deaths per 1,000 children in 2007. Maternal mortality (death as a result of pregnancy or childbirth) is high in Kazakhstan as well. In *Millennium Development Goals in Kazakhstan, 2005*, the UN reports that this rate decreased from 75.8 deaths per 100,000 live births in 1990 to 36.9 deaths per 100,000 in 2004. By 2006, as reported by the UN, in *Millennium Development Goals in Kazakhstan, 2007*, maternal mortality rose to 45.6 deaths per 100,000 live births. This rate is considered unreasonably high, particularly in light of the fact that 99% of births in Kazakhstan were attended by skilled health professionals in 2005. (See Table 5.4.) The MDG maternal mortality rate for Kazakhstan is 19 deaths per 100,000 live births.

Kyrgyzstan/Kyrgyz Republic

Kyrgyzstan, officially known as the Kyrgyz Republic, is a small, mountainous, landlocked country that had 5.3 million people in 2008. (See Table 5.5.) Historically, it was occupied by nomadic peoples, but when it was incorporated into the Soviet Union in 1924, Kyrgyzstan was converted into an agricultural-manufacturing economy. By the time the central Asian republics were granted independence in 1991, Kyrgyzstan's manufacturing sector relied almost entirely on the Soviet military-industrial complex. When this complex collapsed, Kyrgyzstan's manufacturing sector also crumbled, leaving its economy in ruins.

POVERTY AND HEALTH INDICATORS. The Kyrgyzstani government reports in *Kyrgyz Republic: Poverty Reduction Strategy Paper—Country Development Strategy (2007–2010)* (June 2007, http://planipolis.iiep.unesco.org/upload/Kyrgyzstan/PRSP/Kyrgyzstan%20PRSP%202007-2010.pdf) that in 2003 the rural poverty rate was 57.4% and the urban poverty rate was 35.7%. By 2004 this rate had declined slightly to 55.5% for rural dwellers and to 28.3% for urban dwellers. The World Bank indicates in *World Bank Group Data Profile: Kyrgyz Republic* (September 2009, http://ddp-ext.worldbank.org/ext/ddpreports/ViewSharedReport?&CF=&REPORT_ID=9147&REQUEST_TYPE=VIEWADVANCED) that 43.1% of the overall population was living at or below the national poverty line in Kyrgyzstan in 2005.

TABLE 5.5

Selected world development indicators, Kyrgyz Republic, 2000, 2005, 2007, 2008

	2000	2005	2007	2008
World view				
Population, total (millions)	4.92	5.14	5.23	5.28
Population growth (annual %)	1.0	1.0	0.8	0.8
Surface area (sq. km) (thousands)	199.9	199.9	199.9	199.9
GNI per capita, PPP (current international $)	1,250	1,670	1,980	2,140
People				
Life expectancy at birth, total (years)	69	68	68	—
Fertility rate, total (births per woman)	2.4	2.5	2.7	—
Adolescent fertility rate (births per 1,000 women ages 15–19)	34	32	32	—
Contraceptive prevalence (% of women ages 15–49)	—	—	—	—
Births attended by skilled health staff (% of total)	99	98	—	—
Mortality rate, under-5 (per 1,000)	50	42	38	—
Malnutrition prevalence, weight for age (% of children under 5)	—	—	—	—
Primary completion rate, total (% of relevant age group)	95	97	95	—
Ratio of girls to boys in primary and secondary education (%)	101	100	100	—
Prevalence of HIV, total (% of population ages 15–49)	—	0.1	0.1	—
Economy				
GDP (current US$) (billions)	1.37	2.46	3.74	4.42
GDP growth (annual %)	5.4	−0.2	8.2	7.7

GNI = Gross National Income. PPP = Purchasing Power Parity. GDP = Gross Domestic Product. US$ = United States dollars.

SOURCE: Adapted from "Kyrgyz Republic," in *The World Bank Group Data Profile*, The World Bank, April 2009, http://ddpext.worldbank.org/ext/ddpreports/ViewSharedReport?&CF=&REPORT_ID=9147&REQUEST_TYPE= VIEWADVANCED (accessed December 10, 2009). Copyright © International Bank for Reconstruction and Development/The World Bank 2009.

Even though the poverty rate is high in Kyrgyzstan, only 0.7% of the population over the age of 15 was illiterate from 1999 to 2007. (See Table 1.2 in Chapter 1.) All the former Soviet republics have generally high rates of primary-school enrollment and literacy because of the former Soviet Union's compulsory education system. As expected, the rates of enrollment in and completion of primary school in Kyrgyzstan are somewhat high but still need improvement. UNICEF reports in "Kyrgyzstan" (2009, http://www.unicef.org/infobycountry/kyrgyzstan _statistics.html) that the net primary enrollment rate from 2003 to 2008 was 92%. Table 5.5 shows that 95% to 97% of students who were enrolled in primary schooling completed their course of study between 2000 and 2007. According to the UNDP, in the fact sheet "Human Development Report 2009: Kyrgyzstan" (2009, http://hdrstats .undp.org/en/countries/country_fact_sheets/cty_fs_KGZ.html), the combined gross enrollment rate was 77.3% in 2007. The combined gross enrollment rate is the number of students enrolled in primary, secondary, and postsecondary school out of the number of potential students.

In "Kyrgyzstan" (2010, http://www.who.int/countries/ kgz/en/), the WHO states that the life expectancy in Kyrgyzstan was 63 years for males and 70 years for females in 2006. The healthy life expectancy at birth was 52 years for males and 58 years for females in 2003. Kyrgyzstan has a high U5MR, but it has made much progress in reducing it, from 50 deaths per 1,000 children under the age of five in 2000, to 42 deaths per 1,000 children in 2005, to 38 deaths per 1,000 children in 2007. (See Table 5.5.)

Maternal mortality is extremely high in Kyrgyzstan. UNICEF reports that the maternal mortality rate was 100 deaths per 100,000 births in 2008. As in Kazakhstan, this rate is considered unreasonably high, given that 98% of births were attended by skilled health professionals in 2005. (See Table 5.5.)

Tajikistan

After gaining independence in 1991, Tajikistan fell into a civil war that lasted from 1992 to 1994. The conflict seriously deteriorated conditions throughout the country. The U.S. Department of State's Bureau of South and Central Asian Affairs reports in "Background Note: Tajikistan" (October 2009, http://www.state.gov/r/pa/ei/ bgn/5775.htm) that Tajikistan is the poorest of the former Soviet republics—indeed, one of the poorest countries in the world. However, the World Bank notes in *Republic of Tajikistan Poverty Assessment Update* (January 6, 2005, http://www.untj.org/files/reports/Tajikistan%20Poverty% 20Assessment%20Update.pdf) that poverty reduction is occurring in the country. In 2003, 64% of Tajikistanis were living on less than $2.15 per day, down substantially from 81% in 1999. The rate of extreme poverty

(less than $1.08 per day) in 2003 was 19.9%, down from 32.7% in 1999. However, Table 1.2 in Chapter 1 shows that the extreme poverty rate was slightly higher at 21.5% of the population living on less than $1.25 per day from 2000 to 2007 and that the rate of those living on less than $2 per day was 50.8%. The table also shows that 44.4% lived below the Tajikistan national poverty line.

In 2000 the average gross national income (GNI; the total value produced within a country plus income from other countries minus payments made to other countries) per capita in Tajikistan as $800. (See Table 5.6.) The GNI per capita rose to $1,430 in 2005, to $1,700 in 2007, and to $1,860 in 2008. This is slightly lower than the GNI per capita for Kyrgyzstan, which was $2,140 in 2008, and much lower than the GNI per capita for Kazakhstan, which was $9,690 in 2008. (See Table 5.5 and Table 5.4.) In *Investing in Sustainable Development: Millennium Development Goals Needs Assessment* (May 2005, http:// www.undp.tj/files/reports/mdg_eng.pdf), the UN Millennium Development Goals Needs Assessment Team reports that steady economic growth and increased income and consumption have not improved the living standards for most Tajikistanis, even though the rate of poverty was falling. However, this steady growth rate slowed in the face of the world economic crisis, from 7.8% GDP growth rate in 2007, as reported by the World Bank (February 2010, http://www.worldbank.org/tj), to 2% in 2009, as reported by the Bureau of South and Central Asian Affairs.

NUTRITION. Food insecurity and malnutrition are key poverty-related problems for Tajikistanis. The UN Millennium Development Goals Needs Assessment Team notes in *Millennium Development Goals Needs Assessment* that in 2003, 83% of the population suffered from nutrition-related poverty. Families reported cutting down on food consumption and often relying on food given to them as gifts. Unbalanced diets, such as an overdependence on bread, cause a number of nutritional deficiencies in Tajikistan. Children are the demographic group most affected by nutritional deficiencies. In 2003, 36% of children under the age of five were chronically malnourished and 5% had acute malnutrition. Poor maternal nutrition resulted in 15% of Tajikistani babies being born malnourished. Table 5.6 shows that in 2005, 15% of children under the age of five were malnourished, and Table 1.2 in Chapter 1 shows that from 2000 to 2006, 17% of children younger than five years were underweight for their age.

EDUCATION AND LITERACY. According to the Bureau of South and Central Asian Affairs, in "Background Note: Tajikistan," Tajikistan's educational system was slow to recover from the civil war that ended in 1994. Nonetheless, in "World Bank Group Data Profile: Tajikistan" (2007, http://devdata.worldbank.org/edstats/SummaryEducation Profiles/CountryData/GetShowData.asp?sCtry=TJK,

TABLE 5.6

Selected world development indicators, Tajikistan, 2000, 2005, 2007, 2008

	2000	2005	2007	2008
World view				
Population, total (millions)	6.17	6.54	6.73	6.84
GNI per capita, PPP (current international $)	800	1,430	1,700	1,860
People				
Life expectancy at birth, total (years)	64	66	67	67
Fertility rate, total (births per woman)	4.0	3.6	3.5	—
Adolescent fertility rate (births per 1,000 women ages 15–19)	33	30	28	—
Contraceptive prevalence (% of women ages 15–49)	34	38	38	—
Births attended by skilled health staff (% of total)	71	83	—	—
Mortality rate, under-5 (per 1,000)	94	74	67	—
Malnutrition prevalence, weight for age (% of children under 5)	—	15	—	—
Primary completion rate, total (% of relevant age group)	95	102	95	—
Ratio of girls to boys in primary and secondary education (%)	89	88	89	—
Prevalence of HIV, total (% of population ages 15–49)	0.1	0.2	0.3	0.3
Economy				
GDP (current US$) (billions)	0.86	2.31	3.71	5.13
GDP growth (annual %)	8.3	6.7	7.8	7.9

GNI = Gross National Income. PPP = Purchasing Power Parity. GDP = Gross Domestic Product. US$ = United States dollars.

SOURCE: Adapted from "Tajikistan," in *The World Bank Group Data Profile*, The World Bank, April 2009, http://ddp-ext.worldbank.org/ext/ddpreports/ViewSharedReport?&CF=&REPORT_ID=9147&REQUEST_TYPE=VIEWADVANCED (accessed December 10, 2009). Copyright © International Bank for Reconstruction and Development/The World Bank 2009.

Tajikistan), the World Bank reports that net enrollment ratios grew from 76.7% in 1990 to 97.4% in 2005. The World Bank (February 2010, http://web.worldbank.org/) also notes that the primary gross enrollment ratio in Tajikistan was 100% in 2008. The adult (15 years and older) illiteracy rate from 1999 to 2007 was 0.4%. (See Table 1.2 in Chapter 1.)

HEALTH AND MORTALITY. According to the WHO, in "Tajikistan" (2010, http://www.who.int/countries/tjk/en/), life expectancy in Tajikistan was 63 years for males and 66 years for females in 2006. Healthy life expectancy at birth was 53 years for males and 56 years for females in 2003. Much like Kyrgyzstan, Tajikistan has a high U5MR. However, it has made considerable progress in reducing it, from 94 deaths per 1,000 children under the age of five in 2000, to 74 deaths per 1,000 children in 2005, to 67 deaths per 1,000 children in 2007. (See Table 5.6.)

Turkmenistan

Turkmenistan, a nation of over 5 million people in 2008, is considered to be the most closed society in the former Soviet bloc. (See Table 5.7.) For example, in 2004 the last international radio outlet to broadcast in the country—Russia's Mayak radio station—was cut off by Turkmenistan's authoritarian government, leaving the Turkmens with no access to outside information. At that time, Turkmenistan and North Korea were the only countries in the world to retain their Stalinist regimes, meaning that they were ruled by dictators who controlled every aspect of their society. The Turkmen president Saparmurad Niyazov (1940–2006) ruled from 1991, when Turkmenistan gained its independence, until his sudden death in 2006. In 1999 he declared himself "president for life" and adopted the title "Turkmenbashi," which meant "father of all Turkmen."

After Niyazov's death, elections were held that international observers suggested were neither free nor fair. The former president's dentist, Gurbanguly Berdymukhammedov (1957–), was elected, and he officially took office in February 2007. Andrew Osborn indicates in "Oil-Rich Turkmenistan Begins 'New Era' as President Is Sworn In" (*Independent* [London], February 15, 2007) that even though he pledged reform, Berdymukhammedov also highly regarded his predecessor and his ways of thinking.

In "UK Secures Energy Deal with Regime in Turkmenistan" (*Times* [London], November 6, 2007), Robin Pagnamenta notes that by late 2007 Berdymukhammedov vowed to open Turkmenistan to foreign investment and entered into a business arrangement with Great Britain to allow British companies access to Turkmenistan's natural gas reserves. Nonetheless, the Berdymukhammedov government was already being criticized for corruption and a poor record on human rights. The article "Eye on Image, Turkmenistan Overhauls Laws" (Reuters, September 26, 2008) reports that in 2008 Turkmenistan adopted a new constitution that would establish democratic reforms and strengthen its reliability as an economic partner with outside investors. Despite this progress, the article "Turkmen President's Visit to France a Key Opportunity to Urge Improvements" (Reporters without Borders, January 28, 2010) indicates that in early 2010 Turkmenistan was still considered "one of the most repressive countries

TABLE 5.7

Selected world development indicators, Turkmenistan, 2000, 2005, 2007, 2008

	2000	2005	2007	2008
World view				
Population, total (millions)	4.50	4.83	4.96	5.03
Population growth (annual %)	1.3	1.4	1.3	1.3
Surface area (sq. km) (thousands)	488.1	488.1	488.1	488.1
GNI per capita, PPP (current international $)	1,930	4,350	5,650	6,210
People				
Life expectancy at birth, total (years)	63	63	63	—
Fertility rate, total (births per woman)	2.9	2.6	2.5	—
Adolescent fertility rate (births per 1,000 women ages 15–19)	21	21	20	—
Contraceptive prevalence (% of women ages 15–49)	62	—	—	—
Births attended by skilled health staff (% of total)	97	—	—	—
Mortality rate, under-5 (per 1,000)	71	55	50	—
Malnutrition prevalence, weight for age (% of children under 5)	—	—	—	—
Primary completion rate, total (% of relevant age group)	—	—	—	—
Ratio of girls to boys in primary and secondary education (%)	—	—	—	—
Prevalence of HIV, total (% of population ages 15–49)	—	—	0.1	—
Economy				
GDP (current US$) (billions)	2.90	8.10	12.93	18.27
GDP growth (annual %)	18.6	13.0	11.6	9.8

GNI = Gross National Income. PPP = Purchasing Power Parity. GDP = Gross Domestic Product. US$ = United States dollars.

SOURCE: Adapted from "Turkmenistan," in *The World Bank Group Data Profile*, The World Bank, April 2009, http://ddpext.worldbank.org/ext/ddpreports/ViewSharedReport?&CF=&REPORT_ID=9147&REQUEST_TYPE=VIEWADVANCED (accessed December 10, 2009). Copyright © International Bank for Reconstruction and Development/The World Bank 2009.

in the world," in spite of Berdymukhammedov's suggestions of democratic reforms and the country's rich reserves of natural gas, which made it a much sought-after trading partner. Trading partners were expected to put pressure on Berdymukhammedov to make additional progress in human rights in the country

Poverty data for Turkmenistan are difficult to obtain, because the country does not have an established poverty line and because the calculations that the government keeps are not widely available. Despite the country's potential for national wealth, poverty data in Table 1.2 in Chapter 1 show that from 2000 to 2007, 24.8% of the country's people lived on less than $1.25 per day and 49.6% lived on less than $2 per day. In 2009 Turkmenistan was ranked 109 out of 182 countries in the HDI, which is in the medium human development range.

EDUCATION AND LITERACY. From 1999 to 2007 the Turkmen adult (15 years and older) illiteracy rate was low, at 0.5%. (See Table 1.2 in Chapter 1.) UNICEF finds in "Turkmenistan" (2009, http://www.unicef.org/infobycountry/Turkmenistan.html) that the net primary enrollment rate from 2003 to 2008 was 99%. The country's school year is short (150 days) so that teenagers can help in agriculture. Teenagers are also required to work for two years before they can enroll in a post-secondary institution, a requirement that is difficult to achieve because jobs are hard to find in the country. This situation has contributed, in part, to a dramatic decline in university enrollment, from 40,000 in the 1990s to 3,000 in 2004.

HEALTH AND MORTALITY. From 2000 to 2006, 11% of children under five years old were underweight for their age. (See Table 1.2 in Chapter 1.) Progress has been made concerning the U5MR, although the rate in this region is second only to Tajikistan. In 2000 the rate was 71 deaths per 1,000 children under the age of five, and by 2007 the rate had fallen to 50 deaths per 1,000 children. (See Table 5.7.) Infant mortality rates, although still extremely high, have dropped as well. According to UNICEF, in "Turkmenistan," infant mortality rates decreased from 81 deaths per 1,000 live births in 1990 to 43 deaths per 1,000 live births in 2008. Table 5.7 shows that in 2000, 97% of births were attended by skilled health professionals.

The WHO indicates in "Turkmenistan" (2010, http://www.who.int/countries/tkm/en/) that life expectancy for males was 60 years and for females 67 years in 2006. Healthy life expectancy was 52 years for males and 57 years for females in 2003.

Uzbekistan

Uzbekistan is the most populous of the central Asian republics, with 27.3 million people in 2008 (see Table 5.8), compared with 15.7 million in Kazakhstan (see Table 5.4), 6.8 million in Tajikistan (see Table 5.6), 5.3 million in Kyrgyzstan (see Table 5.5), and 5 million in Turkmenistan (see Table 5.7). In *World Factbook: Uzbekistan* (January 19, 2010, https://www.cia.gov/library/publications/the-world-factbook/geos/uz.html), the CIA states that only 37% of the Uzbekistani population lived in urban areas

TABLE 5.8

Selected world development indicators, Uzbekistan, 2000, 2005, 2007, 2008

	2000	2005	2007	2008
World view				
Population, total (millions)	24.65	26.17	26.87	27.31
Population growth (annual %)	1.0	1.2	1.4	1.6
Surface area (sq. km) (thousands)	447.4	447.4	447.4	447.4
GNI per capita, PPP (current international $)	1,420	2,000	2,430	2,660
People				
Life expectancy at birth, total (years)	66	—	67	—
Fertility rate, total (births per woman)	2.6	2.4	2.4	—
Adolescent fertility rate (births per 1,000 women ages 15–19)	25	13	13	—
Contraceptive prevalence (% of women ages 15–49)	67	—	—	—
Births attended by skilled health staff (% of total)	96	—	—	—
Mortality rate, under-5 (per 1,000)	62	46	41	—
Malnutrition prevalence, weight for age (% of children under 5)	—	—	—	—
Primary completion rate, total (% of relevant age group)	95	99	97	—
Ratio of girls to boys in primary and secondary education (%)	98	97	98	—
Prevalence of HIV, total (% of population ages 15–49)	—	0.1	0.1	—
Economy				
GDP (current US$) (billions)	13.76	14.31	22.31	27.92
GDP growth (annual %)	3.8	7.0	9.5	9.0

GNI = Gross National Income. PPP = Purchasing Power Parity. GDP = Gross Domestic Product. US$ = United States dollars.

SOURCE: Adapted from "Uzbekistan," in *The World Bank Group Data Profile*, The World Bank, April 2009, http://ddp-ext.worldbank.org/ext/ddpreports/ViewSharedReport?&CF=&REPORT_ID=9147&REQUEST_TYPE=VIEWADVANCED (accessed December 10, 2009). Copyright © International Bank for Reconstruction and Development/The World Bank 2009.

in 2008. Even though the country is the world's fifth-largest producer and the second-largest exporter of cotton and has large reserves of natural gas and oil, 76.7% of its people lived on less than $2 per day from 2000 to 2007, and 46.3% lived on less than $1.25 per day, higher than the other central Asian republics. (See Table 1.2 in Chapter 1.) Slightly more than a quarter (27.5%) lived below the national poverty line during those years. Meanwhile, the country's GDP grew 9.5% in 2007 and 9% in 2008, surpassing the growth rate of the other central Asian republics with the exception of Turkmenistan, while the rest of the world was struggling with a serious economic recession. (See Table 5.8 and Table 5.7.) Uzbekistan has an authoritarian presidential rule, and the government does not always act in a manner that is economically positive for the country and its people.

In 2009 Uzbekistan ranked 119 out of 182 countries on the HDI, just ahead of Kyrgyzstan at 120 and Tajikistan at 127, but behind Kazakhstan at 82 and Turkmenistan at 109. (See Table 1.2 in Chapter 1.) Uzbekistan was listed as a country having a medium level of human development.

EDUCATION AND LITERACY. From 1999 to 2007 the Uzbekistani adult (aged 15 years and older) illiteracy rate was 3.1%. (See Table 1.2 in Chapter 1.) In "Uzbekistan" (2009, http://www.unicef.org/infobycountry/uzbekistan _statistics.html), UNICEF notes that from 2003 to 2008 the gross enrollment ratio for primary schools was 97% for males and 94% for females. The primary completion rate was 99% in 2005 and 97% in 2007. (See Table 5.8.)

HEALTH AND MORTALITY. From 2000 to 2006, 5% of the children under the age of five in Uzbekistan were underweight for their age. (See Table 1.2 in Chapter 1.) According to the WHO, in "Uzbekistan" (2010, http://www.who.int/countries/uzb/en/), the Uzbekistani life expectancy was 65 years for males and 70 years for females in 2006. Healthy life expectancy in Uzbekistan was 58 years for males and 61 years for females in 2003. The U5MR decreased from 62 deaths per 1,000 children under the age of five in 2000 to 41 deaths per 1,000 children in 2007. (See Table 5.8.)

NORTH KOREA

The peninsula on which both North and South Korea are located was under Japanese rule until the end of World War II (1939–1945). At that point the United States began occupying the southern half, and the Soviet Union took over the northern half. The two countries' inability to agree on unification led to the formation of two separate Korean governments in the north and south. The Korean War broke out between them in 1950 and ended in 1953, but because both sides never signed a peace treaty, the countries are technically still at war. A permanent demilitarized zone separates the two countries, providing a 2.5-mile-wide (4-km) strip of land that serves as a buffer zone. Both sides are heavily patrolled.

From 1948 until his death, Kim Il-Sung (1912–1994) ruled North Korea, which is officially known as the Democratic People's Republic of Korea. Following his death, leadership went to his son Kim Jong-Il (1942–). Between their two periods of leadership, the father and son created a cult of personality and amassed military strength that enriched them and the country's upper class and left North Korea's ordinary citizens in severe poverty. North Korea is known for having one of the worst records in the world for the treatment of its own citizens.

North Korea is a closed society, and even photographs from inside the country are rare. Because everything is so tightly controlled by the government, valid statistics are generally nonexistent. Some worldwide nongovernmental organizations do manage to obtain data about North Korea, and the government of South Korea keeps statistics as well. According to the South Korean Ministry of Unification (February 2010, http://www.unikorea.go.kr/eng/default.jsp?pgname=NORtables), the GNI per capita in North Korea was $1,152 in 2007. By comparison, the World Bank (July 1, 2008, http://www.congre.co.jp/neurosci2009/english/registration/images/gni_per_capita.pdf) reports that in 2007 the GNI per capita for China was $2,360 and for the United States, $45,850. Because poverty numbers and other human development information provided by the North Korean government are known to be inaccurate, the UNDP does not rank North Korea in its HDI.

Food and Nutrition

North Korea operates a rations system, under which all citizens receive food, clothing, medical care, housing, education, and pensions directly from the government. The thinking behind this system is that it will instill gratitude in the people; however, because of the small amount of goods they receive, they will be kept from becoming lazy and frivolous. Food became less available in 1991, following the collapse of the Soviet Union, which had been giving food subsidies to the republic. Shortly thereafter, China decided to withdraw its own food subsidies that it was giving North Korea. With the loss of these food subsidies, North Koreans received less than one-third the amount of food they needed to survive. Then, between 1995 and 1997, the availability of food decreased even further when the country was wracked first by drought and then by devastating floods. People had to acquire their own food by rearing livestock, growing gardens, or collecting edible wild foods or by buying it from black market sources. Those who lacked the resources to buy food or manage on their own faced starvation. Between 1994 and 1998 millions starved to death in one of the largest famines in modern history.

In 2004 the government loosened its control of food supplies by allowing some markets to operate privately and expand their selection of goods. Some farms were also privatized. However, in October 2005 authorities reversed these policies and again prevented the sale of grain in markets. According to the article "Food Aid to North Korea Being Held up in China over Rail Dispute" (Associated Press, October 19, 2007), with an excellent harvest in the fall of 2005, the North Korean government decided that aid organizations were creating an atmosphere of dependence. It requested that the UN World Food Programme (WFP), which supplied food for about 6.5 million North Koreans annually, shift emphasis from food aid to development assistance (social and economic aid). Thus, the WFP reduced its food aid to 1.9 million in 2006. In addition, with tensions escalating over North Korea's pursuit of nuclear weapons, the United States announced in May 2005 that it would suspend all food aid to the country.

According to the article "North Korea Welcomes US Food Aid Offer" (*Seattle Times*, May 17, 2008), widespread flooding destroyed more than 11% of North Korea's crops in 2007. As a result, the United States announced in May 2008 that it would send 500,000 tons (454,000 t) of food to the starving nation. However, by March 2009 tensions between the United States and North Korea had risen due to North Korea's planned launch of a long-range missile in early April 2009 and stalled nuclear disarmament talks between the countries. Despite widespread hunger in North Korea, the government rejected an offer of further food aid from the United States, ordering personnel from U.S. nongovernmental organizations to leave the country. After months of hostility, not only with the United States but also with Japan and South Korea, North Korea accepted an offer of corn from South Korea in January 2010. According to article "North Korea Accepts South Korean Food Aid" (*Asia Pacific News*, January 15, 2010), the WFP estimates that approximately one-third of North Korea's women and children were malnourished in the fall of 2009.

Whether international food aid reaches the intended recipients in North Korea is an unanswered question for the United States and other countries, as well as for aid organizations such as the WFP. The North Korean government will not allow agencies to monitor or report on the progress of their programs within the country. According to the U.S. Committee for Human Rights in North Korea (HRNK), in *The North Korean Refugee Crisis: Human Rights and International Response* (December 2006, http://www.hrnk.org/refugeesReport06.pdf), a survey of North Korean refugees suggests that most food aid does not reach the general North Korean population. Survey results show that only 57% of respondents (North Korean refugees) knew that food aid to North Korea existed. Of those respondents who knew about food aid, only 3% said that they personally received food aid. The HRNK notes that the food aid could have been distributed by the North Korean government without individuals knowing it was aid, but only 21% of the respondents said they received any food from government distribution. Most of the respondents (62%) had to buy food or get food in other ways (16%). Eighteen percent of those who received any food from government distribution had to supplement the food rations themselves because they were insufficient. Various sources suggest that food aid may be sold to vendors for sale in markets and may be diverted to the military or governmental officials.

CHAPTER 6
THE POOR IN DEVELOPED COUNTRIES

Poverty researchers refer to two types of poverty: absolute poverty and relative poverty. Absolute poverty means that a person's income is not sufficient to afford basic goods and services. Relative poverty compares a person's income to the median (average) household income in that country.

Absolute poverty is in decline in the developed world as measured in the 30 member countries of the Organization for Economic Cooperation and Development (OECD). According to Michael Förster and Marco Mira d'Ercole of the OECD, in "Poverty in OECD Countries: An Assessment Based on Static Income" in *Growing Unequal? Income Distribution and Poverty in OECD Countries* (2008, http://browse.oecdbookshop.org/oecd/pdfs/browseit/8108051E.PDF), most measures show that absolute poverty declined approximately 40% in several OECD countries between the mid-1990s and the first few years in the first decade of the 21st century and that it declined 60% or more in a few OECD countries that experienced exceptional economic growth. Relative poverty has not declined in the developed world, however. One benchmark of relative poverty is an income at less than half the median income of that country. Förster and d'Ercole indicate that by about 2005, 11% of people living in most OECD countries were in poverty by this measure.

POVERTY IN WEALTHY COUNTRIES: PSYCHOSOCIAL EFFECTS

Even though the poor in wealthy countries have access to various forms of social assistance and do not experience famine, they may have trouble providing housing and food for themselves and their families. (Homelessness is a multifaceted phenomenon that can have causes other than poverty.) In addition, many poor people in the developed world work full time and earn more money per week than those in the developing world earn per year. Regardless, they are poor relative to others living in their country.

Some researchers and aid workers suggest that the poor in wealthy countries suffer more psychological problems and social isolation than those in low-income countries. In "Psychological Costs of Growing up Poor" (*Annals of the New York Academy of Sciences*, vol. 1136, no. 1, June 2008), Eric Dearing of Boston College summarizes the extensive literature available on the psychological development of youth growing up poor. He notes that "children and adolescents living in poverty often display dysfunction and delay in their cognitive, language, and social-emotional growth. In turn, these developmental problems in early life contribute to reduced earnings, involvement in crime, and mental health problems across the life span." Dearing adds that these problems usually arise when children grow up in extremely poor conditions over a prolonged period, but that living in poverty for even a brief period may result in a child developing mental health problems. Förster and d'Ercole note that by about 2005 one out of every eight children in OECD countries lived in relative poverty.

In his research synopsis, Dearing shows that poverty can affect both the social-emotional functioning and the cognitive (mental) functioning and achievement of youth by two different pathways. According to Dearing, results of studies show that poverty is associated with stress in parents who are poor. The stress of poverty is associated with mental health problems such as depression, which, in turn, is associated with parents being emotionally colder and harsher. These parental behaviors affect the social-emotional development and functioning of children. Likewise, the results of studies show another series of linked effects: poverty is associated with limited materials in the home that foster learning, such as books, and with limited parental involvement in the home learning environment. Thus, poor parents infrequently do things in the home that foster learning, such as reading to their children. The absence of these material, psychological, and social factors affects the cognitive functioning and achievement of children. In addition, the article "Long-Term Poverty Affects Mental Health of Children" (*ScienceDaily*, February 9, 2006) reports that researchers at the University of Alberta find that children who begin life in poverty experience higher levels of antisocial behavior.

THE UNITED STATES
International Comparisons of Poverty

Förster and d'Ercole assess patterns of relative income poverty for the 30 member countries of the OECD. Looking at the relative poverty rates of 40%, 50%, and 60% of the national median income thresholds, the researchers note that the United States, Turkey, and Mexico had the highest rates of relative poverty, with 17% to 18% of their residents living at or below half the national median income by about 2005. Other OECD countries with high levels of relative poverty (approximately 15% living at or below half the national median income) were Spain, Poland, South Korea, Ireland, and Japan. Denmark, Sweden, and the Czech Republic had the lowest rates of relative poverty, with 5% to 6% of their residents living at or below half the national median income. Other OECD countries with low levels of relative poverty (approximately 7% living at or below half the national median income) were Austria, Norway, France, Iceland, Hungary, and Finland.

Figure 6.1 presents another comparative look at poverty internationally. It shows two bar graphs of relative income poverty for the 30 member countries of the OECD. The top graph shows households without children, and the bottom graph shows households with children. Both graphs have two sets of bars: all households (shown by the lighter bars) and households with a single adult (shown by the darker bars). In the top graph, the households shown by the darker bars consist of single people. In the bottom graph, these households consist of single parents with children.

Comparing the lighter bars in both graphs of Figure 6.1 reveals that households with children and households without children in OECD countries face a nearly equal chance of poverty—about a 10% chance on average. Comparing the lighter bars with the darker bars within each graph shows that households consisting of single individuals or single parents with children face a far greater risk of poverty than do households with two adults. On average, single adults living alone in OECD countries face twice the risk of poverty as do two adults living together. Moreover, single parents with children living in OECD countries face about three times the risk of poverty than do two-parent families.

U.S. Poverty Statistics

In 2008, 13.2% of the U.S. population lived below the U.S. poverty thresholds. (See Table 6.1.) The U.S.

poverty thresholds are income thresholds that vary by family size and composition. Under the heading "Family Status" in Table 6.1 are many terms that can be confusing if not defined. The U.S. Census Bureau (November 18, 2008, http://www.census.gov/population/www/cps/cpsdef.html) defines a family as "a group of two people or more (one of whom is the householder) related by birth, marriage, or adoption and residing together.... A subfamily is a married couple with or without children, or a single parent with one or more own never-married children under 18 years old. A subfamily does not maintain their own household, but lives in the home of someone else." Related subfamilies are included in the data for families. An unrelated subfamily, such as a student and his or her spouse living with married friends, are shown separately and are not included with the data for families.

The poverty figure for 2008—13.2%—rose from 12.5% in 2007. (See Table 6.1.) This rise in the percentage of those living in poverty in the United States occurred during a time in which the nation and the world were experiencing an economic recession that began in 2007. Nearly half (46%) of unrelated subfamilies were living in poverty in 2008, up from 38.1% in 2007. One out of every five (20.8%) unrelated individuals was poor in 2008, up from 19.7% in 2007, with poverty affecting women in a higher proportion than men in both 2008 (22.6% versus 18.9%) and 2007 (22.2% versus 17.1%).

Poverty in the United States is related to race and ethnicity. In 2008 the highest percentage of poverty existed in the African-American population at 24.7%. (See Table 6.1.) This means that one out of every four African-Americans living in the United States in 2008 was poor. For Hispanics, nearly one out of every four (23.2%) was in poverty in the United States as well. Poverty affected 11.2% of whites and 11.8% of Asian-Americans.

Poverty is also related to age in the United States, with younger populations experiencing higher rates of poverty than older populations. In 2008, 19% of people younger than the age of 18 were poor, as were 11.7% of those aged 18 to 64 and 9.7% of those 65 years and older. (See Table 6.1.) In addition, people who were foreign born and not U.S. citizens (23.3%) were more likely than U.S. natives (12.6%) or naturalized citizens (10.2%) to be poor in 2008. Not surprisingly, people who did not work at least one week during the year (22%) were more likely to be poor than people who worked regularly part time (13.5%) or full time (2.6%) in 2008.

Figure 6.2 shows U.S. poverty rates by age from 1959 to 2008. People 65 years and older had the highest percentage of poverty from 1959 through 1973. The rates of poverty in all age groups dropped dramatically from 1959 through the early 1970s. As rates somewhat stabilized in the under-18-year-old age group and those aged 18 to 64

FIGURE 6.1

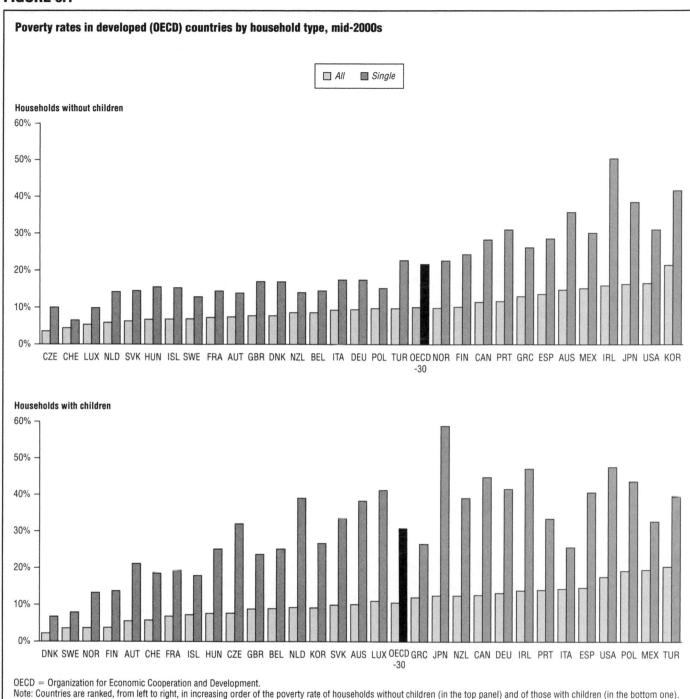

Poverty rates in developed (OECD) countries by household type, mid-2000s

□ All ■ Single

Households without children

OECD = Organization for Economic Cooperation and Development.
Note: Countries are ranked, from left to right, in increasing order of the poverty rate of households without children (in the top panel) and of those with children (in the bottom one).
Data refer to all households, irrespectively of the age of the household head. Poverty thresholds are set at 50% of the median income of the entire population.

SOURCE: "Figure 5.7. Poverty Rates by Household Type, Mid-2000s," in Organization for Economic Co-operation and Development, OECD (2008), *Growing Unequal?: Income Distribution and Poverty in OECD Countries*, p. 133, http://browse.oecdbookshop.org/oecd/pdfs/browseit/8108051E.PDF (accessed December 11, 2009)

during the early 1970s, the percentage of people younger than the age of 18 and in poverty came to match the percentage of people 65 years and older in 1974. Then the percentage of those under the age of 18 and in poverty rose in 1975, making this group the most poverty-stricken of any age group, and this condition remained constant to 2008. Young people under the age of 18 (19%) had the largest percentage living in poverty in 2008. The percent-

age of those 65 years and older continued to fall quite consistently, and by 2008 people in this age bracket had the lowest percentage in poverty (9.7%). Adults aged 18 to 64 years, who had the lowest percentage of people in poverty from 1959 to 1992, had the second-lowest poverty rate (11.7%) in 2008.

People living in the southern United States were more likely to be poor (14.3%) than people living in

TABLE 6.1

People and families in poverty by selected characteristics, United States, 2007 and 2008

(Numbers in thousands. People as of March of the following year.)

Characteristic	Total	2007 Below poverty Number	2007 90 percent C.I.[1](±)	2007 Percentage	2007 90 percent C.I.[1](±)	Total	2008 Below poverty Number	2008 90 percent C.I.[1](±)	2008 Percentage	2008 90 percent C.I.[1](±)	Change in poverty (2008 less 2007)[a] Number	Change in poverty (2008 less 2007)[a] Percentage
People												
Total	**298,699**	**37,276**	**682**	**12.5**	**0.2**	**301,041**	**39,829**	**701**	**13.2**	**0.2**	**2,553**	**0.8**
Family status												
In families	245,443	26,509	587	10.8	0.2	248,301	28,564	607	11.5	0.2	2,055	0.7
Householder	77,908	7,623	184	9.8	0.2	78,874	8,147	192	10.3	0.2	525	0.5
Related children under 18	72,792	12,802	345	17.6	0.5	72,980	13,507	353	18.5	0.5	705	0.9
Related children under 6	24,543	5,101	227	20.8	0.9	24,884	5,295	231	21.3	0.9	194	0.5
In unrelated subfamilies	1,516	577	91	38.1	4.7	1,207	555	89	46.0	5.4	−22	7.9
Reference person	609	222	56	36.5	7.4	452	207	54	45.7	8.9	−15	9.2
Children under 18	819	332	60	40.5	5.7	712	341	61	47.8	6.2	9	7.3
Unrelated individuals	51,740	10,189	221	19.7	0.3	51,534	10,710	228	20.8	0.3	521	1.1
Male	25,447	4,348	131	17.1	0.4	25,240	4,759	139	18.9	0.5	411	1.8
Female	26,293	5,841	156	22.2	0.5	26,293	5,951	158	22.6	0.5	110	0.4
Race[b] and Hispanic origin												
White	239,133	25,120	573	10.5	0.2	240,548	26,990	592	11.2	0.2	1,870	0.7
White, not Hispanic	196,583	16,032	465	8.2	0.2	196,940	17,024	479	8.6	0.2	992	0.5
Black	37,665	9,237	334	24.5	0.8	37,966	9,379	337	24.7	0.8	142	0.2
Asian	13,257	1,349	135	10.2	1.0	13,310	1,576	145	11.8	1.1	227	1.7
Hispanic (any race)	45,933	9,890	333	21.5	0.7	47,398	10,987	348	23.2	0.7	1,097	1.6
Age												
Under 18 years	73,996	13,324	350	18.0	0.5	74,068	14,068	359	19.0	0.5	744	1.0
18 to 64 years	187,913	20,396	516	10.9	0.3	189,185	22,105	536	11.7	0.3	1,709	0.8
65 years and older	36,790	3,556	132	9.7	0.4	37,788	3,656	134	9.7	0.4	100	—
Nativity												
Native born	261,456	31,126	631	11.9	0.2	264,314	33,293	650	12.6	0.2	2,167	0.7
Foreign born	37,243	6,150	335	16.5	0.8	36,727	6,536	345	17.8	0.9	386	1.3
Naturalized citizen	15,050	1,426	162	9.5	1.0	15,470	1,577	171	10.2	1.0	151	0.7
Not a citizen	22,193	4,724	294	21.3	1.2	21,257	4,959	301	23.3	1.3	235	2.0
Region												
Northeast	53,952	6,166	286	11.4	0.5	54,123	6,295	292	11.6	0.5	130	0.2
Midwest	65,403	7,237	308	11.1	0.5	65,589	8,120	319	12.4	0.5	883	1.3
South	109,545	15,501	453	14.2	0.4	110,666	15,862	458	14.3	0.4	361	0.2
West	69,799	8,372	340	12.0	0.5	70,663	9,552	360	13.5	0.5	1,180	1.5
Metropolitan status												
Inside metropolitan statistical areas	251,023	29,921	620	11.9	0.2	253,048	32,570	643	12.9	0.3	2,649	1.0
Inside principal cities	96,731	15,983	465	16.5	0.5	97,217	17,222	481	17.7	0.5	1,240	1.2
Outside principal cities	154,292	13,938	436	9.0	0.3	155,831	15,348	456	9.8	0.3	1,410	0.8
Outside metropolitan statistical areas[3]	47,676	7,355	392	15.4	0.8	47,993	7,259	390	15.1	0.8	−96	−0.3
Work experience												
Total, 16 years and older	233,885	25,297	569	10.8	0.2	236,024	27,216	587	11.5	0.2	1,919	0.7
All workers	158,468	9,089	354	5.7	0.2	158,317	10,085	372	6.4	0.2	996	0.6
Worked full-time, year-round	108,617	2,768	198	2.5	0.2	104,023	2,754	197	2.6	0.2	−14	0.1
Not full-time, year-round	49,851	6,320	297	12.7	0.6	54,294	7,331	319	13.5	0.6	1,011	0.8
Did not work at least one week	75,417	16,208	465	21.5	0.6	77,707	17,131	477	22.0	0.6	923	0.6

other regions of the country in 2008. (See Table 6.1.) Table 6.2 shows the percentage of poverty in each of the 50 states from 2006 to 2008. In 2008, New Mexico (a southwestern state) had the highest percentage of poverty of all U.S. states at 19.3%. Louisiana (18.2%) and Mississippi (18.1%)—both southern states—had the next-highest percentages of poverty in that year. New Hampshire (a northeastern state) had the lowest percentage of poverty, at 7%. Utah, a northwestern state, had the next-lowest poverty rate at 7.6%. The average poverty

rate for the United States in 2008 was 13.2%. States near this poverty average were Michigan (13%), Florida (13.1%), South Dakota (13.1%), and Missouri (13.3%).

These regional variations in poverty across all ages is also reflected in the most poverty-stricken group: those under 18 years of age. Figure 6.3 shows the distribution of youth poverty in the United States in 2007. As can be seen in the map, young people living in the southern United States were more likely to be poor than young people living in other regions of the country in 2007. Figure 6.3

TABLE 6.1

People and families in poverty by selected characteristics, United States, 2007 and 2008 [CONTINUED]

(Numbers in thousands. People as of March of the following year.)

Characteristic		2007				2008					Change in poverty (2008 less 2007)[a]	
			Below poverty					Below poverty				
	Total	Number	90 percent C.I.[1](±)	Percentage	90 percent C.I.[1](±)	Total	Number	90 percent C.I.[1](±)	Percentage	90 percent C.I.[1](±)	Number	Percentage
Families												
Total	77,908	7,623	184	9.8	0.2	78,874	8,147	192	10.3	0.2	525	0.5
Type of family												
Married-couple	58,395	2,849	104	4.9	0.2	59,137	3,261	112	5.5	0.2	412	0.6
Female householder, no husband present	14,411	4,078	127	28.3	1.0	14,482	4,163	128	28.7	1.0	85	0.4
Male householder, no wife present	5,103	696	49	13.6	1.0	5,255	723	50	13.8	1.0	27	0.1

—Represents or rounds to zero.

[a]Details may not sum to totals because of rounding.

[b]Federal surveys now give respondents the option of reporting more than one race. Therefore, two basic ways of defining a race group are possible. A group such as Asian may be defined as those who reported Asian and no other race (the race-alone or single-race concept) or as those who reported Asian regardless of whether they also reported another race (the race-alone-or-in-combination concept). This table shows data using the first approach (race alone). The use of the single-race population does not imply that it is the preferred method of presenting or analyzing data. The Census Bureau uses a variety of approaches. Information on people who reported more than one race, such as white and American Indian and Alaska Native or Asian and black or African American, is available from Census 2000 through American FactFinder. About 2.6 percent of people reported more than one race in Census 2000. Data for American Indians and Alaska Natives, Native Hawaiians and Other Pacific Islanders, and those reporting two or more races are not shown separately.

[3]The "outside metropolitan statistical areas" category includes both micropolitan statistical areas and territory outside of metropolitan and micropolitan statistical areas.

SOURCE: Adapted from Carmen DeNavas-Walt, Bernadette D. Proctor, and Jessica C. Smith, "Table 4. People and Families in Poverty by Selected Characteristics: 2007 and 2008," in *Income, Poverty, and Health Insurance Coverage in the United States: 2008*, U.S. Census Bureau, September 2009, http://www.census.gov/prod/2009pubs/p60-236.pdf (accessed December 6, 2009)

FIGURE 6.2

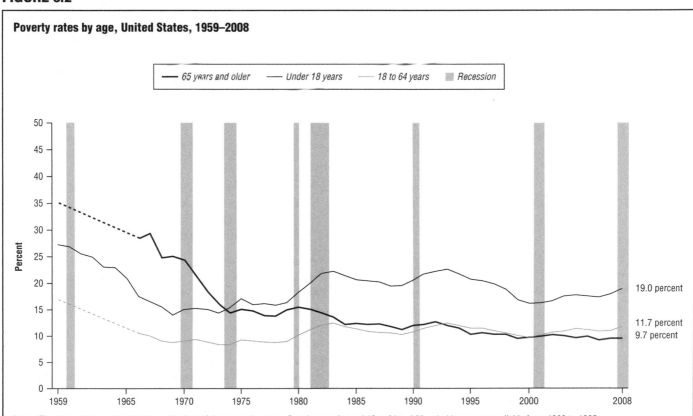

Poverty rates by age, United States, 1959–2008

— 65 years and older — Under 18 years — 18 to 64 years ▇ Recession

19.0 percent
11.7 percent
9.7 percent

Notes: The data points are placed at the midpoints of the respective years. Data for people aged 18 to 64 and 65 and older are not available from 1960 to 1965.

SOURCE: Carmen DeNavas-Walt, Bernadette D. Proctor, and Jessica C. Smith, "Figure 4. Poverty Rates by Age: 1959 to 2008," in *Income, Poverty, and Health Insurance Coverage in the United States: 2008*, U.S. Census Bureau, September 2009, http://www.census.gov/prod/2009pubs/p60-236.pdf (accessed December 6, 2009)

TABLE 6.2

Percent in poverty, by state, United States, 2006–08

State	2008 Percent	2007 Percent	2006 Percent
US	13.2	12.5	12.3
Alabama	14.3	14.5	14.3
Alaska	8.2	7.6	8.9
Arizona	18.0	14.3	14.4
Arkansas	15.3	13.8	17.7
California	14.6	12.7	12.2
Colorado	11.0	9.8	9.7
Connecticut	8.1	8.9	8.0
Delaware	9.6	9.3	9.3
D.C.	16.5	18.0	18.3
Florida	13.1	12.5	11.5
Georgia	15.5	13.6	12.6
Hawaii	9.9	7.5	9.2
Idaho	12.2	9.9	9.5
Illinois	12.3	10.0	10.6
Indiana	14.3	11.8	10.6
Iowa	9.5	8.9	10.3
Kansas	12.7	11.7	12.8
Kentucky	17.1	15.5	16.8
Louisiana	18.2	16.1	17.0
Maine	12.0	10.9	10.2
Maryland	8.7	8.8	8.4
Massachusetts	11.3	11.2	12.0
Michigan	13.0	10.8	13.3
Minnesota	9.9	9.3	8.2
Mississippi	18.1	22.6	20.6
Missouri	13.3	12.8	11.4
Montana	12.9	13.0	13.5
Nebraska	10.6	9.9	10.2
Nevada	10.8	9.7	9.5
New Hampshire	7.0	5.8	5.4
New Jersey	9.2	8.7	8.8
New Mexico	19.3	14.0	16.9
New York	14.2	14.5	14.0
North Carolina	13.9	15.5	13.8
North Dakota	11.8	9.3	11.4
Ohio	13.7	12.8	12.1
Oklahoma	13.6	13.4	15.2
Oregon	10.6	12.8	11.8
Pennsylvania	11.0	10.4	11.3
Rhode Island	12.7	9.5	10.5
South Carolina	14.0	14.1	11.2
South Dakota	13.1	9.4	10.7
Tennessee	15.0	14.8	14.9
Texas	15.9	16.5	16.4
Utah	7.6	9.6	9.3
Vermont	9.0	9.9	7.8
Virginia	10.3	8.6	8.6
Washington	10.4	10.2	8.0
West Virginia	14.5	14.8	15.3
Wisconsin	9.8	11.0	10.1
Wyoming	10.1	10.9	10.0

SOURCE: Adapted from "Table 19. Percent of Persons in Poverty, by State: 2006, 2007, 2008," in *Historical Poverty Tables*, U.S. Census Bureau, 2009, http://www.census.gov/hhes/www/poverty/histpov/perindex.html (accessed December 10, 2009)

also shows pockets of youth poverty within states. Youth poverty was pronounced along the U.S.-Mexican border, and it permeated New Mexico, the state with the highest rate of overall poverty of all the U.S. states. A high rate of youth poverty (25% or higher) also existed in most of Arkansas, Kentucky, Louisiana, Mississippi, and West Virginia. The southern portions of Alabama, Georgia, and Missouri; the central portion of Alaska; and the eastern portion of Arizona (which adjoins New Mexico) also had high rates of youth poverty. Other pockets of high

rates of youth poverty were scattered throughout the continental United States.

Even though the overall U.S. poverty rate in 2008 was high at 13.2%, it had decreased from 22.4% in 1959. (See Figure 6.4.) In 2008 it was higher than, but close to, the lowest rates, which were experienced in 1973, 1974, and 2000. However, because the U.S. population has grown over the years, the number of people affected by poverty is higher in more recent years at a particular rate than in more distant years at that same rate. Thus, in terms of individuals affected by poverty, 39.8 million were poor in 2008, the same as in 1959. The fewest number of people affected by poverty in a single year in the United States was in 1973 at 22.9 million.

Changing the Calculation of U.S. Poverty Thresholds

On August 1, 2007, testimony was heard in the U.S. House of Representatives Subcommittee on Income Security and Family Support about changing the way the poverty thresholds are calculated. According to the press release "McDermott Announces Hearing on Measuring Poverty in America" (July 25, 2007, http://waysandmeans.house .gov/Default.aspx), Representative Jim McDermott (1936–; D-WA), who chaired the subcommittee, provided the following background on this issue:

There is a broad consensus that the poverty measurement has become less accurate in highlighting economic hardship than when it was created more than 40 years ago. For example, the poverty thresholds were created in relation to consumption when the average family of three or more persons spent about one-third of its after-tax income on food. Today, food demands only one-seventh of that family's budget, while the share of income devoted to other expenses, such as housing and health care, has grown. Furthermore, the Federal poverty threshold for a family of four represented about 50 percent of median income when first devised, while it now represents only about 30 percent of median income. Finally, the current poverty measurement fails to count certain benefits, including the Earned Income Tax Credit and food stamps, as well as certain work-related expenses, including child care and transportation.

The witness list for the subcommittee hearings included representatives from the National Academy of Sciences, the University of Maryland at College Park, the National Center for Children in Poverty, the American Enterprise Institute for Public Policy Research, and the Center for American Progress Task Force on Poverty. One method of calculating the poverty thresholds suggested by those giving testimony was to tie the poverty threshold to a percentage of median income, such as 50%, as is done in many countries. In this way the poverty level would fluctuate as the median income fluctuated. It was also suggested that the calculation of poverty thresholds take into account regional cost-of-living differences.

FIGURE 6.3

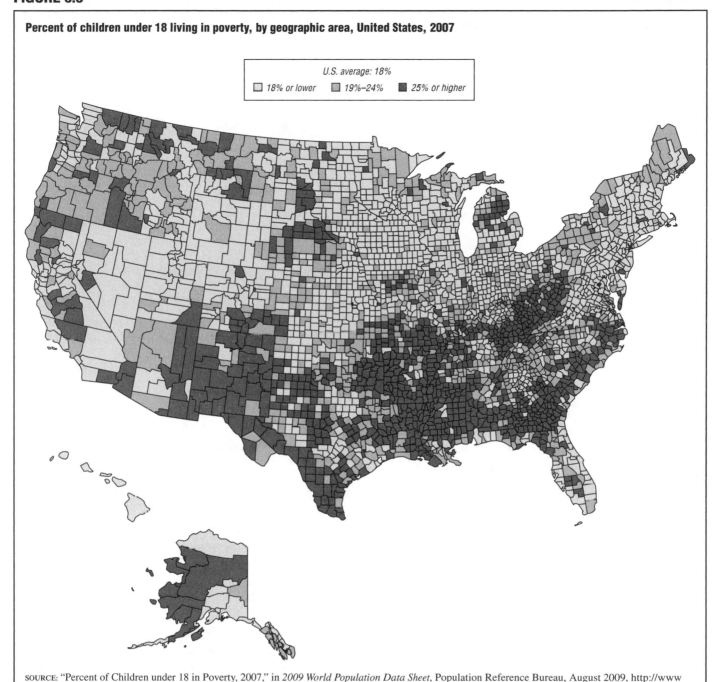

Percent of children under 18 living in poverty, by geographic area, United States, 2007

U.S. average: 18%

☐ 18% or lower ■ 19%–24% ■ 25% or higher

SOURCE: "Percent of Children under 18 in Poverty, 2007," in *2009 World Population Data Sheet*, Population Reference Bureau, August 2009, http://www
.prb.org/pdf09/09wpds_eng.pdf (accessed December 11, 2009)

Two years later the Measuring American Poverty Act was introduced into Congress. Representative McDermott introduced the bill (H.R. 2909) in the House on June 17, 2009, and Senator Christopher J. Dodd (1944–; D-CT) introduced the bill (S. 1625) in the U.S. Senate on August 6, 2009. Senator Dodd explains in the press release "Dodd Introduces Bill to Modernize Poverty Measurement" (August 10, 2009, http://dodd.senate.gov/?q=node/5155) that the bill:

> Would develop a poverty measure based on the current costs of food, clothing, shelter and other basic necessities and include the costs of certain unavoidable expenses

such as medical and necessary work related expenses. The measure would also take into account government programs like the Earned Income Tax Credit, food stamps, and housing assistance. Additionally, the legislation would direct the Census to include geographic differences in the cost of living, both between states and within a state's urban and more rural areas. In order to provide the most accurate picture of geographic variation, the bill also directs the Census to simultaneously examine the impact of state and local taxes and benefit programs on poverty.

As of February 2010, the bill was still in committee in both houses of Congress.

FIGURE 6.4

Number in poverty and poverty rate, United States, 1959–2008

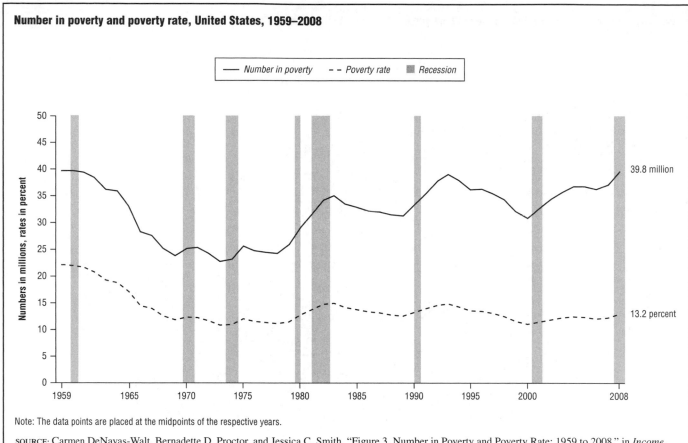

Note: The data points are placed at the midpoints of the respective years.

SOURCE: Carmen DeNavas-Walt, Bernadette D. Proctor, and Jessica C. Smith, "Figure 3. Number in Poverty and Poverty Rate: 1959 to 2008," in *Income, Poverty, and Health Insurance Coverage in the United States: 2008*, U.S. Census Bureau, September 2009, http://www.census.gov/prod/2009pubs/p60-236 .pdf (accessed December 6, 2009)

What Poverty Looks Like in the United States

What does it mean to be poor in the United States? The article "The Mountain Man and the Surgeon: Reflections on Relative Poverty in North America and Africa" (*Economist*, December 20, 2005) compares the lives of an unemployed truck driver in the coal mining industry of eastern Kentucky's Appalachian region (which had a poverty rate of 24.5% in 2004) with a surgeon in the Democratic Republic of Congo in Africa. The article notes that, with incomes of $521 and $250 to $700 per month, respectively, the two men are roughly in the same income bracket, yet the American truck driver is considered desperately poor, whereas the Congolese surgeon is viewed as quite well-off relative to the rest of his country. In 2004 the median annual income in the United States was $44,389, whereas in Congo it was $673. In Congo, basic utilities such as running water and electricity are rare. By contrast, more often than not, impoverished American families have at least one television in their home, their children usually attend school, and they typically do not have to grow their own food to survive.

U.S. poverty is certainly different in nature relative to poverty in the developing world, but there are some similarities. For instance, some people in the United States experience persistent poverty—meaning they live without basic utilities and appropriate sanitation even in the 21st century. Most Americans—even many of those living below the poverty threshold—manage to afford items such as televisions, but a rising number of households have trouble affording food at least once during a given year. This kind of food insecurity is a major indicator of the state of poverty in the United States. Another more visibly extreme indicator of U.S. poverty is homelessness. As the 21st century progresses, both of these situations—food insecurity and homelessness—are occurring with more and more frequency throughout the United States.

FOOD INSECURITY. Food insecurity means that individuals or families do not always have access to enough food for proper nutrition and health. In developing countries food insecurity is often extreme enough to cause fatal malnutrition. In developed countries fatal malnutrition rarely occurs, but food insecurity can result in chronic undernutrition, which can lead to many physical and psychological problems as well as learning disabilities in children.

Mark Nord, Margaret Andrews, and Steven Carlson of the U.S. Department of Agriculture's Economic Research

Service report in *Household Food Security in the United States, 2008* (November 2009, http://www.ers.usda.gov/Publications/ERR83/ERR83.pdf) that 85.4% of U.S. households were food secure in 2008. That is, 85 out of every 100 U.S. households in 2008 always had access to enough food for proper nutrition and health. However, 14.6% of U.S. households were food insecure—8.9% with low food security and 5.7% with very low food security. Households with low food security are those that had trouble getting enough food on multiple occasions but had never or hardly ever had to reduce their food intake because of it. Households with very low food security are those in which there was not enough food for all the family members so on many occasions throughout the year some family members had to reduce their food intake or alter their eating patterns. Nord, Andrews, and Carlson indicate that the proportion of households in 2008 with very low food security was the highest proportion since 1995, when food insecurity began to be measured.

Nord, Andrews, and Carlson report that in food-insecure households in 2008, children were protected from hunger in most cases, with adults cutting back on their own food intake to continue feeding their children. Nonetheless, households with children under the age of 18 had almost twice the rate of food insecurity as households without children: 21% versus 11.3%. (See Table 6.3.) The rate of food insecurity was even higher in households with children under six years old than in households with children under the age of 18: 22.3% versus 21%. Households with children under the age of 18 headed by a married couple had the lowest rate of food insecurity (14.3%), whereas those headed by a female with no spouse had the highest rate (37.2%). Overall, households with elderly (people older than 65) as part of the family experienced the lowest rates of food insecurity in 2008 (8.1%), households of elderly living alone had the next lowest rate of food insecurity (8.8%), and households with more than one adult who were all younger than 65 with no children present had the third-lowest rate (9.1%).

Several household characteristics serve as indicators of high-risk populations—meaning populations with food insecurity and/or hunger rates well above the national average. Nord, Andrews, and Carlson indicate that families with incomes below the poverty threshold (under 1.00 of the income-to-poverty ratio) were particularly vulnerable, with 42.2% of them experiencing food insecurity at some point during 2008. (See Table 6.3.) As income rose, food insecurity fell: 39% of households under 1.3 times the poverty threshold were food insecure in 2008, whereas 33.9% of those under 1.85 times the poverty threshold were food insecure. When income rose to above 1.85 times the poverty threshold, food insecurity plummeted to 7.7%. Non-Hispanic African-American (25.7%) and Hispanic (26.9%) households had rates approaching twice the national average. People living in the South (15.9%) and in principal cities (17.7%) also had higher rates of food insecurity than people living in other demographic areas.

Figure 6.5 is a visual comparison between the data in Table 6.3 for 2008 and the same categories of data for 2007. In all households, food insecurity rose in 2008 from 2007. Food insecurity was also higher in 2008 than in 2007 for all subcategories listed.

HOMELESSNESS. There are many factors that can lead to a person becoming homeless in the United States. The most frequent factors include unemployment or underemployment, mental illness, drug or alcohol addiction, a lack of family support, poor education, and failed social services. However, a primary cause is poverty. The Substance Abuse and Mental Health Services Administration (SAMHSA; February 2010, http://mentalhealth.samhsa.gov/cmhs/homelessness/) estimates that as many as 700,000 people are likely to be homeless in the United States on any given day.

Poor education is one factor that can lead to homelessness, but homelessness can also lead to poor education. Public school enrollment is generally based on the school district in which a child lives, but if a child becomes homeless, what happens to his or her schooling? The McKinney-Vento Homeless Assistance Act of 1987 ensures that homeless children have certain rights regarding school enrollment and attendance:

- Homeless children are permitted to stay in their school even if they move.

- They can enroll in a new school with no proof of residency, immunizations, guardianship papers, or records from former schools.

- They are entitled to transportation to and from school along with other children.

- They can receive all necessary school services.

- They have the right to challenge decisions made by schools and districts.

However, even federal legislation cannot fully protect homeless children. In "Facts about the Education of Children and Youth Experiencing Homelessness" (2009, http://www.naehcy.org/facts.html), the National Association for the Education of Homeless Children and Youth (NAEHCY) reports that during the 2007–08 academic year 794,617 homeless children and youth were enrolled in public schools. This was a 17% increase from the number enrolled during the 2006–07 academic year and a much higher estimate than SAMHSA provides for all homeless children and youth. The NAEHCY suggests that the global economic crisis and an increase in home foreclosures in the United States during that academic year were causal factors involved in the increase of

TABLE 6.3

Prevalence of food security and food insecurity by selected household characteristics, United States, 2008

Category	Total[a] 1,000	Food secure 1,000	Food secure Percent	Food insecure — All 1,000	Food insecure — All Percent	Food insecure — With low food security 1,000	Food insecure — With low food security Percent	Food insecure — With very low food security 1,000	Food insecure — With very low food security Percent
All households	117,565	100,416	85.4	17,149	14.6	10,426	8.9	6,723	5.7
Household composition:									
With children <18 yrs	39,699	31,364	79.0	8,335	21.0	5,718	14.4	2,617	6.6
With children <6 yrs	17,503	13,595	77.7	3,908	22.3	2,818	16.1	1,090	6.2
Married-couple families	26,705	22,887	85.7	3,818	14.3	2,735	10.2	1,083	4.1
Female head, no spouse	9,639	6,057	62.8	3,582	37.2	2,296	23.8	1,286	13.3
Male head, no spouse	2,782	2,013	72.4	769	27.6	569	20.5	200	7.2
Other household with child[b]	572	405	70.8	167	29.2	118	20.6	49	8.6
With no children <18 yrs	77,866	69,052	88.7	8,814	11.3	4,708	6.0	4,106	5.3
More than one adult	45,772	41,610	90.9	4,162	9.1	2,409	5.3	1,753	3.8
Women living alone	17,934	15,266	85.1	2,668	14.9	1,284	7.2	1,384	7.7
Men living alone	14,160	12,177	86.0	1,983	14.0	1,015	7.2	968	6.8
With elderly	28,211	25,927	91.9	2,284	8.1	1,402	5.0	882	3.1
Elderly living alone	11,148	10,168	91.2	980	8.8	552	5.0	428	3.8
Race/ethnicity of households:									
White non-Hispanic	82,935	74,041	89.3	8,894	10.7	5,154	6.2	3,740	4.5
Black non-Hispanic	14,441	10,732	74.3	3,709	25.7	2,251	15.6	1,458	10.1
Hispanic[c]	13,504	9,873	73.1	3,631	26.9	2,439	18.1	1,192	8.8
Other	6,686	5,772	86.3	914	13.7	582	8.7	332	5.0
Household income-to-poverty ratio:									
Under 1.00	13,117	7,576	57.8	5,541	42.2	3,014	23.0	2,527	19.3
Under 1.30	20,383	12,427	61.0	7,956	39.0	4,403	21.6	3,553	17.4
Under 1.85	29,680	19,622	66.1	10,058	33.9	5,731	19.3	4,327	14.6
1.85 and over	70,433	65,038	92.3	5,395	7.7	3,595	5.1	1,800	2.6
Income unknown	17,452	15,755	90.3	1,697	9.7	1,101	6.3	596	3.4
Area of residence:[d]									
Inside metropolitan area	98,189	83,790	85.3	14,399	14.7	8,757	8.9	5,642	5.7
In principal cities[e]	32,808	27,006	82.3	5,802	17.7	3,634	11.1	2,168	6.6
Not in principal cities	48,239	42,125	87.3	6,114	12.7	3,650	7.6	2,464	5.1
Outside metropolitan area	19,375	16,625	85.8	2,750	14.2	1,669	8.6	1,081	5.6
Census geographic region:									
Northeast	21,341	18,616	87.2	2,725	12.8	1,610	7.5	1,115	5.2
Midwest	26,370	22,671	86.0	3,699	14.0	2,254	8.5	1,445	5.5
South	43,542	36,621	84.1	6,921	15.9	4,216	9.7	2,705	6.2
West	26,311	22,507	85.5	3,804	14.5	2,346	8.9	1,458	5.5

[a]Totals exclude households whose food security status is unknown because they did not give a valid response to any of the questions in the food security scale. In 2008, these represented 366,000 households (0.3 percent of all households.)
[b]Households with children in complex living arrangements, e.g., children of other relatives or unrelated roommate or boarder.
[c]Hispanics may be of any race.
[d]Metropolitan area residence is based on the 2003 Office of Management and Budget delineation. Prevalence rates by area of residence are comparable with those for 2004 and later years but are not precisely comparable with those of earlier years.
[e]Households within incorporated areas of the largest cities in each metropolitan area. Residence inside or outside of principal cities is not identified for about 17 percent of households in metropolitan statistical areas.

SOURCE: Mark Nord, Margaret Andrews, and Steven Carlson, "Table 2. Households by Food Security Status and Selected Household Characteristics, 2008," in *Household Food Security in the United States, 2008*, U.S. Department of Agriculture (USDA), Economic Research Service (ERS), November 2009, http://www.ers.usda.gov/Publications/ERR83/ERR83.pdf (accessed December 6, 2009)

homelessness among school students. Nonetheless, the organization notes that a trend in the decrease in affordable housing and an increase in severe poverty in the United States has been instrumental in increasing the population of school children experiencing homelessness even before the economic crisis hit the United States.

Tumaini R. Coker et al. analyze in "Prevalence, Characteristics, and Associated Health and Health Care of Family Homelessness among Fifth-Grade Students" (*American Journal of Public Health*, vol. 99, no. 8, August 2009) data from a survey conducted from 2004 to 2006 by the Centers for Disease Control and Prevention. The data were collected from the parents of 5,147 fifth-grade students living in three major U.S. cities. The researchers indicate that 7% of respondents had experienced homelessness, with more than one-third (37%) of that group having spent over one year homeless. Having ever been homeless was most prevalent for parents aged 18 to 34, with only a high school education, who were African-American, who were single parents, and with an income of less than $20,000 per year. Coker et al. also find an association between a history of family homelessness and parental emotional, developmental, and behavioral problems.

FIGURE 6.5

Prevalence of food insecurity, by selected characteristics, 2007 and 2008

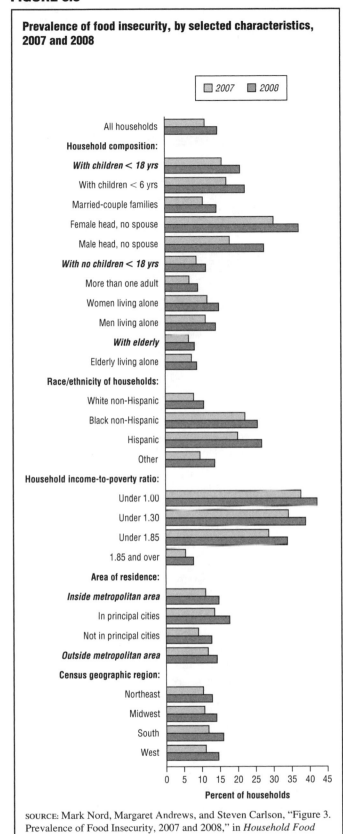

☐ 2007   ■ 2008

SOURCE: Mark Nord, Margaret Andrews, and Steven Carlson, "Figure 3. Prevalence of Food Insecurity, 2007 and 2008," in *Household Food Security in the United States, 2008*, U.S. Department of Agriculture (USDA), Economic Research Service (ERS), November 2009, http://www.ers.usda.gov/Publications/ERR83/ERR83.pdf (accessed December 6, 2009)

WESTERN EUROPE: POVERTY IN THE UNITED KINGDOM AND GERMANY

The United Kingdom (UK) and Germany are two of the largest economies in the European Union (EU), yet they have a portion of their residents living in poverty as do all countries. According to the Poverty Site, in "Numbers in Low Income" (February 3, 2010, http://www.poverty.org.uk/01/index.shtml), the UK had 22% of its residents living below 60% of the average income in 2007–08. Germany had similar poverty statistics. Tristana Moore explains in "New Report Reveals the Depth of German Poverty" (*Time*, May 25, 2009) that the average poverty rate in Germany, also measured as a percentage of its residents living below 60% of the average income, ranged from 7.4% to 27% in 2007, depending on the location.

According to Steve Schifferes, in "Is the UK a Model Welfare State?" (BBC News, August 4, 2005), Western countries address the problems of the poor with three different models of social welfare programs: social demo-cratic, liberal, and corporatist. The social democratic model exists mainly in the Scandinavian countries (Norway, Sweden, and Denmark) and is paid for mostly through taxes, which allows the government to provide a high level of services for all. The liberal model, which is reflected in the practices of the United Kingdom (UK) and the United States, provides a low level of benefits, but also lower taxes; it relies on the private sector to supplement aid to the poor and encourages the unemployed to take whatever work is available. The corporatist model is used in most other countries in continental Europe, including France and Germany, with benefits coming through employers from individual contributions.

Poverty is a global issue: it exists everywhere to some degree, regardless of what welfare model a country uses. Even Scandinavian countries have not eradicated poverty entirely, but they do have the lowest poverty rates in the EU and among developed countries. The country with the lowest rank on the Human Poverty Index is Sweden, followed by Norway and then the Netherlands. (See Table 1.3 in Chapter 1.)

The United Kingdom

Kevin Watkins of the United Nations Development Programme (UNDP) notes in *Human Development Report 2005—International Cooperation at a Crossroads: Aid, Trade, and Security in an Unequal World* (2005, http://hdr.undp.org/en/media/HDR05_complete.pdf) that by the late 1990s the UK (the state consisting of the countries England, Wales, Scotland, and Northern Ireland) had one of the highest rates of child poverty in Europe and among developed countries. In 1998 an estimated 4.6 million children—one out of every three—were living in low-income households. The overall low-income rate was double what it had been in the late 1970s. According to Watkins, this situation was the result of government policies during the 1980s that caused income inequality to increase at a remarkable rate: the wealthiest 20% of UK society saw their annual incomes increase 10 times more than those of the poorest 20%.

In response, the British government initiated a radical antipoverty campaign in 1999, the main goal of which was to eradicate child poverty in Great Britain entirely by 2020. The results have been encouraging. Evan Davis reports in "UK Poverty Line Is Moving Target" (BBC News, March 9, 2006) that the program of tax credits and new jobs successfully moved about 100,000 British children per year out of poverty. However, due to the nature of relative poverty, if the average income increases, then the poverty line also increases, resulting in even more people living in relative poverty. The answer and the challenge for the government, suggests Davis, lay in increasing the incomes of poor people at a faster rate than the incomes of the wealthier members of the society. According to Guy Palmer, Tom MacInnes, and Peter Kenway, in *Monitoring Poverty and Social Exclusion 2006* (2006, http://www.poverty.org.uk/reports/mpse%202006.pdf), in 2004–05 approximately 3.4 million children were living in the low-income bracket in Great Britain, down from 4.1 in 1998–99. The researchers note that in 2004–05 adults without children made up the largest low-income group in Great Britain at 31% (3.5 million adults), children made up the next largest group at 30% (3.4 million children), adults with dependent children represented 24% (2.7 million people), and old-age pensioners accounted for 16% (1.8 million).

One result of poverty is living in overcrowded housing. Figure 6.6 compares the percentage of children living in overcrowded housing in five developed countries from 1999 to 2006. In the UK, 10% of children of native-born families lived in overcrowded housing, which was slightly higher than in Australia, where 9% of children of native-born families lived in overcrowded housing, but lower than in the United States (11%), France (19%), and Italy (43%). In all five countries, children of immigrant families from low- or middle-income countries were more likely to live in overcrowded housing than children of native-born families. In the UK, 33% of children of immigrant families from low- or middle-income countries lived in overcrowded housing. Nonetheless, compared with the other four affluent countries, the UK was faring well.

However, Tom MacInnes, Peter Kenway, and Anushree Parekh indicate in *Monitoring Poverty and Social Exclusion 2009* (2009, http://www.jrf.org.uk/sites/files/jrf/monitoring-poverty-social-exclusion-2009-full.pdf) that by 2007–08 the news on poverty in the UK was not as good as it had been in 2004–05. The researchers report that 13.4 million people were living in low-income households

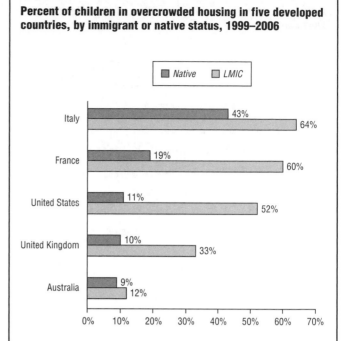

FIGURE 6.6

Percent of children in overcrowded housing in five developed countries, by immigrant or native status, 1999–2006

Legend: ■ Native ■ LMIC

Italy — Native 43%, LMIC 64%
France — Native 19%, LMIC 60%
United States — Native 11%, LMIC 52%
United Kingdom — Native 10%, LMIC 33%
Australia — Native 9%, LMIC 12%

LMIC = children of immigrant families from low- or middle-income countries.

SOURCE: "Figure 12.1. Children in Overcrowded Housing, Five Affluent Countries," in *Children in Immigrant Families in Eight Affluent Countries: Their Family, National and International Context*, United Nations Children's Fund (UNICEF) Innocenti Research Centre, Florence, August 2009, http://www.unicef-irc.org/publications/pdf/ii_immig_families.pdf (accessed December 7, 2009)

in 2007–08, which was an increase from 12.1 million in 2004–05. The number of children living in poverty increased as well, from 3.4 million in 2004–05 to 4 million in 2007–08. The percentage of children in poverty in 2007–08 was 31%, one percentage point higher than in 2004–05. MacInnes, Kenway, and Parekh note that tax credits helped lift children out of poverty during the initial years of the UK's antipoverty campaign, but that the number of households needing tax credits increased. They suggest that the causes behind the three-year trend of rising poverty are not clear nor are the effects that the global recession will have on poverty rates for the future.

Germany

Even though Germany has one of the largest economies in the world and was extraordinarily successful in recovering from the economic, infrastructural, and social disasters wrought by World War II (1939–1945), the country fell into economic stagnation during the first few years of the first decade of the 21st century. The article "German Jobless Rate at New Record" (BBC News, March 1, 2005) states that by early 2005 the unemployment rate was 12.6%, the highest it had been since the 1930s. However, the rate had decreased by 2008. According to IndexMundi, in "Germany Unemployment Rate"

(October 10, 2009, http://www.indexmundi.com/germany/unemployment_rate.html), the International Labour Office placed Germany's overall unemployment rate at 9% for 2008 and 7.8% for 2009. The International Monetary Fund differed, with unemployment rates of 7.4% for 2008 and 8% for 2009. In spite of these differences, Germany's unemployment had decreased significantly since 2005, but it was still relatively high, compared with previous years.

The unemployed are not the only people who are poor. The article "Germany Serious about Minimum Wage" (*Deutsche Welle*, February 24, 2006) indicates that 2 million poor Germans have full-time jobs, but they are so poorly paid that their income falls below the poverty line. As of February 2010, Germany did not have a minimum-wage law, but collective bargaining agreements set minimum wages by job classification for each industry and region. The idea of instituting a national minimum wage in Germany had the nation split: many union leaders were calling for a high minimum wage, whereas others argued this would result in the loss of more jobs.

In *World Factbook: Germany* (February 16, 2010, https://www.cia.gov/library/publications/the-world-factbook/geos/gm.html), the Central Intelligence Agency notes that as of 2001, 11% of Germans were estimated to be living below the nation's poverty line, which is a relatively low proportion. Child poverty in Germany is a serious issue, but it is not as acute as in the UK or the United States. Figure 6.7 presents a comparative overview of child poverty in five developed countries from 1999 to 2006. Germany had the second-lowest child poverty rate in its native-born population (8%), second only to France (6%), and the lowest child poverty rate in its immigrant population (15%). In contrast, the United States had the highest child poverty rate in its native-born population (20%) and the highest child poverty rate in its immigrant population (33%).

EASTERN EUROPE: THE RUSSIAN FEDERATION

The Russian Federation is the largest country by land area in the world, at 6.6 million square miles (17.1 million sq km). (See Table 6.4.) It is a loose federation of 89 separate republics, territories, and other political subdivisions, each of which has two delegates in the Russian parliament and varying degrees of political and economic autonomy. Its population, which was 141.8 million in 2008, is extremely diverse culturally and ethnically. There are believed to be more than 100 distinct ethnic groups throughout the country. This diversity has fueled violent conflicts since the dissolution of the Soviet Union in 1991. The Russian Federation is more commonly referred to as Russia. Before the Soviet Union was dissolved, Russia was the name of the largest of its republics. As a part of the Soviet Union, Russia accounted for more than half of the country's population and at least 60% of its gross domestic

FIGURE 6.7

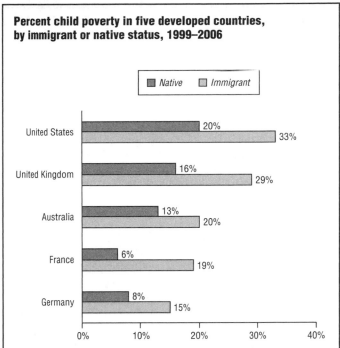

Percent child poverty in five developed countries, by immigrant or native status, 1999–2006

SOURCE: "Figure 11.3. Child Poverty Rate Based on Market Income and Including the Effect of Social Transfers, Five Affluent Countries," in *Children in Immigrant Families in Eight Affluent Countries: Their Family, National and International Context*, United Nations Children's Fund (UNICEF) Innocenti Research Centre, Florence, August 2009, http://www.unicef-irc.org/publications/pdf/ii_immig_families.pdf (accessed December 7, 2009)

product (GDP; the total value of all goods and services produced by a country in a year).

The Transition from Soviet Control to Free Market

The Russian Federation emerged as an independent nation late in 1991, when the Soviet Union collapsed. The Soviet Union was a communist country with a centrally planned and tightly controlled economy. In theory, this system ensured that all citizens would receive the basic necessities of life and that there would be no poverty. In reality, however, the Soviet system struggled for decades to meet the basic needs of its citizens. Mikhail Gorbachev (1931–), who led the Soviet Union from 1985 to 1991, introduced the concepts of *glasnost* (openness) and *perestroika* (reconstruction) in an attempt to reform and repair the Soviet system.

The pace of reform under Gorbachev proved too slow to satisfy critics of the Soviet system, and too fast to be satisfactory to its defenders. In August 1991 communist hard-liners launched a coup d'état in an attempt to remove Gorbachev and end his reforms. They were resisted and defeated by reformers, most notably by Boris Yeltsin (1931–2007), the president of the Russian state within the Soviet Union. Having defeated the hard-line communists, the reformers were left as the most powerful

TABLE 6.4

Selected world development indicators, Russian Federation, 2000, 2005, 2007, 2008

	2000	2005	2007	2008
World view				
Population, total (millions)	146.30	143.15	142.10	141.80
Population growth (annual %)	0.0	−0.5	−0.3	−0.2
Surface area (sq. km) (thousands)	17,098.2	17,098.2	17,098.2	17,098.2
GNI per capita, PPP (current international $)	1,086.35	1,655.78	2,036.49	2,216.33
People				
Life expectancy at birth, total (years)	65	65	68	—
Fertility rate, total (births per woman)	1.2	1.3	1.4	—
Adolescent fertility rate (births per 1,000 women ages 15–19)	31	26	25	—
Contraceptive prevalence (% of women ages 15–49)	—	—	—	—
Births attended by skilled health staff (% of total)	—	9	—	—
Mortality rate, under-5 (per 1,000)	24	17	15	—
Malnutrition prevalence, weight for age (% of children under 5)	—	—	—	—
Primary completion rate, total (% of relevant age group)	94	—	93	—
Ratio of girls to boys in primary and secondary education (%)	—	9	98	—
Prevalence of HIV, total (% of population ages 15–49)	0.3	1.1	1.1	—
Economy				
GDP (current US$) (billions)	259.71	764.53	1,290.08	1,607.82
GDP growth (annual %)	10.0	6.4	8.1	7.3

GNI = Gross National Income. PPP = Purchasing Power Parity. GDP = Gross Domestic Product. US$ = United States dollars.

SOURCE: Adapted from "Russian Federation," in *The World Bank Group Data Profile*, The World Bank, April 2009, http://ddp-ext.worldbank.org/ext/ddpreports/ViewSharedReport?&CF=&REPORT_ID=9147&REQUEST_TYPE=VIEWADVANCED (accessed December 10, 2009). Copyright © International Bank for Reconstruction and Development/The World Bank 2009.

force in the country, and they moved quickly to end the Soviet Union.

The Soviet Union was officially dissolved on December 21, 1991. Yeltsin became the president of an independent Russia. He had already embarked on a program of radical economic reforms, known as shock therapy, to end the communist economic system and force the country into a Western-style free-market economy. The result of these major changes was massive economic disruption. Inflation soared, wages for Russians fell, manufacturing output declined, and many Russians became unemployed. Some Russians were able to take advantage of the new system to become quite wealthy, but many more sank into poverty. In subsequent years the economy recovered somewhat, but poverty remained a serious problem.

Russian Poverty since the 1990s

According to the World Bank, in *Russian Federation: Reducing Poverty through Growth and Social Policy Reform* (February 8, 2005; http://194.84.38.65/mdb/upload/PAR_020805_eng.pdf), poverty in Russia was reduced by half, from 41.5% in 1999 to 19.6% in 2002, with an estimated 30 million people lifted above the poverty line during this period. In *Russian Economic Report* (April 2006, http://ns.worldbank.org.ru/files/rer/RER_12.1_eng.pdf), the World Bank notes that the Russian Ministry of the Economy projected that the percentage of those living below the country's poverty line had declined even further, from 17.8% in 2004 to 15.8% in 2005. However, the country felt the effects of the global recession that began

in 2007 and the World Bank projected in "Russian Federation: Country Brief 2009" (September 22, 2009, http://go.worldbank.org/3D0BHTWAG0) that the poverty rate would rise to 17.4% by the end of 2009.

According to the World Bank, in *Russian Federation*, the unemployment rate dropped dramatically in the Russian Federation, from a high of 13.2% in 1998 to 8.6% in 2002. The World Bank indicates in *Russian Economic Report* that the unemployment rate for 2005 was down to 7.6%. However, because of the global recession the World Bank projected in "Russian Federation: Country Brief 2009" that the Russian Federation unemployment rate would rise to 13% by the end of 2009.

The World Bank notes in *Russian Federation* that poverty in Russia is "shallow," meaning that most of the poor have incomes somewhere near the poverty line, with many people living just above it. Even though this makes for less depth of poverty, it also means that a greater number of people are vulnerable to economic fluctuations: the risk of falling into, or deeper into, poverty is greater for far more people.

The World Bank also indicates that certain segments of the Russian population are more likely to be poor than others. For children younger than the age of 16 the poverty rate was quite high, at 26.7% in 2002. People living in rural areas in the central and eastern parts of the Russian Federation had a poverty rate of 30.4%, compared with 15.7% for urban dwellers in 2002. Nonetheless, because the population is concentrated in urban areas, the number of poor people is actually higher in urban areas than in rural areas.

The Russian Federation also experiences greater disparities in regional income because the country is so large and has such a diversity of geographical features and varying degrees of remoteness, ranging from the huge metropolitan city of Moscow to the most isolated, inhospitable parts of southern Siberia. The World Bank points out that urban and rural Russians live with very different basic services, which are an indicator of poverty and standards of living. Even though at least 60% of all five income categories in urban areas had access to most infrastructural and utilities services in 2002, in rural areas access ranged from less than 20% of the poorest with access to hot water to barely 70% of the richest with running water.

The World Bank shows in "Macroeconomic Indicators: Russian Federation" (July 12, 2006, http://siteresources .worldbank.org/INTRUSSIANFEDERATION/Resources/ macromay2006.pdf) that the share of people living below the national subsistence level in 2005 was 15.8%, down from 27.3% in 2001. Table 1.2 in Chapter 1 indicates that from 2000 to 2006 a higher percentage (19.6%) of the people of the Russian Federation lived below the national poverty line, but this value spans a wide time frame during which poverty rates fell. The table also shows that less than 2% of the population of the Russian Federation lived on less than US $2 per day or US $1.25 per day from 2000 to 2007.

The article "Education in the Russian Federation" (*World Education News and Reviews*, December 2005, http://www.wes.org/ewenr/05dec/practical.htm) states that education in the Russian Federation in the post-Soviet years has seen a slight decline. During the Soviet years literacy was near 100%, and free, compulsory education was open to all. In 2003 the literacy rate had fallen from 100% to 99.6%. Prior to 1984 there were 10 years of compulsory schooling, beginning at the age of seven. By 2005 there were nine years of compulsory schooling, beginning at the age of six or seven. The Russian constitution guarantees tuition-free higher education, but since the early 1990s the federal budget has been unable to provide full public support. In addition, Kevin Watkins of the UNDP indicates in *Human Development Report 2006—Beyond Scarcity: Power, Poverty, and the Global Water Crisis* (2006, http://hdr.undp.org/en/media/HDR06-complete.pdf) that government spending on education in Russia, when measured as a percent of GDP, has fallen behind several former-Soviet countries in central and eastern Europe. In 2002–04, for example, Russia spent 3.7% of its GDP on education, whereas Estonia spent 5.7%; Latvia, 5.4%; and Lithuania, 5.2%.

According to the United Nations Children's Fund (UNICEF), in "Russian Federation" (2009, http://www .unicef.org/infobycountry/russia_statistics.html), the net primary school enrollment ratio (the percentage of students enrolled of all students of primary school age) was 91% for both boys and girls from 2003 to 2008. The gross primary school enrollment ratio (the percentage of students enrolled of any age) was 96% for both boys and girls. Table 6.4 shows that the net primary completion rate of students fell slightly from 94% in 2000 to 93% in 2007. Slightly fewer girls than boys completed primary school in the Russian Federation in 2005 (99 girls for every 100 boys) and in 2007 (98 girls for every 100 boys).

Perhaps most troubling is the decline in overall Russian health and its link to poverty since the economic transition. According to the World Health Organization (WHO), in "Russian Federation" (2010, http://www.who.int/countries/ rus/en/), life expectancy in the Russian Federation was 60 years for males and 73 years for females in 2006. Healthy life expectancy was 53 years for males and 64 years for females in 2003. Oleksiy Ivaschenko of the World Bank states in *Longevity in Russia's Regions: Do Poverty and Low Public Health Spending Kill?* (June 2004, http://www .wider.unu.edu/publications/working-papers/research-papers/ 2004/en_GB/rp2004-040/_files/78091744559563942/default/ rp2004-040.pdf) that life expectancy throughout the Russian Federation declined substantially between 1990 and 2000, by as much as seven years in some of the regions hit hardest by the depression into which the country sank following the 1991 collapse of the Soviet Union. Working-age men accounted for the majority of premature deaths—an estimated 1.3 million to 1.6 million between 1990 and 1995. Ivaschenko cites studies linking the rise in premature deaths to stress related to unemployment, low wages, poor diet, increased crime rates, and a dramatic rise in alcoholism—all associated with low income.

In *Global Tuberculosis Control: Surveillance, Planning, Financing* (2007, http://www.who.int/tb/publications/ global_report/2007/pdf/full.pdf), the WHO reports that Russia has also experienced an increase in the incidence of tuberculosis since 1991. The emergence of drug-resistant strains in particular has caused concern among health care professionals worldwide. The WHO notes in *Global Tuberculosis Control: A Short Update to the 2009 Report* (2009, http://www.who.int/tb/publications/global_report/ 2009/update/tbu_9.pdf) that in 2008, 20,888 people in the Russian Federation died of tuberculosis, 97,644 were living with the disease, and 150,898 new cases were diagnosed. The WHO refers to the Russian Federation as a "high burden" country with respect to tuberculosis infection.

In "Russian Federation" (December 2005, http:// www.who.int/hiv/HIVCP_RUS.pdf), the WHO explains that the incidence of HIV/AIDS has also increased, rising from 3,623 cases diagnosed in 1997 to 327,899 in 2005. UNICEF reports in "Russian Federation" that approximately 940,000 people in the Russian Federation were living with HIV/AIDS in 2007. Analysts point to the breakdown of the health care and social services systems, along with an increase in stress-related risky behavior, in the post-Soviet era.

ALCOHOLISM IN RUSSIA. Vodka has played an important role in Russian culture for centuries. Even before the economic crash of the 1990s and the shaky recovery during the first decade of the 21st century, alcoholism was common throughout the country. However, according to David A. Leon et al., in "Hazardous Alcohol Drinking and Premature Mortality in Russia: A Population Based Case-Control Study" (*Lancet*, vol. 369, no. 9578, June 16, 2007), leading up to the economic downturn in 2000, Russians turned to cheap counterfeit alcohol, homemade moonshine, and even deicing solvent and cologne as substitutes for vodka. The researchers suggest that this hazardous drinking contributed to "almost half of all deaths in working age men in a typical Russian city" between October 2003 and October 2005. Alex Rodriguez reports in "Alcohol Destroying Rural Russia" (*Chicago Tribune*, December 15, 2005) that as many as 40,000 Russians die of alcohol poisoning each year and that one-third of all deaths in the country are related in some way to alcohol abuse.

Rodriguez explains that poverty is one of the root causes of this problem: "Fifteen years of post-Soviet capitalism has left rural Russia straggling far behind. Russians in collective farms across the country's 11 time zones could count on a safety net of free housing and health care—and on regular paychecks—during the Soviet era. In today's Russia, those same villagers live day-to-day, shivering through stretches of winter without heat, cringing at the sight of their children in tattered school clothes."

CHAPTER 7
WOMEN AND CHILDREN IN POVERTY

Under-investing in women limits economic growth and slows down poverty reduction, which is one reason that countries with greater gender equality tend to have lower poverty rates. Evidence links increases in women's productivity and earnings to lower household poverty.

—World Bank, "The World Bank and Gender Equality" (October 2009)

Study after study shows that educated women are better equipped to earn income to support their families, more likely to invest in their children's health care, nutrition and education, and more inclined to participate in civic life and to advocate for community improvements.

—Her Majesty Queen Rania Al Abdullah of Jordan, United Nations Children's Fund's Eminent Advocate for Children, in *The State of the World's Children, 2009: Maternal and Newborn Health* (December 2008)

Most groups that study poverty—from international organizations such as the United Nations Children's Fund (UNICEF) and the World Bank to small local charities—agree that the most effective way to reduce poverty is to improve the social, economic, educational, and political situation of women and, by extension, children. Women's levels of health, education, and security affect those of their families. When a mother suffers the effects of poverty, future generations of her family do as well, creating a cycle of impoverishment that is difficult to escape.

GLOBAL CONVENTIONS ON THE RIGHTS OF WOMEN AND CHILDREN
Convention on the Rights of the Child

In November 1989 the United Nations (UN) adopted the treaty Convention on the Rights of the Child (CRC; http://www2.ohchr.org/english/law/crc.htm). Considered to be one of the most wide-ranging and important human rights documents the global community had ever agreed on, the CRC was charged with establishing "norms" and standards for the lives of children to which all countries would hold themselves accountable, including:

- Protection from violence, abuse, and abduction

- Protection from hazardous employment and exploitation

- Adequate nutrition

- Free compulsory primary education

- Adequate health care

- Equal treatment regardless of gender, race, or cultural background

The UN reports in the press release "Committee on Rights of Child to Hold Forty-sixth Session in Geneva from 17 September to 5 October 2007" (September 13, 2007, http://www.unog.ch/) that the CRC has become the most widely ratified human rights treaty in history. According to the UN (February 3, 2010, http://treaties.un.org/Pages/ViewDetails.aspx?src=TREATY&mtdsg_no=IV-11&chapter=4&lang=en), the CRC has been ratified by 193 countries. Only two countries have not ratified it: Somalia and the United States. Ratification by the United States has been hampered by the fact that the CRC forbids capital punishment of minors. Before the U.S. Supreme Court outlawed it in *Roper v. Simmons* (543 U.S. 551 [2005]), several states had allowed the death penalty for those who were between 16 and 18 years old at the time they committed their crime.

The United States signed the Treaty on the Rights of the Child (gave preliminary endorsement) in February 1995, which signified that the country would, in good faith, avoid practices that countered the purpose and ideals of the treaty. Ratification is a country's consent to be legally bound by the treaty. As of February 2010, in spite of the 2005 Supreme Court ruling forbidding the capital punishment of minors, the treaty had not yet been ratified by the U.S. Senate.

Beijing Declaration and Platform for Action

In September 1995 at the UN Fourth World Conference on Women in Beijing, China, representatives from 189 countries unanimously adopted a program intended to promote gender equality around the world, which became known as the *Beijing Declaration* (http://www.un.org/womenwatch/daw/beijing/beijingdeclaration.html) and the *Platform for Action* (http://www.un.org/womenwatch/daw/beijing/platform/index.html). One of the main goals outlined by the *Platform for Action* was addressing the enormous increase of women living in poverty in the late 20th century—a trend that has come to be known as the "feminization of poverty." The platform sought to:

- Review, adopt, and maintain macroeconomic policies and development strategies that address the needs and efforts of women in poverty

- Revise laws and administrative practices to ensure women's equal rights and access to economic resources

- Provide women with access to savings and credit mechanisms and institutions

- Develop gender-based methodologies and conduct research to address the feminization of poverty

The *Platform for Action* also required the 189 countries that adopted the platform to each develop a National Plan of Action to implement the platform locally. In June 2000, five years after the 1995 conference, the UN General Assembly adopted a political declaration (http://www.stopvaw.org/sites/3f6d15f4-c12d-4515-8544-26b7a3a5a41e/uploads/Political_Dec_Beijing.pdf) that reaffirmed the member states' commitment to the objectives in the *Beijing Declaration* and the *Platform for Action*. It also agreed to regularly assess progress on these objectives.

For the 10th anniversary of the *Beijing Declaration* and the *Platform for Action* (often called Beijing +10), the UN Department of Economic and Social Affairs Commission of the Status of Women (http://www.un.org/womenwatch/daw/csw/csw49/documents.html), during its 49th session from February to March 2005, reviewed and appraised progress that had been made.

In the press release "Beijing at Ten: Achieving Gender Equality, Development, and Peace" (January 31, 2005, http://www.un.org/womenwatch/daw/Review/documents/Beijing%20Press%20Eng_1.pdf), the UN quotes Rachel Mayanja, the special adviser to the secretary-general on gender issues and advancement of women, on Beijing +10: "A lot of progress has been made since Beijing. We are seeing more equitable laws that protect women from discrimination, abuse, and violence. However, there is much more that needs to be done to put the *Platform for Action* into practice, especially in terms of alleviating poverty, improving health, creating opportunity for economic advancement and political leadership, and reducing human

rights violations." Moving forward, priority themes were adopted for upcoming years and included the elimination of discrimination and violence against female children, financing for gender equality and the empowerment of women, and the equal sharing of responsibilities between women and men. Beijing +15 was held in March 2010. According to the UN Division for the Advancement of Women (February 25, 2010, http://www.un.org/womenwatch/daw/beijing15/regional_review.html), "Each of the five UN regional commissions is preparing regional review reports, and intergovernmental meetings are being organized to contribute to the global review process in the Commission on the Status of Women."

Millennium Development Goals

In September 2000 all member countries of the UN pledged to meet eight human development goals outlined in the Millennium Campaign, an international effort to eradicate extreme poverty, along with its causes and consequences. (See Table 2.6 in Chapter 2.) These Millennium Development Goals (MDGs) include four that specifically address the needs and challenges of women and children affected by poverty:

- Achieve universal primary education

- Promote gender equality and empower women

- Reduce child mortality

- Improve maternal health

The standards of the CRC, the *Beijing Declaration*, the *Platform for Action*, and the Millennium Campaign together have led to a global acknowledgment that the protection of children and the eradication of gender disparities are essential to combating poverty. Throughout this book, progress toward the MDGs has been reviewed in various contexts, and Chapter 10 does a final review. This chapter will focus on progress being made toward MDGs that affect women and children. MDG data will be supplemented with data from other sources to provide a global view of progress in the economics, health, and education of women and children and in combating abuse and violence toward them.

Another view of the progress of countries on gender issues is the Gender-Related Development Index (GDI). The GDI ranks for 155 countries for 2007 are shown in Table 7.1. In *Human Development Report 2006—Beyond Scarcity: Power, Poverty, and the Global Water Crisis* (2006, http://hdr.undp.org/en/media/HDR06-complete.pdf), Kevin Watkins of the UN Development Programme (UNDP) explains the GDI in a way that clarifies its purpose well: "The GDI is not a measure of *gender inequality*. Rather, it is a measure of *human development* that adjusts the human development index (HDI) to penalize for disparities between women and men in the three dimensions of the HDI: a long and healthy life, knowledge

TABLE 7.1

Gender-related development index ranks for 155 countries and areas, 2007

1 Australia	41 Chile	81 Jamaica	121 Kenya
2 Norway	42 Lithuania	82 Paraguay	122 Yemen
3 Iceland	43 Croatia	83 Sri Lanka	123 Bangladesh
4 Canada	44 Latvia	84 Tunisia	124 Pakistan
5 Sweden	45 Uruguay	85 Gabon	125 Tanzania (United Republic of)
6 France	46 Argentina	86 Philippines	126 Ghana
7 Netherlands	47 Costa Rica	87 Jordan	127 Sudan
8 Finland	48 Mexico	88 Algeria	128 Mauritania
9 Spain	49 Cuba	89 El Salvador	129 Cameroon
10 Ireland	50 Bulgaria	90 Fiji	130 Djibouti
11 Belgium	51 Panama	91 Bolivia	131 Uganda
12 Denmark	52 Romania	92 Mongolia	132 Lesotho
13 Switzerland	53 Trinidad and Tobago	93 Indonesia	133 Nigeria
14 Japan	54 Libyan Arab Jamahiriya	94 Viet Nam	134 Malawi
15 Italy	55 Venezuela (Bolivarian Republic of)	95 Honduras	135 Benin
16 Luxembourg	56 Oman	96 Guyana	136 Zambia
17 United Kingdom	57 Belarus	97 Moldova	137 Côte d'Ivoire
18 New Zealand	58 Malaysia	98 Syrian Arab Republic	138 Eritrea
19 United States	59 Russian Federation	99 Uzbekistan	139 Rwanda
20 Germany	60 Saudi Arabia	100 Kyrgyzstan	140 Senegal
21 Greece	61 Albania	101 Cape Verde	141 Gambia
22 Hong Kong, China (SAR)	62 Macedonia (the Former Yugoslav Rep. of)	102 Equatorial Guinea	142 Liberia
23 Austria	63 Brazil	103 Guatemala	143 Guinea
24 Slovenia	64 Colombia	104 Vanuatu	144 Ethiopia
25 Korea (Republic of)	65 Peru	105 Botswana	145 Mozambique
26 Israel	66 Kazakhstan	106 Nicaragua	146 Burundi
27 Cyprus	67 Mauritius	107 Tajikistan	147 Burkina Faso
28 Portugal	68 Armenia	108 Namibia	148 Guinea-Bissau
29 Brunei Darussalam	69 Ukraine	109 South Africa	149 Chad
30 Barbados	70 Turkey	110 Sao Tome and Principe	150 Congo (Democratic Republic of the)
31 Czech Republic	71 Lebanon	111 Morocco	151 Central African Republic
32 Malta	72 Thailand	112 Lao People's Democratic Republic	152 Sierra Leone
33 Bahrain	73 Azerbaijan	113 Bhutan	153 Mali
34 Kuwait	74 Dominican Republic	114 India	154 Afghanistan
35 Qatar	75 China	115 Congo	155 Niger
36 Estonia	76 Iran (Islamic Republic of)	116 Cambodia	
37 Hungary	77 Maldives	117 Comoros	
38 United Arab Emirates	78 Tonga	118 Swaziland	
39 Poland	79 Suriname	119 Nepal	
40 Slovakia	80 Samoa	120 Madagascar	

SOURCE: Jeni Klugman, "GDI Ranks for 155 Countries and Areas," in *Human Development Report 2009—Overcoming Barriers: Human Mobility and Development*, United Nations Development Programme (UNDP), published 2009, Palgrave Macmillan, http://hdr.undp.org/en/media/HDR 2009 EN Complete .pdf (accessed November 22, 2009). Reproduced with permission of Palgrave Macmillan.

and a decent standard of living (as measured by estimated earned income)." Per Table 7.1, developed countries have the highest GDI ranks and less developed countries have the lowest. For 2007 Australia ranked highest, Canada was fourth, and the United States was 19th.

WAGES

The UN Development Fund for Women (UNIFEM) explains in *Progress of the World's Women 2008/2009: Who Answers to Women?—Gender and Accountability* (October 2008, http://www.unifem.org/progress/2008/ media/POWW08_Report_Full_Text.pdf) that even though globalization has brought new opportunities in the workplace:

> Gender biases in labour markets have meant that women's productive potential is less effectively tapped than men's and that women have been more concentrated than men in informal, subsistence and vulnerable employment. In the last decade, more than 200 million women have joined the global labour force. In 2007,

there were 1.2 billion women in paid work, compared with 1.8 billion men. An indicator of the accountability challenge they continue to face in formal employment is the gender wage gap, standing at a global average of about 17 per cent, and which tends to be higher in private than in public sector employment.

Figure 7.1 shows average female earnings as a percentage of male earnings in selected occupations. In central and eastern Europe and the Commonwealth of Independent States (CIS) wages are about equal for men and women (shown at the 100% mark) who are primary school teachers, hotel receptionists, or nurses. In these parts of the world, female computer programmers make about 18% more than men do and female accountants make about 65% more than men do. However, in central and eastern Europe and the CIS, as well as in industrialized economies and developing economies, women generally make less money than men for the same jobs.

UNIFEM notes that globalization has led to a demand for women in jobs that are labor intensive, such

FIGURE 7.1

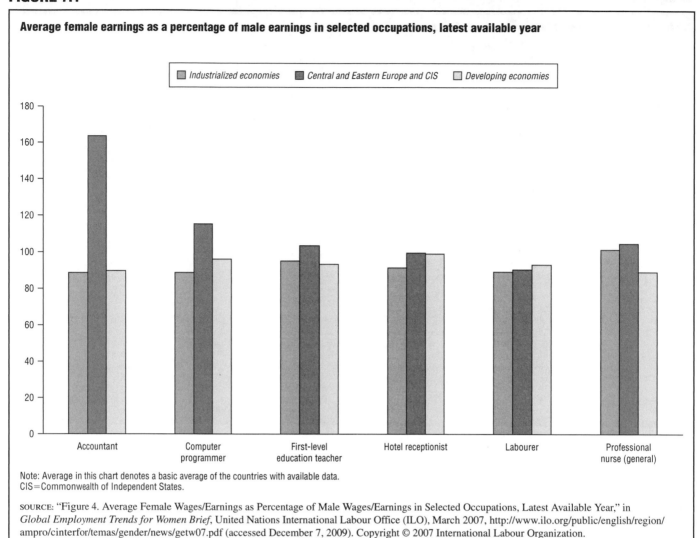

Average female earnings as a percentage of male earnings in selected occupations, latest available year

☐ *Industrialized economies*　　■ *Central and Eastern Europe and CIS*　　☐ *Developing economies*

Note: Average in this chart denotes a basic average of the countries with available data.
CIS=Commonwealth of Independent States.

SOURCE: "Figure 4. Average Female Wages/Earnings as Percentage of Male Wages/Earnings in Selected Occupations, Latest Available Year," in *Global Employment Trends for Women Brief*, United Nations International Labour Office (ILO), March 2007, http://www.ilo.org/public/english/region/ampro/cinterfor/temas/gender/news/getw07.pdf (accessed December 7, 2009). Copyright © 2007 International Labour Organization.

as those in agriculture and clothing. Furthermore, the outsourcing of services has opened up new opportunities for women in call centers of various types. Women are used as a flexible labor force that is hired or fired as market needs change. They are attractive to employers because they can usually be hired without being paid benefits. Moreover, employers find it easy to justify paying women low wages because they are often thought of as just making extra income. Thus, gender discrimination in the workplace continues, with many women working without job security or benefits. UNIFEM states that "there is a strong link between insecure informal employment, especially home-based work, and poverty" and adds that it has become increasingly difficult for governments to play a role in overseeing the global marketplace and its workers' rights due to the international nature of large corporations and restrictions of international trade agreements.

Martha Chen et al. identify in *Progress of the World's Women 2005: Women, Work, and Poverty* (August 2005, http://www.un-ngls.org/women-2005.pdf) four dimensions that create the relationship between work (paid and unpaid) and poverty for women:

• The temporal dimension: Because women spend more time doing unpaid work within the home, performing housework and child care, they have less time to spend doing paid work outside the home, even though studies show that women spend more time working overall than men do. This means that women tend to do more part-time paid work, which in turn means that they earn less money. In developing countries women spend much of their unpaid time performing heavier physical chores such as collecting water and fuel and growing and harvesting crops, leaving them even less time for paid work and for child care.

• The spatial dimension: Women in both developing and developed countries are sometimes forced to migrate to other areas, regions, or even countries to find paid work. This might mean leaving a rural home to work in a city (or vice versa) or migrating from, for example, a country such as Mexico to perform seasonal farm work in a country such as the United States. In either case, a woman who migrates for work will have to find someone to care for her family while she is away. At the same time, women who have children are often not able to migrate to regions with better work opportunities.

- The employment segmentation dimension: Women's traditional role as caretakers within the home has led to a narrow choice of work outside the home. Without specific training or education, women in almost every culture tend to fall into the same occupations: domestic servants, clothing and textile workers, teachers, and care workers. These occupations are relatively unstable, informal, lower paying, and, in some cases (such as in the textile industry), more dangerous than other jobs.

- The valuation dimension: The value placed on work that is seen as traditionally female is related to employment segmentation. "Women's work," meaning the kind of work that women typically do for free within their home and community, is generally considered less valuable than work that is perceived to require more training or education. Therefore, it is less regulated and brings in lower pay.

Gender is not the only factor that determines women's greater likelihood of impoverishment and difficulty obtaining and holding on to work. In different cultures religion, race, and especially class play a role. However, as the previously described dimensions of work demonstrate, women in general—in nearly every culture—experience living and working conditions that make economic advancement difficult.

The United States

According to the U.S. Bureau of Labor Statistics (BLS), in *Women in the Labor Force: A Databook* (September 2009, http://www.bls.gov/cps/wlf-databook-2009.pdf), the median (average) weekly full-time earnings of females in the United States 16 years and older in 2008 were 79.9% of the earnings of males of the same age group. In 2008 African-American and Hispanic women had median earnings of 89.4% and 89.6%, respectively, of what men of their ethnicities earned, and white and Asian-American women had median earnings of 79.3% and 78%, respectively, of what men of their ethnicities earned. This pay inequity exists in spite of the Equal Pay Act of 1963, which outlaws unequal pay for equal work. However, these figures do not compare earnings job for job, but simply the median full-time earnings across full-time jobs. Job-for-job comparisons are shown in Figure 7.1 for selected jobs, but these comparisons are not specific to the United States. The United States is included in the bars showing percentages for industrialized economies.

The BLS notes in *A Profile of the Working Poor, 2007* (March 2009, http://www.bls.gov/cps/cpswp2007.pdf) that among U.S. workers active in the labor force for at least 27 weeks during 2007, a slightly higher percentage of women (5.8%) than men (4.6%) lived in poverty. However, for working families (those with at least one family member in the labor force for half the year or more) the rates displayed a wider gap, with families headed by women (23.6%) experiencing a significantly higher poverty rate than families headed by men (11.7%).

Canada

In "Average Earnings by Sex and Work Pattern" (June 2, 2009, http://www40.statcan.ca/l01/cst01/labor01a-eng.htm), Statistics Canada reports that as of 2007 the earnings ratio of women working full time for the full year to men working the same was 65.7%—that is, for every dollar of income for men, women made only $0.66. In 2007 men working in Canada earned an average income of CAD $44,400, whereas women earned an average income of CAD $29,200.

Statistics Canada uses the phrase "low income after tax" to refer to its national line of relative poverty. The statistical agency reports in *Income in Canada 2007* (June 2009, http://www.statcan.gc.ca/pub/75-202-x/75-202-x2007000-eng.pdf) that unmarried women under the age of 65 had an incidence of low income after tax (relative poverty) of 35.1% in 2007, down from 39.3% in 2004 and 45.8% in 1998.

Children under the age of 18 who lived in a household headed by a single female parent suffered a much higher incidence of relative poverty (26.6%) than children living in two-parent families (6.5%). However, this percentage had dropped as well, from 40.4% in 2004 and 46.2% in 1998. Statistics Canada notes in "Average Total Income by Economic Family Types" (June 2, 2009, http://www40.statcan.gc.ca/l01/cst01/famil05a-eng.htm) that the average total income in families headed by single women (CAD $42,900) was significantly less in 2007 than in families headed by single men (CAD $63,000).

The European Union

The European Union (EU) is a confederation of 27 sovereign states that allows people to move and trade freely among member countries. The EA (Economic Area) 16 is a group of member countries that have adopted the euro as their common currency. The EA-16 consists of Austria, Belgium, Cyprus, Finland, France, Germany, Greece, Ireland, Italy, Luxembourg, Malta, the Netherlands, Portugal, Slovakia, Slovenia, and Spain. The EU-27 consists of the EA-16 plus Bulgaria, Denmark, the Czech Republic, Estonia, Hungary, Latvia, Lithuania, Poland, Romania, Sweden, and the United Kingdom. In *The Social Situation in the European Union, 2008* (May 2009), the European Commission indicates that in 2007 women's earnings averaged 17% lower than men's in the EU-27 and in the EA-16.

UNEMPLOYMENT

The International Labour Office (ILO) reports in *Global Employment Trends for Women* (March 2009, http://www.ilo.org/wcmsp5/groups/public/—dgreports/—dcomm/documents/publication/wcms_103456.pdf) that not only are women paid less than men in the workplace but also they have, in general, higher rates of unemployment. Worldwide, the average unemployment rate for women (6.3%) was only slightly higher than that for men (5.9%) in 2008. (See Table 7.2.) However, the disparities in male-female unemployment rates vary throughout the world. The largest gap in 2008 was in the Middle East and North Africa, where the unemployment rates for men were 8.2% and 8.5%, respectively, whereas the unemployment rates for women were 13.4% and 16.1%, respectively. Thus, the unemployment rate gaps were 5.2 percentage points in the Middle East and 7.6 percentage points in North Africa.

Table 7.2 shows that the next largest unemployment gap in 2008 was in Latin America and the Caribbean, with the unemployment rate for men at 5.8% and the rate for women at 9.3%—a gap of 3.5 percentage points. The differences in male-female unemployment rates were small in the developed economies and the EU, central and southeastern Europe (non-EU) and the CIS, East Asia, Southeast Asia and the Pacific, South Asia, and sub-Saharan Africa. Central and southeastern Europe (non-EU) and the CIS and East Asia were the only regions of the world in which the unemployment rates of men were above the rates for women in 2008, but the differences were small.

WOMEN'S REPRODUCTIVE HEALTH AND POVERTY

It is not surprising that poor people suffer from more health problems and receive a lower quality of health care than their nonpoor counterparts. Women, however, suffer disproportionately: first, because there simply are more poor women than poor men in the world; and second, as the bearers of children, women face an increased set of

TABLE 7.2

Percent unemployed, world and regions, by sex, 1998–2008

	1998	1999	2000	2001	2002	2003	2004	2005	2006	2007	2008*
Both sexes											
World	6.1	6.2	6.1	6.1	6.1	6.3	6.3	6.2	6.0	5.7	6.0
Developed Economies and European Union	7.1	6.9	6.7	6.7	7.4	7.3	7.2	6.9	6.3	5.7	6.7
Central and South Eastern Europe (non-EU) & CIS	12.1	12.4	10.5	10.2	9.9	9.9	9.6	9.2	9.1	8.4	8.7
East Asia	4.3	4.3	4.1	4.1	4.0	3.9	3.8	3.8	3.6	3.4	3.9
South-East Asia and the Pacific	4.8	5.1	5.0	5.8	6.1	6.2	6.4	6.1	6.2	5.5	5.6
South Asia	3.7	4.0	4.5	3.8	3.3	4.5	5.3	5.4	5.4	5.4	5.4
Latin America and the Caribbean	8.2	8.5	8.3	8.3	8.6	8.5	8.2	7.9	7.3	7.0	7.3
Middle East	11.1	10.6	10.1	11.6	11.7	11.8	9.2	9.8	9.8	9.4	9.4
North Africa	13.0	13.6	14.3	13.8	13.6	13.2	12.4	11.6	10.5	10.8	10.7
Sub-Saharan Africa	7.3	8.1	8.2	8.4	8.2	8.1	8.4	8.3	8.2	8.1	8.0
Males											
World	5.9	6.0	5.9	5.9	5.9	6.1	6.1	6.0	5.8	5.5	5.9
Developed Economies and European Union	6.6	6.5	6.2	6.4	7.2	7.2	6.9	6.6	6.0	5.5	6.6
Central and South Eastern Europe (non-EU) & CIS	11.9	12.1	10.3	10.2	10.1	10.3	9.8	9.4	9.3	8.6	9.0
East Asia	4.9	4.9	4.7	4.7	4.5	4.4	4.4	4.3	4.1	3.9	4.5
South-East Asia and the Pacific	4.5	4.8	5.0	5.6	5.7	5.7	5.9	5.6	5.7	5.3	5.3
South Asia	3.6	3.9	4.4	3.7	3.1	4.3	5.0	5.1	5.1	5.1	5.2
Latin America and the Caribbean	6.7	7.0	6.9	6.8	7.1	6.9	6.5	6.3	5.7	5.6	5.8
Middle East	9.8	9.4	9.0	10.3	10.3	10.7	8.0	8.5	8.5	8.2	8.2
North Africa	11.3	12.0	12.4	11.8	11.5	11.1	10.2	9.4	8.4	8.7	8.5
Sub-Saharan Africa	7.3	7.7	7.9	8.1	8.2	8.1	8.1	8.0	7.9	7.7	7.7
Females											
World	6.4	6.6	6.3	6.4	6.4	6.5	6.7	6.6	6.3	6.0	6.3
Developed Economies and European Union	7.8	7.5	7.3	7.1	7.6	7.5	7.5	7.2	6.6	6.0	6.8
Central and South Eastern Europe (non-EU) & CIS	12. 3	12.7	10.8	10.2	9.6	9.4	9.4	9.0	8.9	8.1	8.4
East Asia	3.6	3.6	3.4	3.4	3.3	3.2	3.2	3.2	3.0	2.9	3.3
South-East Asia and the Pacific	5.2	5.5	4.9	6.1	6.6	7.0	7.2	6.9	6.8	5.8	6.0
South Asia	4.1	4.4	4.6	4.2	3.7	4.9	6.0	6.1	6.0	6.0	6.0
Latin America and the Caribbean	10.8	11.0	10.7	10.7	10.9	11.0	10.7	10.3	9.4	9.1	9.3
Middle East	16.1	15.2	14.1	16.6	16.6	15.9	13.1	14.1	14.0	13.4	13.4
North Africa	18.3	18.5	19.7	19.4	19.5	19.1	18.3	17.6	15.9	16.3	16.1
Sub-Saharan Africa	7.3	8.7	8.5	8.9	8.3	8.0	8.9	8.7	8.6	8.4	8.3

*2008 are preliminary estimates
CIS = Commonwealth Independent States.
EU = European Union.

SOURCE: "Table A2. Unemployment Rate, World and Regions," in *Global Employment Trends for Women*, International Labour Office (ILO), March 2009, http://www.ilo.org/wcmsp5/groups/public/--dgreports/--dcomm/documents/publication/wcms_103456.pdf (accessed December 7, 2009). Copyright © 2009 International Labour Organization.

health issues related to their reproductive systems and to childbearing.

The MDG of improving maternal health, as opposed to women's health, points to the significance of reproduction in the overall picture of women's health and to the social and economic status of their families. Included in reproductive rights are issues such as violence against women, as well as the right to marry voluntarily, to time the birth of children as desired, to receive clear and accurate information about the reproductive process, and to benefit from scientific progress. For women living in low-income countries, these rights cannot be taken for granted. In fact, many women are prohibited from using contraception—or from even receiving information about it—and must marry whomever their families choose for them. In some cultures going against these conventions can place the woman in a position that results in physical and emotional violence. The inability to decide how many children to have or how many years apart to have them can easily overwhelm a family's finances, particularly a family that is already poor.

Maternal Death

The World Health Organization (WHO) lists causes of maternal death in *World Health Report 2005: Make Every Mother and Child Count* (2005, http://www.who.int/whr/ 2005/whr2005_en.pdf). These causes include severe bleeding, infections, obstructed labor, unsafe abortion, and eclampsia (seizures brought on by seriously high blood pressure during pregnancy). The World Bank adds in *World Development Indicators 2007* (April 2007, http://web.world bank.org/) that malnutrition, frequent pregnancies, and inadequate health care during pregnancy and delivery also contribute to maternal mortality.

Table 7.3 shows numbers of maternal deaths and death ratios (deaths per 100,000 live births) for world regions. The difference in maternal death ratios between developed regions and developing regions is striking. In 2005 there were 9 maternal deaths per 100,000 live births in developed regions, compared with 450 maternal deaths per 100,000 live births in developing regions. In developed regions the lifetime risk of maternal death was 1 in 7,300. In developing regions the lifetime risk was 1 in 75—a 100-fold difference. Sub-Saharan Africa had the highest maternal death ratio in the world at 900 maternal deaths per 100,000 live births and the highest lifetime risk of maternal death at 1 in 22.

Because most maternal deaths occur in already impoverished countries that are clustered together geographically, their regional impact is particularly acute. At the most personal level, children who lose their mother tend to experience emotional problems that may make

TABLE 7.3

Maternal mortality rates, number, and lifetime risk, by world region, 2005

Region	MMR[a] (maternal deaths per 100,000 live births)[b]	Number of maternal deaths[b]	Lifetime risk of maternal death[b]: 1 in:	Range of uncertainty on MMR[a] estimates	
				Lower estimate	Upper estimate
World total	400	536,000	92	220	650
Developed regions[c]	9	960	7,300	8	17
Countries of the Commonwealth of Independent States (CIS)[d]	51	1,800	1,200	28	140
Developing Regions	450	533,000	75	240	730
Africa	820	276,000	26	410	1,400
Northern Africa[e]	160	5,700	210	85	290
Sub-Saharan Africa	900	270,000	22	450	1,500
Asia	330	241,000	120	190	520
Eastern Asia	50	9,200	1,200	31	80
South Asia	490	188,000	61	290	750
South-Eastern Asia	300	35,000	130	160	550
Western Asia	160	8,300	170	62	340
Latin America and the Caribbean	130	15,000	290	81	230
Oceania	430	890	62	120	1,200

[a]MMR = maternal mortality rates.
[b]The MMR and lifetime risk have been rounded according to the following scheme: < 100, no rounding; 100–999, rounded to nearest 10; and >1,000, rounded to nearest 100. The numbers of maternal deaths have been rounded as follows: <1,000, rounded to nearest 10,1,000–9,999, rounded to nearest 100; and >10,000, rounded to nearest 1,000.
[c]Includes Albania, Australia, Austria, Belgium, Bosnia, and Herzegovina, Bulgaria, Canada, Croatia, Czech Republic, Denmark, Estonia, Finland, France, Germany, Greece, Hungary, Iceland, Ireland, Italy, Japan, Latvia, Lithuania, Luxembourg, Malta, the Netherlands, New Zealand, Norway, Poland, Portugal, Romania, Serbia, Montenegro (Serbia and Montenegro became separate independent entities in 2006), Slovakia, Slovenia, Spain, Sweden, Switzerland, the former Yugoslav Republic of Macedonia, the United Kingdom, and the United States of America.
[d]The CIS countries are Armenia, Azerbaijan, Belarus, Georgia, Kazakhstan, Krygystan, Tajikistan, Turkmenistan, Uzbekistan, the Republic of Moldova, the Russian Federation and Ukraine.
[e]Excludes Sudan, which is included in sub-Saharan Africa.

SOURCE: Joy Moncrieffe, "Table 1. Estimates of MMR Number of Maternal Deaths, Lifetime Risk, and Range of Uncertainty by United Nations MDG Regions, 2005," in *The State of the World Population 2008: Reaching Common Ground: Culture, Gender and Human Rights*, United Nations Population Fund (UNFPA), 2008, http://www.unfpa.org/upload/lib_pub_file/816_filename_en-swop08-report.pdf (accessed December 9, 2009). Non-UN agency data from The World Bank, 2007.

them less productive as adults, and households lose valuable income without an adult female wage earner. In fact, many families, in the time leading up to a mother's death, are pushed over the brink of poverty as a result of the high cost of health care when a mother becomes sick. Communities feel the loss because women in developing countries perform so many essential unpaid tasks, such as caring for children and elders, growing and harvesting food, and gathering fuel and water. High rates of maternal deaths affect the overall economic situation in a region in terms of lost productivity and lost potential for economic, cultural, and technological expansion.

Access to Skilled Reproductive Health Care

Many maternal deaths can be prevented with increased access to skilled health care before, during, and after childbirth. However, poor women are far less likely to have a skilled attendant present during the births of their children. For example, in Latin America and the Caribbean nearly 100% of the births of the wealthiest women were attended by a skilled health professional from 1998 to 2006, whereas just under 50% of the births of the poorest women were. (See Figure 7.2.) The disparity was similar

in the Asia/North Africa region, where over 90% of the births of the wealthiest women were attended by a skilled health professional and 50% of the births of the poorest women were attended. The situation for poor women in sub-Saharan Africa was even more dire: just under 90% of the births of the wealthiest women were attended by a skilled health professional, whereas only 27% of the births of the poorest women were. Clearly, the world's poorest women do not have reproductive rights equal to those of their nonpoor counterparts.

Not only do women living in poverty have less access to skilled health care during childbirth but also the proportion of women who see skilled health care professionals during their pregnancies is low. Both UNICEF and the WHO recommend that pregnant women see a skilled health professional at least four times during pregnancy to detect and treat possible health problems and to receive prenatal education and vitamins. Figure 7.3 shows the proportion of women who were attended four or more times during their pregnancy by a skilled health professional by world region from 2003 to 2008. Overall, in the developing regions of the world slightly less than half (47%) of women saw a health professional four times or more during their pregnancy. The percentage was lowest in southern Asia, at 36%, and highest in Latin America and the Caribbean, at 83%.

Contraception

The lack of appropriate reproductive health care, reproductive rights, and family planning options most strongly affects poor young women, who may not be prepared for pregnancy and parenthood physically, emotionally, or financially. The availability of contraceptives and education about reproductive processes and contraceptive use are necessary factors for young women to help them control their reproduction. Figure 7.4 shows the average level of unmet need and the total demand for family planning (contraception) by level of household wealth and world region. The figure shows that as household wealth increases, the demand for contraception increases and the unmet need for contraception decreases. That is, a lower proportion of poor women seek out contraception compared with women with greater monetary resources, and a lower proportion of poor women have their contraceptive needs met than women having greater monetary resources. The demand for contraception is lowest among women of all levels of household wealth in sub-Saharan Africa, compared with women of all levels of household wealth in Asia/ northern Africa and Latin America and the Caribbean. Likewise, the unmet need for contraception is greater overall in sub-Saharan Africa.

Even though much progress is still to be made in meeting contraceptive need, contraceptive use increased between 1990 and 2005 in the developing world. Figure 7.5 reveals that contraceptive use in developing regions increased

FIGURE 7.2

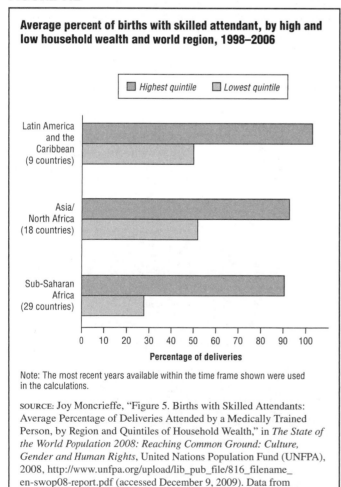

Average percent of births with skilled attendant, by high and low household wealth and world region, 1998–2006

Note: The most recent years available within the time frame shown were used in the calculations.

SOURCE: Joy Moncrieffe, "Figure 5. Births with Skilled Attendants: Average Percentage of Deliveries Attended by a Medically Trained Person, by Region and Quintiles of Household Wealth," in *The State of the World Population 2008: Reaching Common Ground: Culture, Gender and Human Rights*, United Nations Population Fund (UNFPA), 2008, http://www.unfpa.org/upload/lib_pub_file/816_filename_en-swop08-report.pdf (accessed December 9, 2009). Data from *Proportion of Births Attended by a Skilled Attendant—2007 Updates*, World Health Organization, 2007.

FIGURE 7.3

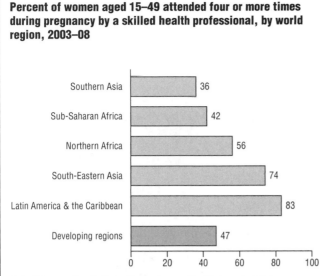

Percent of women aged 15–49 attended four or more times during pregnancy by a skilled health professional, by world region, 2003–08

Note: Data are not available for the Commonwealth of Independent States, Eastern Asia, Western Asia or Oceania. The most recent years available within the time frame shown were used in the calculations.

SOURCE: "Proportion of Women (15–49 Years Old) Attended Four or More Times during Pregnancy by Skilled Health Personnel, 2003/2008," in *The Millennium Development Goals Report 2009*, © United Nations, 2009, http://www.un.org/millenniumgoals/pdf/MDG_Report_2009_ENG.pdf (accessed December 5, 2009). The United Nations is the author of the original material. Reproduced with permission.

from 50% of married women aged 15 to 49 in 1990 to 62% in 2005. The greatest increase was 16 percentage points in northern Africa, from 44% of women using contraception in 1990 to 60% using contraception in 2005. Close behind in increase of contraceptive use was southern Asia, with an increase of 15 percentage points, from 39% in 1990 to 54% in 2005. Eastern Asia had the lowest increase in the use of contraception at eight percentage points, from 78% in 1990 to 86% in 2005. Contraceptive use in developed regions of the world remained unchanged at 67% between 1990 and 2005.

Childbearing in Young Women

Figure 7.4 shows a positive correlation between household wealth and contraceptive demand: as one rises, so does the other. Thus, poorer women ask for contraceptives less and the needs they express are not as often met. Figure 7.6 shows the average number of children born per woman by region and level of household wealth from 1990 to 2005. As expected from the contraceptive data, a positive correlation also exists between household wealth and average number of children per woman. Women who have the lowest level of household wealth have more children than women who have the highest level of household wealth. That is, those who can afford children the least, have the most children. In sub-Saharan Africa the poorest women had, on average, from six to

seven children, whereas women with higher household incomes had an average of four children from 1990 to 2005. In Latin American and the Caribbean the disparity was even greater: the poorest women had an average of six children, whereas women of better financial means had an average of two.

Figure 7.7 shows the number of births per 1,000 women aged 15 to 19 in 1990 and 2006 for various regions of the world. The birth rate in this adolescent age group is an indicator of the burden of fertility on young women. In addition, women who are adolescents and become pregnant are more likely to die or experience complications during pregnancy and childbirth than are older females. Their babies are at higher risk of dying before the age of one as well.

The birth rate estimated for adolescents in developed regions of the world was 22 per 1,000 women aged 15 to 19 in 2006, down from 35 per 1,000 women in 1990. (See Figure 7.7.) For adolescents in developing regions, the birth rate was 53 per 1,000 women in 2006, down from 67 per 1,000 women in 1990. In 2006 the adolescent birth rate was the highest in sub-Saharan Africa (an under-developed region) at 123 per 1,000 women, down from 131 per 1,000 women in 1990. Eastern Asia (an emerging and transition region) had the lowest adolescent birth rate in both 1990 and 2006. In 2006 the adolescent birth rate in Eastern Asia was 5 per 1,000 women, down from 21 per 1,000 women in 1990.

Figure 7.8 depicts how pregnancy early in a girl's life might affect the ability of her and those in her household to move out of poverty. Factors that affect populations, such as child-rearing norms, are shown at the top of the figure, while household and individual factors are shown lower in the figure. The direction of the arrow indicates the direction of the link. For example, labor markets affect incomes, and adolescent pregnancy brings with it a higher risk of pregnancy-related complications, such as infant mortality. Thus, factors such as these examples are linked with arrows and create interconnected pathways that bear on a family's resources (income and consumption).

Obstetric Fistula

One of the most serious health and social consequences of childbirth in poor countries—particularly in sub-Saharan Africa and South Asia—is the development of obstetric fistula. This childbirth-related injury is caused by exceptionally long labor—often as long as five to seven days—that cuts off blood flow to the vagina, bladder, and/or rectum. Areas of tissue that are severely deprived of oxygen die due to the lack of blood flow. The resulting holes in the tissue leave women unable to control the flow of urine and feces, which leak out constantly. Nerve damage to the legs, severe infections, and kidney disease are also common among fistula sufferers.

FIGURE 7.4

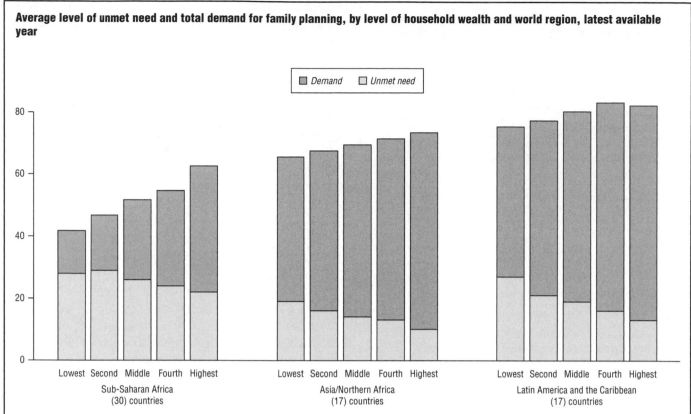

Average level of unmet need and total demand for family planning, by level of household wealth and world region, latest available year

Legend: ■ Demand □ Unmet need

Note: Unweighted averages based on the most recent available survey for each country.

SOURCE: Joy Moncrieffe, "Figure 3. Mean Level of Unmet Need and Total Demand for Family Planning, by Region and Quintiles of Household Wealth," in *The State of the World Population 2008: Reaching Common Ground: Culture, Gender and Human Rights*, United Nations Population Fund (UNFPA), 2008, http://www.unfpa.org/upload/lib_pub_file/816_filename_en-swop08-report.pdf (accessed December 9, 2009). Data from C. F. Westoff, *New Estimates of Unmet Need and the Demand for Family Planning*, DHS Comparative Reports no. 14, USAID, 2006.

In "Fistula Fast Facts and Frequently Asked Questions" (2009, http://www.fistulafoundation.org/aboutfistula/faqs.html), the Fistula Foundation and the WHO state that about 2 million women in the developing world are known to suffer from obstetric fistula, which was virtually eradicated in wealthier countries when cesarean sections (the delivery of a fetus by surgical incision through the abdominal wall and uterus) became commonplace in the late 19th century and skilled health care became available to treat birthing emergencies immediately. The actual number of women who live with this condition is believed to be much higher than reported, because it is rarely discussed, most women who suffer from it never get medical help, and it most often occurs in remote areas of the world (estimates are based on the numbers of women who seek treatment). Approximately 100,000 new cases of obstetric fistula occur each year.

EDUCATION: TO HELP LIFT WOMEN OUT OF POVERTY

The *Beijing Declaration* and the *Platform for Action* state that education is an essential human right that contributes to economic development at all levels of society—a statement that has been supported by the UN, the UN Educational, Scientific, and Cultural Organization, the World Bank, and most nongovernmental organizations. However, according the Central Intelligence Agency (CIA), in *World Factbook: World* (February 12, 2010, https://www.cia.gov/library/publications/the-world-factbook/geos/xx.html), an estimated 785 million adults over the age of 15—one-fifth of the world's adult population—could not read or write at a functional level in 2005; two-thirds of them were women. The CIA notes that extremely low rates of literacy exist primarily in three regions of the world: the Arab states, South and West Asia, and sub-Saharan Africa.

Table 7.4 shows illiteracy percentages for males and females worldwide, for the more and less developed regions and countries, and for geographical regions. From 1995 to 2007 one out of every five (20.6%) of the world's women over the age of 15 were illiterate, whereas slightly more than one out of 10 (11.6%) men over the age 15 of were illiterate. Illiteracy rates were highest in Africa, where 27.6% of men and 45.3% of women were illiterate. Illiteracy rates were also high in the Arab states, where 18.9% of men and 37.4% of women were illiterate. South central Asia also had high

FIGURE 7.5

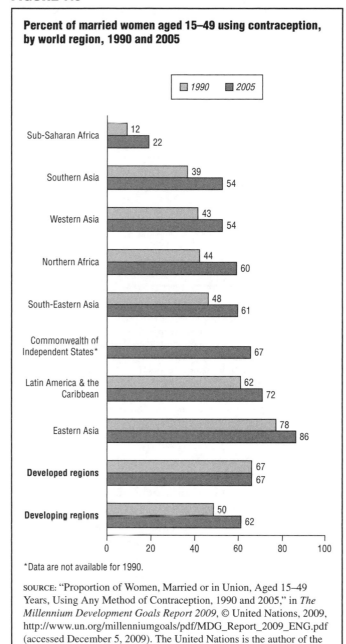

Percent of married women aged 15–49 using contraception, by world region, 1990 and 2005

*Data are not available for 1990.

SOURCE: "Proportion of Women, Married or in Union, Aged 15–49 Years, Using Any Method of Contraception, 1990 and 2005," in *The Millennium Development Goals Report 2009*, © United Nations, 2009, http://www.un.org/millenniumgoals/pdf/MDG_Report_2009_ENG.pdf (accessed December 5, 2009). The United Nations is the author of the original material. Reproduced with permission.

FIGURE 7.6

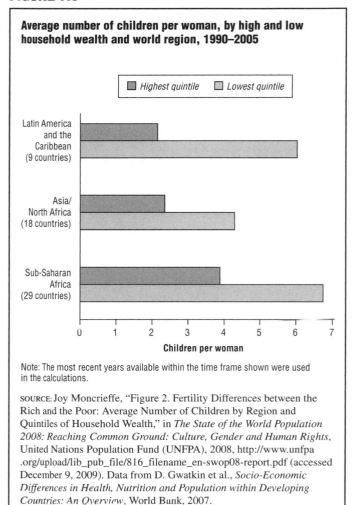

Average number of children per woman, by high and low household wealth and world region, 1990–2005

Note: The most recent years available within the time frame shown were used in the calculations.

SOURCE: Joy Moncrieffe, "Figure 2. Fertility Differences between the Rich and the Poor: Average Number of Children by Region and Quintiles of Household Wealth," in *The State of the World Population 2008: Reaching Common Ground: Culture, Gender and Human Rights*, United Nations Population Fund (UNFPA), 2008, http://www.unfpa.org/upload/lib_pub_file/816_filename_en-swop08-report.pdf (accessed December 9, 2009). Data from D. Gwatkin et al., *Socio-Economic Differences in Health, Nutrition and Population within Developing Countries: An Overview*, World Bank, 2007.

illiteracy rates at 24.7% for men and 45% for women. The gender gap in illiteracy rates was highest in south central Asia, at 20.3 percentage points of difference between illiteracy rates of men and women. The illiteracy gender gap was 18.5 percentage points difference in the Arab states and 17.7 percentage points difference in Africa.

There are many reasons for these literacy gender gaps, and poverty is chief among them. The costs associated with educating girls are generally not seen as worthwhile in the three regions of the world in which illiteracy is high, because girls are not expected to continue their education or earn a living when they grow up. More simply, in many cultures girls are not valued in the same way that boys are,

so to many impoverished families educating them seems like a waste of time and money—and in some places it is even forbidden. In addition, many poor families keep daughters at home to help tend and harvest crops, do housework, and care for elders and young siblings.

Girls' safety is another factor in not sending them to school in developing regions of the world. In rural areas many families fear their daughters will be sexually assaulted on the long walk to and from school. In some regions sexual exploitation comes another way: wealthy men offer to pay for girls' schooling in exchange for sex. Early marriage and pregnancy also cause millions of girls to drop out of school every year.

Barbara Herz and Gene B. Sperling of the Council on Foreign Relations report in *What Works in Girls' Education: Evidence and Policies from the Developing World* (2004, http://www.cfr.org/content/publications/attachments/Girls_Education_full.pdf) that education for girls in developing countries is essential for economic success at all levels of society. The benefits of educating girls are seen from families to nations, in the form of higher wages, faster economic growth, and more productive farming.

FIGURE 7.7

Birth rate for women aged 15–19, by world region, 1990 and 2006

[Per 1,000 women in age group]

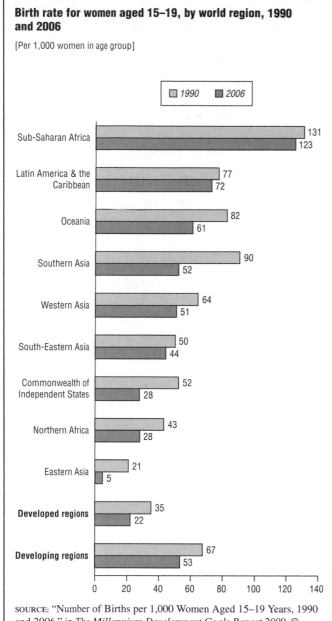

SOURCE: "Number of Births per 1,000 Women Aged 15–19 Years, 1990 and 2006," in *The Millennium Development Goals Report 2009*, © United Nations, 2009, http://www.un.org/millenniumgoals/pdf/MDG_Report_2009_ENG.pdf (accessed December 5, 2009). The United Nations is the author of the original material. Reproduced with permission.

FIGURE 7.8

Channels linking early pregnancy and childbearing to poverty

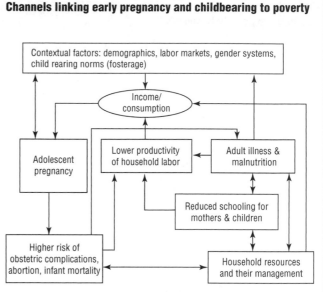

SOURCE: Margaret E. Greene and Thomas Merrick, "Figure 2. Channels Linking Early Pregnancy and Childbearing to Poverty," in *Poverty Reduction: Does Reproductive Health Matter?* The International Bank for Reconstruction and Development/The World Bank, July 2005, http://siteresources.worldbank.org/HEALTHNUTRITIONAND POPULATION/Resources/281627-1095698140167/GreenePoverty ReductionFinal.pdf (accessed January 16, 2009). Copyright © The International Bank for Reconstruction and Development/World Bank 2005.

This in turn results in decreased levels of malnutrition; women having smaller, healthier, and more educated families; reducing the spread of the human immunodeficiency virus (HIV) and the acquired immunodeficiency syndrome (AIDS); decreasing rates of violence against women; and fostering democratic participation in society.

According to Herz and Sperling, when girls attend school just one year beyond the average, they eventually earn 10% to 20% more than average as adults. Even modest increases in the number of women receiving a secondary education can lead to an increase of 0.3% in their nation's annual per capita (per person) income. As per capita growth continues, more girls achieve higher levels of education—a cycle that is ultimately beneficial for everyone. In addition, the more education women have, the lower their rates of fertility. For example, in Brazil illiterate women have an average of six children, whereas literate women average 2.5 children. Lower overall fertility rates lead to healthier, better-educated children. In fact, infant mortality rates are between 5% and 10% lower among girls who stay in school just one year longer than average. In countries where girls receive as many years of schooling as boys, infant mortality rates are 25% lower than in countries without educational gender parity (equality).

Herz and Sperling conclude that governments of low-income countries can encourage families to educate their daughters and increase overall educational gender parity by eliminating school fees, providing local schools with flexible schedules that are safe for girls, and focusing on providing a quality education that takes into account the needs of girls and their families.

Table 7.4 shows the gross primary school enrollment ratio for boys and girls from 1995 to 2007. The gross enrollment ratio (GER) is the number of students of any age enrolled in a level of education as a percentage of the total population of the relevant age group for that level of schooling. For example, if the GER is 90%, this means that

TABLE 7.4

Gender parity in education, by world region, 1995–2007

World and regional data	Education		
	Primary enrollment (gross) Male/female	Secondary enrollment (gross) Male/female	% Illiterate (>15 years) Male/female
World total	109/104	68/65	11.6/20.6
More developed regions[a]	101/101	98/98	0.5/0.8
Less developed regions[b]	110/104	63/60	14.4/26.2
Least developed countries[c]			
Africa[d]	104/94	43/36	27.6/45.3
Eastern Africa	108/103	33/27	31.1/48.9
Middle Africa[e]	110/92	35/22	23/47.4
Northern Africa[f]	101/93	65/63	23.8/42.9
Southern Africa	105/102	89/93	11.9/12.9
Western Africa[g]	97/84	36/27	32.4/50.2
Arab States[h]	99.8/90.2	71.6/65.2	18.9/37.4
Asia	110/106	67/62	12.2/23.7
Eastern Asia[i]	111/111	79/80	3.2/8.7
South Central Asia	110/105	60/49	24.7/45
South-Eastern Asia	111/109	71/73	5.8/11.3
Western Asia	104/94	78/66	8.2/22
Europe	103/102	98/98	0.6/1
Eastern Europe	98/98	90/89	0.4/0.8
Northern Europe[j]	102/102	100/102	0.2/0.3
Southern Europe[k]	106/104	102/103	1.3/2.6
Western Europe[l]	107/106	107/105	0.4/0.4
Latin America & Caribbean	119/115	85/92	8.3/9.7
Caribbean[m]	107/104	68/73	13.3/11.8
Central America	116/113	81/84	8.2/11.6
South America[n]	122/117	89/97	7.8/8.7
Northern America[o]	99/99	95/95	0.2/0.2
Oceania	93/90	145/141	6.4/7.6
Australia-New Zealand	107/106	145/141	0/0

[a]More-developed regions comprise North America, Japan, Europe and Australia-New Zealand.
[b]Less-developed regions comprise all regions of Africa, Latin America and Caribbean, Asia (excluding Japan), and Melanesia, Micronesia and Polynesia.
[c]Least-developed countries according to standard United Nations designation.
[d]Including British Indian Ocean Territory and Seychelles.
[e]Including Sao Tome and Principe.
[f]Including Western Sahara.
[g]Including St. Helena, Ascension and Tristan da Cunha.
[h]Comprising Algeria, Bahrain, Comoros, Djibouti, Egypt, Iraq, Jordan, Kuwait, Lebanon, Libyan Arab Jamahiriya, Mauritania, Morocco, Occupied Palestinian Territory, Oman, Qatar, Saudi Arabia, Somalia, Sudan, Syria, Tunisia, United Arab Emirates and Yemen. Regional aggregation for demographic indicators provided by the UN Population Division. Aggregations for other indicators are weighted averages based on countries with available data.
[i]Including Macau.
[j]Including Channel Islands, Faeroe Islands and Isle of Man.
[k]Including Andorra, Gibraltar, Holy See and San Marino.
[l]Including Leichtenstein and Monaco.
[m]Including Anguilla, Antigua and Barbuda, Aruba, British Virgin Islands, Cayman Islands, Dominica, Grenada, Montserrat, Netherlands Antilles, Saint Kitts and Nevis, Saint Lucia, Saint Vincent and the Grenadines, Turks and Caicos Islands, and United States Virgin Islands.
[n]Including Falkland Islands (Malvinas) and French Guiana.
[o]Including Bermuda, Greenland, and St. Pierre and Miquelon
Note: The most recent years available within the time frame shown were used in the calculations. Gross enrollment ratios indicate the number of students enrolled in a level in the education system per 100 individuals in the appropriate age group. They do not correct for individuals who are older than the level-appropriate age due to late starts, interrupted schooling or grade repetition.

SOURCE: Adapted from Robert Engelman, "Monitoring ICPD Goals: Selected: Indicators," in *The State of the World Population 2009: Facing a Changing World: Women, Population and Climate*, United Nations Population Fund (UNFPA), 2009, http://www.unfpa.org/swp/2009/en/pdf/EN_SOWP09.pdf (accessed December 9, 2009). Data from the UNESCO Institute for Statistics and the UN Population Division.

90 students out of 100 primary school–aged students are enrolled in primary school. If the GER is more than 100%, it means that more students are enrolled than the total of those of primary school age. That is, students younger or older than primary school age are enrolled in primary school along with the students of primary school age.

The GERs shown in Table 7.4 were high and indicate that in most instances students older than primary age were attending primary school from 1995 to 2007. Additionally, in most regions the GER for boys was higher than that for girls. The exceptions were Eastern Asia, eastern Europe, northern Europe, and North America, where the GERs were equal for boys and girls. The GERs for eastern Europe and North America were lower than the rest because students generally enrolled in primary school were of primary school age, so the GER was not inflated with older students as in other regions of the world.

Figure 7.9 compares girls' primary school enrollment with boys' (girls per 100 boys) for the academic years 1998–99 and 2006–07. Overall, developed regions of the world show gender parity in primary schooling while developing regions do not. However, developing regions have made progress in primary schooling parity since the academic year 1998–99. During that academic year, 91 girls for every 100 boys were enrolled in primary school in the developing world. By academic year 2006–07, 95 girls for every 100 boys were enrolled. In spite of the progress made in gender parity, the UN points out in *Millennium Development Goals Report 2009* (2009, http://www.un.org/millenniumgoals/pdf/MDG_Report_2009_ENG.pdf) that 2005 was the target date for gender parity to be achieved in primary education, and that date was missed. Nonetheless, gender parity gaps in primary school enrollment are falling rapidly.

Figure 7.10 shows secondary school net attendance ratios for males and females in developing countries between 1998 and 2007 by place of residence and household wealth. The net attendance ratio is the number of students who attend school who are of the relevant age group for that level as a percentage of the total population in the relevant age group for that level. Thus, the net attendance ratio can never be over 100%, because only students of the relevant age level are included. The figure shows that boys and girls living in rural locations have an educational disadvantage compared with boys and girls living in urban locations. In addition, there is a positive correlation between secondary education and household wealth: as household wealth increases, the secondary school net attendance ratio increases. Thus, children of poverty are at a distinct disadvantage in acquiring a secondary education. Moreover, girls of all household incomes and places of residence are at a disadvantage over boys,

FIGURE 7.9

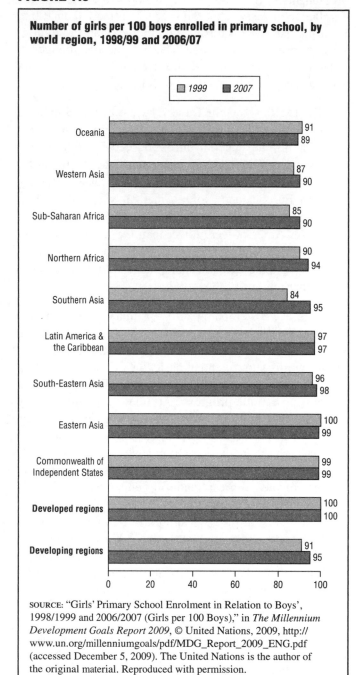

Number of girls per 100 boys enrolled in primary school, by world region, 1998/99 and 2006/07

SOURCE: "Girls' Primary School Enrolment in Relation to Boys', 1998/1999 and 2006/2007 (Girls per 100 Boys)," in *The Millennium Development Goals Report 2009*, © United Nations, 2009, http://www.un.org/millenniumgoals/pdf/MDG_Report_2009_ENG.pdf (accessed December 5, 2009). The United Nations is the author of the original material. Reproduced with permission.

FIGURE 7.10

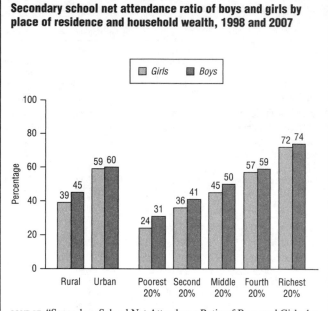

Secondary school net attendance ratio of boys and girls by place of residence and household wealth, 1998 and 2007

SOURCE: "Secondary School Net Attendance Ratio of Boys and Girls, by Place of Residence and Household Wealth, 1998/2007 (Percentage)," in *The Millennium Development Goals Report 2009*, © United Nations, 2009, http://www.un.org/millenniumgoals/pdf/MDG_Report_2009_ENG.pdf (accessed December 5, 2009). The United Nations is the author of the original material. Reproduced with permission.

especially girls living in poverty and in rural locations. For example, only one out of four (24%) girls living in the lowest household-income family was enrolled in secondary school between 1998 and 2007, whereas one out of three (31%) boys in this same category was enrolled. For those living in rural areas, 39% of girls were enrolled in secondary school, whereas 45% of boys were enrolled.

Figure 7.11 compares girls' secondary school enrollment with boys' for the academic years 1998–99 and 2006–07. Overall, gender parity exists in developed regions of the world but not in developing regions. During the 1998–99 academic year 89 girls were enrolled in secondary school for every 100 boys in developing regions. The situation improved during the 2006–07 academic year, when 94 girls for every 100 boys were enrolled in secondary school. Over this time span, there was an increase in gender parity in western Asia, southern Asia, northern Africa, Eastern Asia, and Southeastern Asia. In Eastern Asia and in the CIS the balance of gender parity changed, so that in 2006–07 more girls than boys (101 girls for every 100 boys) were enrolled in secondary school in Eastern Asia, but more boys than girls (98 girls for every 100 boys) were enrolled in secondary school in the CIS. In Latin America and the Caribbean more girls than boys (107 girls for every 100 boys) were enrolled in secondary school during the 1998–99 academic year, and this disparity remained during the 2006–07 academic year. Gender parity decreased over time in sub-Saharan Africa, Oceania, and the CIS.

Figure 7.12 shows that girls outnumber boys in postsecondary education in developed regions, but not in developing regions, although girls are close to gender parity there. During the 2006–07 academic year, girls outnumbered boys in higher education in northern Africa, Southeastern Asia, Latin America and the Caribbean, and the CIS. However, in sub-Saharan Africa, southern Asia, Oceania, western Asia, and Eastern Asia boys far outnumbered girls in advancing to postsecondary education.

FIGURE 7.11

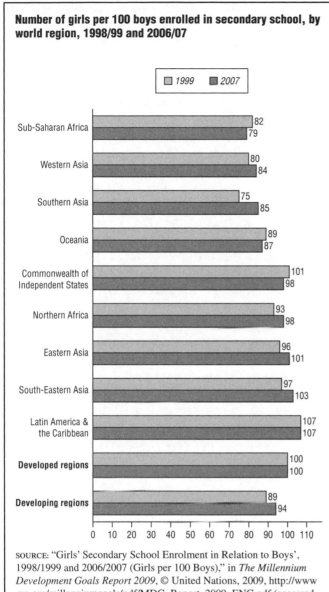

Number of girls per 100 boys enrolled in secondary school, by world region, 1998/99 and 2006/07

▢ 1999　■ 2007

Region	1999	2007
Sub-Saharan Africa	82	79
Western Asia	80	84
Southern Asia	75	85
Oceania	89	87
Commonwealth of Independent States	101	98
Northern Africa	93	98
Eastern Asia	96	101
South-Eastern Asia	97	103
Latin America & the Caribbean	107	107
Developed regions	100	100
Developing regions	89	94

SOURCE: "Girls' Secondary School Enrolment in Relation to Boys', 1998/1999 and 2006/2007 (Girls per 100 Boys)," in *The Millennium Development Goals Report 2009*, © United Nations, 2009, http://www.un.org/millenniumgoals/pdf/MDG_Report_2009_ENG.pdf (accessed December 5, 2009). The United Nations is the author of the original material. Reproduced with permission.

FIGURE 7.12

Number of girls per 100 boys enrolled in postsecondary school, by world region, 1998/99 and 2006/07

▢ 1999　■ 2007

Region	1999	2007
Sub-Saharan Africa	69	67
Southern Asia	64	77
Oceania	69	85
Western Asia	82	93
Eastern Asia	55	96
Northern Africa	68	104
South-Eastern Asia	92	111
Latin America & the Caribbean	112	119
Commonwealth of Independent States	121	129
Developed regions	119	129
Developing regions	78	96

SOURCE: "Girls' Tertiary School Enrolment in Relation to Boys', 1998/1999 and 2006/2007 (Girls per 100 Boys)," in *The Millennium Development Goals Report 2009*, © United Nations, 2009, http://www.un.org/millenniumgoals/pdf/MDG_Report_2009_ENG.pdf (accessed December 5, 2009). The United Nations is the author of the original material. Reproduced with permission.

VIOLENCE AGAINST WOMEN

In *Addressing Violence against Women and Achieving the Millennium Development Goals* (2005, http://www.who.int/gender/documents/MDGs&VAWSept05.pdf), the WHO cites two main reasons poor women are more vulnerable to violence than their nonpoor counterparts: fewer resources—in terms of both money and support services—to help women avoid or escape violence; and the stressors of poverty, such as hunger, unemployment, and lack of education, that may lead some men to become violent or worsen an already violent situation. In addition, women who work in unregulated, informal employment are often subject to physical, sexual, or psychological abuse by their employers. In both developing and developed countries social standards and enforced gender roles contribute to the incidence of violence.

The WHO recommends several global economic actions that can affect women who are routine victims of violence:

• Promote increased access to postprimary, vocational, and technical education for women.

• Address gender gaps in earnings as well as barriers to accessing credit for women.

• Extend and upgrade childcare benefits to enable women's full participation in the paid labor market.

• Address issues of occupational segregation that often translate into inferior conditions of employment for women.

- Ensure social protection and benefits for women in precarious employment situations—often those involved in informal employment.

Violence against Women in the United States

In the United States domestic violence is conclusively linked to homelessness among women and children. The American Civil Liberties Union (ACLU) reports in the fact sheet "Domestic Violence and Homelessness" (March 2006, http://www.aclu.org/pdfs/dvhomelessness032106.pdf) that domestic violence was cited by 50% of U.S cities surveyed in 2005 as a primary cause of homelessness. Furthermore, the ACLU notes that 50% of homeless women in San Diego, California, reported being the victims of domestic violence and that in Minnesota one-third of homeless women indicated that they left their home to escape domestic violence.

In December 2005 both the U.S. Senate and the U.S. House of Representatives passed the Violence against Women Act (VAWA). President George W. Bush (1946–) signed the VAWA into law in January 2006. A reauthorization of the 1994 VAWA, the 2005 VAWA enhanced the provisions of its earlier version, with increased funding for violence-prevention programs, emergency shelter for women and children, and long-term housing solutions for low-income women and their children. The act also mandates that abused women be allowed to take 10 days off from work each year to attend court or to look for housing, and it provides greater access to law enforcement and the justice system for abused immigrant women who would otherwise have no legal recourse and might have to leave the country with abusive partners.

POVERTY'S YOUNGEST VICTIMS

Children who live in poverty face special challenges. Because childhood—particularly the first few months of life—is a time of key developmental changes physically, emotionally, and intellectually, neglect in any of these areas can be a permanent detriment to future well-being. Impoverished children become transmitters of poverty to the next generation when they become parents themselves, and the cycle of poverty continues.

As was shown earlier in this chapter, there is a positive correlation between the level of wealth and the number of children a woman has: as the income level increases, the number of children a woman bears decreases. Thus, the poorest women have the most children, and the least developed and poorest countries in the world are home to the greatest number of children. According to the Population Reference Bureau (PRB), in *2009 World Population Data Sheet* (August 2009, http://www.prb.org/pdf09/09wpds_eng.pdf), the growth of the world population is concentrated in the world's poorer countries. In *2008 World Population Data Sheet* (August 2008, http://www .prb.org/pdf08/08WPDS_Eng.pdf), the PRB indicates that from 2003 to 2007, 41% of the population of the least developed countries was under 15 years of age, whereas only 17% of the population of the most developed countries was under the age of 15.

Child poverty is not limited to low-income or low human development countries. Michael Förster and Marco Mira d'Ercole of the Organization for Economic Cooperation and Development (OECD) list in "Poverty in OECD Countries: An Assessment Based on Static Income" in *Growing Unequal? Income Distribution and Poverty in OECD Countries* (2008, http://browse .oecdbookshop.org/oecd/pdfs/browseit/8108051E.PDF) the 30 member countries of the OECD and the percentage of children in poverty in each by 2005. All 30 OECD countries had a ranking level of very high or high on the Human Development Index in 2009. (See Table 1.2 and Table 1.3 in Chapter 1.) The OECD country with the highest level of child poverty was Turkey, at 25%. Turkey had a high level of human development and was ranked 79 out of 182 countries on the HDI index. Both Mexico (HDI rank 53) and Poland (HDI rank 41) had the next highest rate of child poverty at 22%, followed by the United States (HDI rank 13) at 21%. The OECD countries with the lowest rates of child poverty were the Scandinavian countries of Denmark (HDI rank 16) with a 3% rate of child poverty, Sweden (HDI rank 7) and Finland (HDI rank 12) with a 4% rate each, and Norway (HDI rank 1) with 5%.

Children's Health and Mortality

Improving children's health and reducing rates of child mortality is an implicit factor of the CRC and is explicitly listed as one of the MDGs. The most fundamental and important indicators of poverty among children are the state of their health and their rates of mortality. Child mortality rates are also a major indicator of the overall social and economic stability of nations. How much a country invests—or does not invest—in measures to cut back preventable deaths and diseases of children is ultimately indicative of its commitment to its own economic development.

An important health factor in children is whether they grow properly during their first years of life. Breast-feeding is important to children in the first six months of life because not only does it provide appropriate nutrition for the developing infant but also it provides passive resistance to disease by means of the mother's antibodies. This nutrition and protection is particularly important in areas of the world where the water is unsafe to drink, where rates of disease are high, where rates of immunization are low, and where poverty prevents a family from providing a safe and nutritionally appropriate substitute. Vitamin A supplementation is important in reducing childhood deaths due to vitamin A deficiency. This problem is prevalent in areas in which children do not receive proper nutrition. Iodized salt helps avoid iodine deficiency, the effects of which include irreversible mental retardation, goiter (enlargement of the thyroid gland), reproductive failure, and increased child mortality.

One way to measure child growth is to determine whether a child's weight meets established norms for age and height. In developed countries the percentage of children younger than five years old exhibiting moderate to severe levels of underweight is negligible, whereas in developing countries the rate is high, as is shown in Figure 3.2 in Chapter 3. In 1990, 31% of children under the age of five were underweight in developing countries. By 2007 the rate had declined but was still high at 26%.

In 1990 southern Asia had the highest percentage of underweight children under the age of five. (See Figure 3.2 in Chapter 3.) At 54%, over half of the young South Asian children were underweight. By 2007 nearly half (48%) of children were still underweight. Sub-Saharan Africa (28%) and Southeastern Asia (25%) had the next highest percentages of underweight children under five in 2007. Eastern Asia, northern Africa, and Latin America and the Caribbean had relatively low proportions of underweight children younger than five in their populations, at 6% to 7% in 2007.

INFANT MORTALITY. The global distribution of infant mortality (deaths of infants under 12 months old per 1,000 live births) is shown in Table 7.5 for 2007–08 or the most recent year available. There is a negative correlation between infant mortality rate and the level of development of a region. That is, as development increases, infant mortality decreases. Overall, the more developed regions of the world had an infant mortality rate of 6 deaths per 1,000 live births. By contrast, less developed regions had an infant mortality rate of 50 deaths per 1,000 live births and the least developed regions had an infant mortality rate of 80 deaths per 1,000 live births. The highest rates of infant deaths were in Africa (74 deaths per 1,000 live births), especially in sub-Saharan Africa (80 deaths per 1,000 live births), with middle Africa having the highest infant mortality rate of the sub-Saharan region (95 deaths per 1,000 live births). South central Asia was another region with high infant mortality, at 57 deaths per 1,000 live births. Europe and Northern America each had low infant mortality rates at 6 deaths per 1,000 live births.

Infant deaths are dramatically reduced by access to clean water and sanitation. When clean water and toilets are available, the incidence of diarrheal diseases is reduced. Diarrhea is the second-most cause of death of children in the world. According to Figure 7.13, 17% of deaths of children worldwide in 2006 were caused by

TABLE 7.5

Infant mortality rate, by world region, 2007–08 or most recent year available

	Infant Mortality Rate
World	46
More developed	6
Less developed	50
Less developed (excluding China)	55
Least developed	80
Africa	74
Sub-Saharan Africa	80
Northern Africa	38
Western Africa	80
Eastern Africa	76
Middle Africa	95
Southern Africa	48
Americas	18
Northern America	6
Latin America/Caribbean	23
Central America	21
Caribbean	34
South America	23
Asia	43
Asia (excluding China)	48
Western Asia	38
South Central Asia	57
Southeast Asia	30
East Asia	20
Europe	6
Northern Europe	4
Western Europe	4
Eastern Europe	8
Southern Europe	5
Oceania	22

Note: All rates shown are estimates.

SOURCE: Adapted from "Population, Health, and Environment Data and Estimates for the Countries and Regions of the World," in *2009 World Population Data Sheet*, Population Reference Bureau, August 2009, http://www.prb.org/pdf09/09wpds_eng.pdf (accessed December 11, 2009)

diarrheal diseases. A slightly higher percentage (19%) of childhood deaths was caused by pneumonia.

MORTALITY OF CHILDREN UNDER THE AGE OF FIVE. In 2006 the number-one cause of death of children under the age of five worldwide was pneumonia, causing 19% of deaths. (See Figure 7.13.) Diarrhea was the second-leading cause of death under the age of five, claiming 17% of deaths. Neonatal severe infections and preterm birth (being born before development is complete) were the third-leading cause of death under the age of five, each causing 10% of childhood deaths. According to the UNDP, high rates of such deaths occur primarily in the developing world, where they account for one-third of all deaths. In industrialized countries, such as the United States, they account for less than 1%.

In *The State of the World's Children 2008: Child Survival* (December 2007, http://www.unicef.org/sowc08/docs/SOAC_2008_EN_A4.pdf), UNICEF explains that even though the developing and least developed countries

FIGURE 7.13

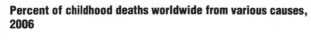

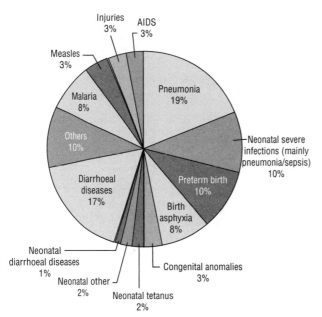

Percent of childhood deaths worldwide from various causes, 2006

Note: Undernutrition is implicated in up to 50 per cent of all deaths of children under five.

SOURCE: "Figure 1.8. Global Distribution of Cause-Specific Mortality among Children under Five," in *The State of the World's Children 2008: Child Survival*, United Nation's Children's Fund (UNICEF), December 2007, http://www.unicef.org/sowc08/docs/Figure-1.8.pdf (accessed December 11, 2009). Copyright © UNICEF. Data from World Health Organization (WHO) and UNICEF.

child labor is among the worst, resulting in physical and psychological damage and, frequently, premature death. The UN, the ILO, and other nongovernmental organizations distinguish, however, between the terms *child work* (economic activity by children at least 12 years old that is not hazardous and does not interfere with their education) and *child labor* (all work by children under the age of 12, hazardous work by children aged 12 to 14, and all work defined as "worst forms of child labor"). According to the ILO, in "C182 Worst Forms of Child Labour Convention, 1999" (2006, http://www.ilo.org/ilolex/cgi-lex/convde.pl? C182), "worst forms of child labor" include:

- All forms of slavery or practices similar to slavery, such as the sale and trafficking of children, debt bondage and serfdom and forced or compulsory labor, including forced or compulsory recruitment of children for use in armed conflict.

- The use, procuring or offering of a child for prostitution, for the production of pornography or for pornographic performances.

- The use, procuring or offering of a child for illicit activities, in particular for the production and trafficking of drugs as defined in the relevant international treaties.

- Work which, by its nature or the circumstances in which it is carried out, is likely to harm the health, safety or morals of children.

Figure 7.15 shows the percentage of children aged five to 14 engaged in labor worldwide, comparing child labor in various regions of the world from 1999 to 2007. Nearly half the proportion of young children worked in developing countries (16%), compared with the proportion in least developed countries (30%). That progression can be seen with specific regions in the figure. In the least developed areas of Africa shown at the top, over one-third (34% to 36%) of all children aged five to 14 worked. That proportion dropped to approximately one-tenth in the developing countries (6% to 13%).

Not only is it important to know what proportion of young children work throughout the world but also it is important to know how much they work. Time spent in employment affects the time available to attend school, do homework, and benefit from rest and leisure. Federico Blanco Allais of the International Programme on the Elimination of Child Labour discusses in *Assessing the Gender Gap: Evidence from SIMPOC Surveys* (July 2009, http:// www.ilo.org/ipecinfo/product/viewProduct.do?productId= 10952) the hours per week that five- to 15-year-old males and females work in a variety of countries. In some countries girls work more hours per week than boys, whereas in other countries the reverse is true. Allais notes

of the world have a great deal of work to do in decreasing the mortality rate of under-age-five children, rates improved nearly everywhere in the world between 1990 and 2006. During that time the child mortality rate worldwide fell by almost a quarter (23%), from 93 under-five deaths per 1,000 live births in 1990 to 72 deaths per 1,000 live births in 2006. Figure 7.14 shows that East Asia and the Pacific, Latin America and the Caribbean, and central and eastern Europe and the CIS made great progress in reducing their under-five mortality rates by nearly half. The industrialized (developed) nations collectively reduced their rates by 40%, from 10 under-five deaths per 1,000 live births in 1990 to 6 deaths per 1,000 live births in 2006. However, much more work needs to be done in most of Africa, especially in sub-Saharan Africa, where under-five deaths were 187 per 1,000 live births in 1990 and only dropped 14% to 160 deaths per 1,000 live births in 2006.

Child Labor

Children from poor families must frequently go to work to contribute income to their household, and of all the poverty-related abuses and deprivations children suffer,

FIGURE 7.14

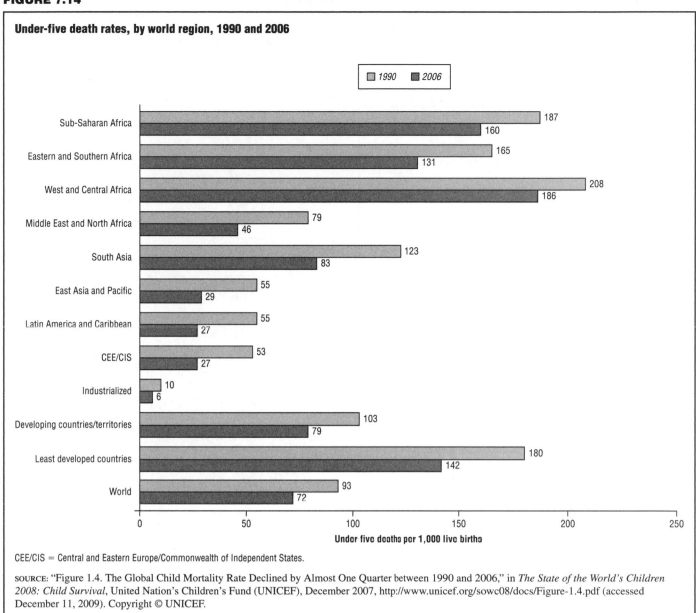

Under-five death rates, by world region, 1990 and 2006

□ 1990   ■ 2006

Region	1990	2006
Sub-Saharan Africa	187	160
Eastern and Southern Africa	165	131
West and Central Africa	208	186
Middle East and North Africa	79	46
South Asia	123	83
East Asia and Pacific	55	29
Latin America and Caribbean	55	27
CEE/CIS	53	27
Industrialized	10	6
Developing countries/territories	103	79
Least developed countries	180	142
World	93	72

Under five deaths per 1,000 live births

CEE/CIS = Central and Eastern Europe/Commonwealth of Independent States.

SOURCE: "Figure 1.4. The Global Child Mortality Rate Declined by Almost One Quarter between 1990 and 2006," in *The State of the World's Children 2008: Child Survival*, United Nation's Children's Fund (UNICEF), December 2007, http://www.unicef.org/sowc08/docs/Figure-1.4.pdf (accessed December 11, 2009). Copyright © UNICEF.

that the average number of hours boys and girls work overall is quite similar: 20.2 hours per week for boys and 19.2 hours per week for girls. (See Figure 7.16.)

Injuries and impairments of individual children are not the only risks of child labor. Working as a child can affect the child's entire life and has far-reaching repercussions. The more hours children spend working, the less time they spend in school, which in turn affects their ability to improve their economic status later in life. Thus, UNICEF states in *Progress for Children: A Report Card on Child Protection* (September 2009, http://www.unicef.org/protection/files/Progress_for_Children-No.8_EN_081309(1).pdf) that "child labour is both a cause and a consequence of poverty, and it perpetuates impoverishment by severely compromising children's education. With early entry into the labour force, most children delay entry to school, fail to complete a basic education or never attend school at all. Where girls who labour are in school, they carry a 'triple burden' of housework, schoolwork and work outside the home, paid or unpaid, which inevitably reduces their educational attainment and achievement." This in effect traps these children—and later their children—in the cycle of poverty and prolongs the economic instability of poor countries.

FIGURE 7.15

FIGURE 7.16

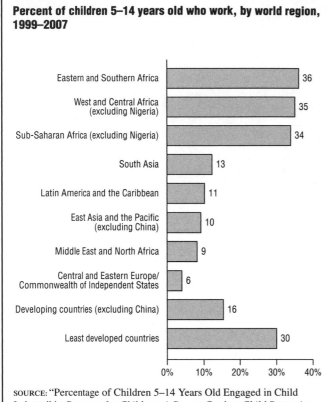

Percent of children 5–14 years old who work, by world region, 1999–2007

SOURCE: "Percentage of Children 5–14 Years Old Engaged in Child Labour," in *Progress for Children: A Report Card on Child Protection*, United Nations Children's Fund (UNICEF), September 2009, http://www.unicef.org/protection/files/Progress_for_Children-No.8_EN _081309(1).pdf (accessed January 12, 2010). Copyright © UNICEF.

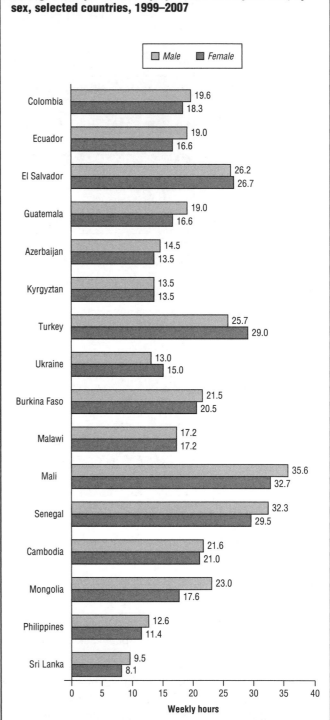

Average weekly hours in employment, 5-to-14-year-olds, by sex, selected countries, 1999–2007

Note: Average male weekly hours in employment = 20.2, average female weekly hours in employment = 19.2.

SOURCE: Federico Blanco Allais, "Chart 10: Average Weekly Hours in Employment, 5 to 14 Years Age Group, by Sex and Country," in *Assessing the Gender Gap: Evidence from SIMPOC Surveys*, International Labour Organization, International Programme on the Elimination of Child Labour, Statistical Information and Monitoring Programme on Child Labour, July 2009, http://www.ilo.org/ipecinfo/ product/viewProduct.do?productId=10952 (accessed December 7, 2009). Copyright © 2009 International Labour Organization.

CHAPTER 8
POVERTY AND ENVIRONMENTAL HAZARDS

Conditions in the environment that have a negative impact on the health and well-being of a population are known as environmental hazards. These can be natural events, such as an overabundance of insects that destroys crops; a weather pattern that causes a drought or flood; or a sudden, violent disaster such as an earthquake or volcanic eruption. Environmental hazards can also be human-caused problems such as air and water pollution, chemical toxicity, or a poor use of resources that brings about environmental degradation. These events can have an immediate, devastating impact, or they can have more extended consequences. For example, a famine might cause hundreds of thousands of people to starve to death over a number of months, or exposure to pollution might be associated with long-term health effects over several generations.

THE EFFECTS OF ENVIRONMENTAL HAZARDS ON THE POOR

Throughout the world the poor are more often and more severely affected by environmental hazards, including both daily pollutants and large-scale disasters. In "Housing and Health: Intersection of Poverty and Environmental Exposures" (*Annals of the New York Academy of Sciences*, vol. 1136, no. 1, June 2008), Virginia A. Rauh, Philip J. Landrigan, and Luz Claudio find that people living in economically disadvantaged communities are more likely to be exposed, and exposed at higher levels, to pollutants and other risks in their homes, schools, and workplaces. For example, flaking lead-based paint, which is a particular danger to children, is more prevalent in the poorly-maintained, older houses of low-income neighborhoods than in newly-constructed homes or carefully-maintained, older dwellings. Rauh, Landrigan, and Claudio note that poverty, poor housing, and degraded environments are all risk factors for ill health. Steven Woolf, Robert Johnson, and H. Jack Geiger agree in "The Rising Prevalence of Severe Poverty in America:

A Growing Threat to Public Health" (*American Journal of Preventive Medicine*, vol. 31, no. 4, October 2006) and note that "the public health implications of increasing poverty are profound."

In underdeveloped and developing countries environmental risks are generally many times greater because health and safety regulations, if they exist at all, are less stringent. According to Annette Prüss-Üstün and Carlos Corvalán, in "How Much Disease Burden Can Be Prevented by Environmental Interventions?" (*Epidemiology*, vol. 18, no 1, January 2007), an estimated 24% of diseases globally are due to modifiable environmental risk factors. Furthermore, in *Preventing Disease through Healthy Environments: Towards an Estimate of the Environmental Burden of Disease* (2006, http://www.who.int/quantifying_ehimpacts/publications/preventingdisease.pdf), Prüss-Üstün and Corvalán determine that people in developing countries lose more years of healthy life due to environmental causes of disease than do people living in developed countries. For example, the researchers find that the loss of healthy life years from infectious diseases due to environmental causes (such as unsafe water and inadequate sanitation) is 15 times higher in developing countries than in developed countries. The risk of environmentally related unintentional injuries (accidents) is twice as high. (Conversely, however, the per capita [per person] rates for cancer and heart disease are twice as high in developed countries than they are in developing countries.)

Natural disasters affect the poor disproportionately because they so often occur in rural regions and in high-risk zones where poor people live out of tradition or necessity. In addition, high-income countries are often better prepared for emergencies than low-income countries. The World Bank notes in "Natural Disasters: Counting the Cost" (March 2, 2004, http://econ.world bank.org/) that developed countries tend to have early warning systems and emergency response plans, as well as emergency medical care and insurance coverage. In low-income countries and remote areas communications systems are less reliable, if they exist at all, making it difficult to implement early warning systems. After a disaster, victims must often wait for outside help from international organizations, and any money targeted for local development plans must be diverted to relief and rebuilding efforts, which is often a significant setback to human development projects.

Besides the absence of early warning systems, P. C. Kesavan and M. S. Swaminathan suggest in "Managing Extreme Natural Disasters in Coastal Areas" (*Philosophical Transactions of the Royal Society: Mathematical, Physical, and Engineering Sciences*, vol. 364, no. 1845, August 15, 2006) that a "low level of technology development in the rural areas together with social, economic and gender inequities enhance the vulnerability of the largely illiterate, unskilled, and resource-poor fishing, farming and landless labour communities. Their resilience to bounce back to pre-disaster level of normality is highly limited."

WHICH AREAS ARE MOST VULNERABLE TO NATURAL DISASTERS?

In *Natural Disaster Hotspots: A Global Risk Analysis* (2005, http://www.proventionconsortium.org/themes/default/pdfs/Hotspots.pdf), Maxx Dilley et al. report that 3.4 billion people—more than half the global population—are vulnerable to natural disasters, especially in Bangladesh, Nepal, the Dominican Republic, Burundi, Haiti, Taiwan (the Republic of China), Malawi, El Salvador, and Honduras. The regions that statistically face the greatest risks are Central America, East and South Asia, parts of the Mediterranean, and the Middle East.

FAMINE

Famine is the phenomenon of large-scale starvation in a population due to a severe shortage of food or a lack of access to food. It can be caused by natural occurrences such as drought, flooding, or pestilence (diseases of food crops or infestations by organisms, such as locusts). Famine can also occur during war, when access to food is disrupted, or be the result of government policies, as in the case of North Korea. (See Chapter 5.) It is one of the most devastating events human beings can experience and one of the most dramatic and emotional from the point of view of spectators worldwide. For centuries, periodic famines were a more or less normal part of human existence, mostly because of crop failure. However, since the 19th century some famines have occurred as a result of economic and political manipulations. For example, the Irish Potato Famine (1845–1849), which killed an estimated 500,000 to 1 million people, was

caused by a combination of factors, including a naturally occurring potato fungus that ruined crops, Irish property law, and British import-export practices that had some Irish food producers exporting crops to England while the Irish were starving.

Famines in modern times almost exclusively hurt the poor, and, in general, they afflict those who are the poorest with the greatest frequency and the most serious effects. Developed countries have sufficient wealth and infrastructure that they do not suffer from famines except under the most extraordinary of circumstances. The most recent famine in a developed country was in the Netherlands in 1944, when an exceptionally difficult winter combined with the destruction caused by World War II (1939–1945) caused at least 30,000 Dutch to starve to death. By contrast, underdeveloped regions have suffered many famines since that time. People in these areas may have difficulty meeting their basic needs during the best of times, and when disaster strikes it can become impossible for them to find enough food to eat. This is especially true for the poorest members of these societies.

In "Famine Intensity and Magnitude Scales: A Proposal for an Instrumental Definition of Famine" (*Disasters*, vol. 28, no. 4, December 2004), Paul Howe and Stephen Devereux of the University of Sussex provide a measurement of famine with scales for both intensity and magnitude. Their article has proven to be quite influential, and their scales are used by many international relief organizations to help differentiate among crises and respond appropriately.

Table 8.1 is the famine intensity scale. The designations range from level 0, in which food security conditions exist, to level 5, in which extreme famine conditions exist. The crude mortality rate (total number of deaths per 10,000 people per day) is 0.2—or 2 people per 100,000 per day—at level 0. Child wasting (a gauge of a child's vitality and strength) is at less than 2.3%. Prices are stable and coping strategies are not needed. As the scale rises from 0 to 5, the mortality and malnutrition indicators rise and the food security descriptors show more stress in the social system and food markets. At level 5 (extreme famine conditions), the crude mortality rate is 15 per 10,000 per day, or 150 dying each day per 100,000 people. There is a complete social breakdown with food scarcity identified as the dominant problem.

Table 8.2 is the famine magnitude scale, which focuses not on the rate of death, but on the total number of deaths. This five-level scale ranges from category A (minor famine) to category E (catastrophic famine). When 0 to 999 deaths occur due to famine, it is considered a minor famine. When 1 million or more deaths occur due to famine, it is considered a catastrophic famine. These scales of intensity and magnitude are used together because areas of famine have different-sized

TABLE 8.1

Famine intensity scale

Levels	Phrase designation	'Lives': malnutrition and mortality indicators	'Livelihoods': food-security descriptors
0	Food-security conditions	CMR < 0.2/10,000/day and wasting < 2.3%	Social system is cohesive; prices are stable; negligible adoption of coping strategies.
1	Food-insecurity conditions	CMR >= 0.2 but < .5/10,000/day and/or wasting >=2.3 but <10%	Social system remains cohesive; price instability, and seasonal shortage of key items; reversible 'adaptive strategies' are employed.
2	Food crisis conditions	CMR >=.5 but < 1/10,000/day and/or wasting >=10 but < 20% and/or prevalence of edema	Social system significantly stressed but remains largely cohesive; dramatic rise in price of food and other basic items; adaptive mechanisms start to fail; increase in irreversible coping strategies.
3	Famine conditions	CMR >=1 but < 5/10,000/day and/or wasting >=20% but < 40% and/or prevalence of edema	Clear signs of social breakdown appear; markets begin to close or collapse; coping strategies are exhausted and survival strategies are adopted; affected population identify food as the dominant problem in the onset of the crisis.
4	Severe famine conditions	CMR >5= but <15/10,000/day and/or wasting >=40% and/or prevalence of edema	Widespread social breakdown; markets are closed or inaccessible to affected population; survival strategies are widespread; affected population identify food as the dominant problem in the onset of this crisis.
5	Extreme famine conditions	CMR >=15/10,000/day	Complete social breakdown; widespread mortality; affected population identify food as the dominant problem in the onset of the crisis.

CMR = Crude mortality rate.
Wasting: proportion of child population (six months to five years old) who are below 80 percent of the median weight-for-height.

SOURCE: Paul Howe and Stephen Devereux, "Table 2. Intensity Scale," in "Famine Intensity and Magnitude Scales: A Proposal for an Instrumental Definition of Famine," *Disasters*, vol. 28, no. 4, 2004, http://www.blackwell-synergy.com/toc/disa/28/4 (accessed December 11, 2009). Copyright © 2004 Blackwell Publishing. Reprinted by permission of Wiley-Blackwell.

TABLE 8.2

Famine magnitude scale

Category	Phrase designation	Mortality range
A	Minor famine	0–999
B	Moderate famine	1,000–9,999
C	Major famine	10,000–99,999
D	Great famine	100,000–999,999
E	Catastrophic famine	1,000,000 and over

SOURCE: Paul Howe and Stephen Devereux, "Table 3. Magnitude Scale," in "Famine Intensity and Magnitude Scales: A Proposal for an Instrumental Definition of Famine," *Disasters*, vol. 28, no. 4, 2004 http://www.blackwell-synergy.com/toc/disa/28/4, (accessed December 11, 2009). Copyright © 2004 Blackwell Publishing. Reprinted by permission of Wiley-Blackwell.

populations. Thus, in an area with a small population, the famine may be minor in magnitude because there are fewer than 1,000 deaths total, but it may be extreme in intensity with a high rate of death and a complete social breakdown in a small population.

Ethiopia: The "Face of Famine"

The Ethiopian famine in 1984–85, which is considered to be one of the most devastating in recent history, was the result of nearly all the contributing factors to famine—drought, war, politics, and pestilence—coalescing in a single country. By 1986 over 1 million people had starved to death. Perhaps the most remarkable thing about Ethiopia's famine was the international outrage it provoked and the public response it elicited, ushering in a period of international charitable donation that continued more than 20 years later.

WAR AND POLITICS IN ETHIOPIA. Engaged in a civil war with its northern province of Eritrea since 1960, Ethiopia was taken over in 1974 by a pro-Soviet military junta called the Derg. During the early 1970s the country had experienced a drought and subsequent famine, from which it had not fully recovered by the end of the decade. With the Derg focusing on insurgencies that had sprung up in all of Ethiopia's regions by 1976, government spending was directed toward increasing military power rather than addressing crop failure. By the late 1970s another drought was beginning, and by the early 1980s famine was inevitable. The war with Eritrea cut off relief supplies through the north, and anti-Soviet Eritrean rebels, backed by the United States, took control of all of Ethiopia's sea ports, further isolating the country's hungry citizens and damaging its economy. Complicating matters was Ethiopia's agricultural economy, which had focused for many years on growing crops for export, especially coffee, rather than for its own subsistence.

IMAGES OF DEATH BROADCAST AROUND THE WORLD. Kate Milner reports in "Flashback 1984: Portrait of a Famine" (BBC News, April 6, 2000) that by March 1984 the Ethiopian government appealed to the international community for aid, but Western leaders were reluctant to send money to a pro-Soviet country that was known for its military spending. In the summer of 1984 European countries had surplus crops, but none of the food was sent to Ethiopia. Then in October 1984, with 200,000 people already dead and 8 million more at risk of starving, a Canadian Broadcasting Corporation news crew traveled to Tigray province in northern Ethiopia and covered the story, taking photographs and footage of the dead and dying and broadcasting them to the world. (The original television segment can be viewed online at http://archives.cbc.ca/arts_entertainment/music/topics/1568-10600/.) One image in particular, of a little girl named Birhan Woldu who was apparently about to die, caught the public's attention and became known as the "face of famine." Even though the girl survived and has become an international symbol for hope, the image of her emaciated face, delirious from hunger, motivated people around the world to donate to emergency relief funds for the country. According to Milner, relief agencies received donations totaling nearly £5 million in just three days from the United Kingdom (UK) alone.

THE ETHIOPIAN GOVERNMENT'S SOLUTION. By December 1984 the situation had become completely chaotic. Even though international aid was beginning to enter the country, Ethiopian leaders were intercepting the supplies, first to keep them away from insurgents in the regions fighting for independence, and second to divert them to their own soldiers. Thousands of starving Ethiopians—refugees from both the war and the famine—were fleeing to Sudan every day. The arrival of relief supplies in villages set off riots, with people desperate to get food for their children. In 1985–86 the government imposed a policy of resettlement, with the military forcibly moving those in the northern portions of the country south and relocating peasants into planned villages around services such as water, utilities, medical care, and schools. However, the services promised by Ethiopian leaders were rarely provided, and food production throughout the country actually declined. In 1985–86 Ethiopian crops were hit with a wave of locusts, which destroyed much of the harvest.

BAND AID AND LIVE AID. According to the article "Band Aid: Pop's Global Mission" (BBC News, October 21, 2004), on October 23, 1984, British Broadcasting Corporation journalist Michael Buerk reported on the famine from Ethiopia. Among his television audience was the Irish pop singer Bob Geldof (1951–). That night Geldof telephoned James Ure (1953–), another British pop musician, with a plan to record a song about the famine and donate all the proceeds to relief efforts. Just over a month later more than 40 of the UK's most famous pop musicians—including U2's lead singer Bono (1960–), who would go on to become one of the most visible celebrities to campaign for poverty relief—were assembled under the name Band Aid in a recording studio to produce the single "Do They Know It's Christmas?" Gil Kaufman notes in "Live Aid: A Look Back at a Concert That Actually Changed the World" (MTV.com, June 29, 2005) that the song became the best-selling single in UK history at the time and generated more than US$10 million for Ethiopian famine relief. The song was rerecorded by different sets of popular singers once in 1985 (Band Aid II) and again in 2004 (Band Aid 20), with the proceeds going to poverty relief through Geldof's organization, Band Aid Trust.

Kaufman states that in July 1985 Geldof and Ure organized Live Aid, a set of worldwide simultaneous concerts with venues in London, Philadelphia, Sydney, and Moscow that featured some of the best-known pop musicians of the time. Live Aid was broadcast in 160 countries to an estimated 1.4 billion viewers. The concerts raised more than $200 million for famine relief and ushered in a new era of charity events with celebrity participants. Prior to the U.S. concert, a group of 46 musicians called USA for Africa produced the single "We Are the World," written by Michael Jackson (1958–2009) and Lionel Ritchie (1949–), to benefit Ethiopia's famine relief. The U.S. concert concluded with this song. On February 2, 2010—25 years after "We Are the World" was first recorded—the song was rerecorded by 100 celebrities in Hollywood, California, to provide economic assistance for Haiti, which had been hit with a powerful earthquake on January 12, 2010.

The Ongoing Story of Famine

In 2006 the entire Horn of Africa region, which includes Ethiopia, Kenya, Somalia, and Djibouti, experienced another food crisis. The United Nations (UN) Food and Agriculture Organization (FAO) indicates in "Millions of People Are on the Brink of Starvation in the Horn of Africa" (January 6, 2006, http://www.fao.org/newsroom/en/news/2006/1000206/index.html) that in 2006 an estimated 11 million people in these countries were at risk of starvation due to drought and ongoing violent conflict. The FAO notes that at least 8 million people in Ethiopia, 2.5 million in Kenya, 2 million in Somalia, and 150,000 in Djibouti were expected to be dependent on food aid at least through the summer of 2006. The drought lasted through October 2006, and the ongoing pattern of drought is expected to get worse. According to the article "Climate Change Will Worsen Drought, Hunger in Africa" (Mongabay.com, April 10, 2007), the Intergovernmental Panel on Climate Change reports that climate change is likely to bring with it an increased incidence of extreme weather that could worsen droughts and flooding in Africa. The FAO emphasizes in "Climate Change and Bioenergy Challenges for Food and Agriculture" (October 2009, http://www.fao.org/fileadmin/templates/wsfs/docs/Issues_papers/HLEF2050_Climate.pdf) that climate change will affect agriculture and food production not only in Africa but also in all developing countries prone to droughts, floods, and cyclones "and that have low incomes and high incidence of hunger and poverty." The FAO concludes that "adaptation of the agriculture sector to climate change will be costly but necessary for food security [and] poverty reduction."

By late 2009 the story of worldwide hunger and famine intensified as donor countries slashed aid funding to countries in need of food. The roots of the problem lay in a deepening global economic crisis that began in 2007 and that was exacerbated by increasing oil and food prices. In addition, crops were destroyed in Africa and Southeast Asia due to severe weather-related events. John Vidal reports in "Millions Will Starve as Rich Nations Cut Food Aid Funding, Warns UN" (*Observer* [London], October 11, 2009) that "tens of millions of the world's poor" were to be affected. According to Vidal, Josette Sheeran, the head of the UN's World Food Programme (WFP), characterized the situation as "a silent tsunami" and an unrolling "humanitarian disaster." Even though donor countries gave record amounts of money to the WFP in 2008 to avert a global food crisis that year, contributions in 2009 were considerably less.

MAJOR NATURAL DISASTERS OF 2004 AND 2005

Between 2004 and 2005 there were three natural disasters that were so devastating that they shocked the world. All of them had an especially powerful impact on the poor. One was in a high-poverty area that was also a popular tourist destination for the wealthy; the second was in a desperately impoverished zone with treacherous terrain and little outside contact; and the third, in one of the world's richest nations, exposed a long-ignored underclass. These disasters and their impact demonstrate how natural catastrophes tend to push the poor deeper into poverty.

Asian Tsunami

Marsha Walton reports in "Scientists: Sumatra Quake Longest Ever Recorded" (CNN.com, May 20, 2005) that on December 26, 2004, an undersea earthquake with a magnitude of 9.1 to 9.3 on the Richter scale (a measure of an earthquake's magnitude) occurred in the Indian Ocean off the coast of Sumatra, Indonesia. Unlike most earthquakes, which last from less than 1 second to several seconds, the Sumatran earthquake lasted 500 to 600 seconds (8 to 10 minutes) and briefly shook the entire planet, triggering other, less powerful, earthquakes around the world and a massive tsunami (a series of rolling tidal waves) that devastated 12 countries in and along the Indian Ocean and caused deaths as far away as South Africa. In "Sumatran Quake Sped up Earth's Rotation" (*Nature*, December 30, 2004), Michael Hopkin explains that the earthquake was so powerful that it caused the Earth to shake on its axis and even slightly accelerated its rotation.

The countries directly affected by the earthquake and tsunami included Bangladesh, India, Indonesia, Kenya, Madagascar, Malaysia, Maldives, Myanmar, Seychelles, Somalia, South Africa, Sri Lanka, Tanzania, Thailand, and Yemen. The affected areas in these countries included some of the poorest in the world. The U.S. Geological Survey (USGS) estimates in the press release "2004 Deadliest in Nearly 500 Years for Earthquakes" (February 10, 2005, http://www.usgs.gov/newsroom/article.asp?ID=672)

that the final death toll was 275,950. Thousands of tourists enjoying the region's spectacular beaches were among those killed.

In all, the earthquake and tsunami are believed to be one of the deadliest and costliest natural disasters on record. In *After the Tsunami: Rapid Environmental Assessment* (February 2005, http://www.unep.org/tsunami/tsunami_rpt.asp), the UN Environment Programme estimates damage to the region at more than $10 billion. Nearly every living creature was affected, including the wildlife in ecosystems that were destroyed. Many mangrove forests, coral reefs, sand dunes, and sea grasses were devastated, even while serving as a buffer against the strongest impact of the waves and preventing even more destruction. Fishermen lost their boats, fishing equipment, and livelihoods. Farmers lost the farm animals that are necessary to their survival, and their rice, fruit, and vegetable crops were destroyed because of saltwater contamination.

More women than men were killed because many men were out fishing on the sea, where their boats managed to survive the waves, or were working in the fields or selling crops at inland markets. By contrast, the women and children were either at home or on the beach awaiting the fishermen's return. In addition, many women lost their lives while trying to save children who were in their care at the time of the disaster. In the press release "Three Months On: New Figures Show Tsunami May Have Killed up to Four Times as Many Women as Men" (November 1, 2005, http://www.oxfam.org/node/297), the international relief and development organization Oxfam observes that this disproportion of men to women could have significant socioeconomic consequences in these societies, causing long-term demographic changes and potentially altering women's home, work, marriage, childbearing, property ownership, and education patterns, possibly over the course of generations.

Northern Pakistan Earthquake

On October 8, 2005, an earthquake with a magnitude of about 7.6 on the Richter scale hit South Asia. According to Akhtar Naeem et al., in "A Summary Report on Muzaffarabad Earthquake, Pakistan" (November 7, 2005, http://www.reliefweb.int/), more than 80,000 people were killed, 200,000 were injured, and 4 million were left homeless. The earthquake set off a series of landslides that buried entire villages and blocked roadways in the mountains, impeding rescue efforts. Afghanistan and northern India suffered some damage from the earthquake, but Pakistan sustained the most, particularly the Pakistan-controlled portion of Kashmir, whose capital city, Muzaffarabad, was partially destroyed.

In *Human Development Report 2007/2008—Fighting Climate Change: Human Solidarity in a Divided World*

(2007, http://hdr.undp.org/en/media/HDR_20072008_EN _Complete.pdf), the UN Development Programme notes that in 2004 only 59% of Pakistan's population had access to improved sanitation, half its population was literate, and 40% of its children attended school. From 1990 to 2005 nearly three-quarters (73.6%) lived below the US $2-per-day poverty line. Already in deep poverty, Pakistan had stockpiles of food destroyed in the rubble. Due to postquake landslides, the remote Himalayan villages became even more isolated. In "World Vision Aids Pakistan Victims in Forbidden Quake Zone" (March 1, 2006, http://www.reliefweb.int/rw/rwb.nsf/db900sid/ KKEE-6MGS9T?OpenDocument), Andy Goss notes that relief efforts were further complicated because certain areas of Kashmir are part of the "forbidden tribal belt." These areas are ruled by tribal leaders who forbid outsiders to visit. With more than 13,000 families in these villages in desperate need of help after the earthquake, tribal leaders contacted a trusted Pakistani aid organization that managed to send help to the area. Other aid organizations were warned not to enter the area because of the possibility of armed attack.

By March 2006 millions of people in the mountains were still living in tents, with no water, electricity, or communications systems. Snow in the high elevations and heavy rains in the valleys hampered relief efforts, as helicopters were grounded and roadways blocked. The World Health Organization (WHO) reports in "Health Situation Report #34" (http://www.who.int/hac/crises/ international/pakistan_earthquake/Pakistan_situation _report_34_14_28Feb2006.pdf) that in February 2006 the region was seeing many cases of acute respiratory infection, acute diarrhea, fevers, and earthquake-related injuries. There were also reported cases of measles, meningitis, and acute hepatitis.

The article "UN: 300,000 Quake Survivors at Risk" (*China Daily*, December 5, 2006) states that as the winter of 2006–07 came upon this region, more than 300,000 survivors of the quake were continuing to need food aid. Many families who had lost everything they had in the quake were still living in tents in the mountains in extremely harsh conditions. Refugee camps housed some of the victims, whose homes and land had been washed away by landslides and floods. However, the Canadian Red Cross reports in the press release "From Rubble to Recovery in Two Years" (October 4, 2007, http://www .redcross.ca/article.asp?id=24359&tid=001) that by October 2007 the tents were gone, people were back in homes in their villages, and reconstruction continued.

Hurricane Katrina

On August 29, 2005, one of the strongest, costliest, and deadliest hurricanes in U.S. history made landfall on the Gulf Coast states of Louisiana, Mississippi, and Alabama.

According to the article "FOX Facts: Hurricane Katrina Damage" (FOX News, August 29, 2006), an estimated 1,833 people were killed and nearly 93,000 square miles (241,000 sq km) of land were affected. The damage was estimated at $96 billion. Much of New Orleans, Louisiana, lies below sea level and is protected by a system of levees, which were breached by the rising water; more than 80% of the city was flooded. Residents trapped in their homes climbed to their attics and then to their roofs, but many drowned as they tried to reach safety.

In the aftermath of the storm, much of the world's attention was focused on two factors. First, the administration of President George W. Bush (1946–) and the Federal Emergency Management Agency (FEMA) came under scathing criticism for their handling of the crisis. Critics charged that the federal preparations for the storm were inadequate, that warnings about its danger were ignored or came too late, and that rescue efforts were uncoordinated and often ineffective. However, other critics laid fault with state and local governments, especially Louisiana's governor, Kathleen Blanco (1942–), and the mayor of New Orleans, Ray Nagin (1956–), for poorly coordinating overall rescue and recovery efforts. Still other critics looked at Congress for not providing sufficient funding (through organizations such as the U.S. Army Corps of Engineers) on adequate levee protection and for perpetuating ineptness in government agencies. Second, the catastrophe highlighted the extreme poverty of the residents in the areas hardest hit by the storm, many of whom did not have telephone service or own cars with which to escape. Because many of the residents of the devastated areas were African-American, the exposure of their poverty and the inadequate response by FEMA engendered charges of racism and brought to light issues of racial inequality that still persist in the United States.

POVERTY BEFORE THE HURRICANE. In "Essential Facts about the Victims of Hurricane Katrina" (September 19, 2005, http://www.cbpp.org/9-19-05pov.htm), Isaac Shapiro and Arloc Sherman of the Center on Budget and Policy Priorities report that in 2005 the hurricane-affected states of Mississippi, Louisiana, and Alabama had the first, second, and eighth highest rates of poverty in the country, respectively. More than 1 million of the 5.8 million people who lived in areas affected by Hurricane Katrina were poor before the disaster. Mississippi's poverty rate in 2004 was 21.6%; Louisiana's was 19.4%; and Alabama's was 16.1%. In contrast, the poverty rate for the United States as a whole was approximately 13% in 2004.

According to Shapiro and Sherman, 27.9% of the total population in New Orleans lived in poverty before Hurricane Katrina, and 34.9% of the city's African-American population lived in poverty. In addition, the National Center for Children in Poverty (NCCP) indicates in the fact sheet "Child Poverty in States Hit by Hurricane Katrina" (September 2005, http://www.nccp.org/publications/pdf/text_622.pdf) that in 2004, 38% of children in New Orleans lived in poverty, as did 23% of children in Louisiana as a whole, 24% of children in Mississippi, and 21% in Alabama. For African-American children in these states, the situation was even worse: 44% of African-American children in Louisiana lived in poor families, as did 42% in Alabama and 41% in Mississippi.

KATRINA PERSPECTIVES YEARS LATER. According to Oxfam America, in "US Gulf Coast Recovery Program Fact Sheet" (August 22, 2008, http://www.oxfamamerica.org/files/usgulfcoast-factsheet.pdf), as of April 2007—nearly two years after the devastation of Katrina—more than 100,000 families were still living in temporary housing. In addition, repair of approximately 82,000 rental units in Louisiana and 21,000 in Mississippi had yet to be prioritized. (Before the storm 45% of the families affected by Hurricane Katrina had been renters.) Oxfam also determines that "despite poverty rates that topped 30 percent in some storm-devastated communities, state officials sought and the federal government approved waivers reducing—and in several cases eliminating—the share of recovery grants required to benefit low- and moderate-income communities. Though Louisiana and Mississippi have $16 billion in housing and community development grants to distribute, the states are not consistently sharing information about how much of that money is reaching low-income residents. Very little data is available publicly for evaluating the effectiveness and equity of the grant program."

The editorial "FEMA's Formaldehyde Foul-Up" (*New York Times*, February 15, 2008) notes that in February 2008 the Centers for Disease Control and Prevention announced that several of the trailers provided by FEMA to many who had lost their homes contained unacceptably high levels of formaldehyde, a suspected cancer-causing substance that can also produce serious breathing problems in healthy individuals. The editorial indicates that those who were most vulnerable to the effects of the formaldehyde were the ones still living in the trailers, unable to move "for reasons of age, illness or poverty."

Becky Bohrer reports in "Fewer Katrina, Rita Trailers but Challenges Left" (Associated Press, December 24, 2009) that as of December 2009, approximately 1,600 families were still living in FEMA trailers in Louisiana and Mississippi. Meanwhile, property owners from the Lower Ninth Ward and St. Bernard Parish—areas that were devastated by flooding during Katrina—were claiming a bittersweet court victory against the U.S. Army Corps of Engineers. According to Campbell Robertson, in "Ruling on Katrina Flooding Favors Homeowners" (*New York Times*, November 18, 2009), Judge Stanwood R. Duval Jr.

(1942–) ruled in November 2009 that the Corps had not properly maintained the Mississippi River–Gulf Outlet, a navigation channel that runs 76 miles (122 km) from the Gulf of Mexico to New Orleans harbor. Robertson notes that "the corps' actions, [the plaintiffs] said, brought salt water into the New Orleans area, killing off marshes; eroded the banks on which levees sat; and more than doubled the channel in width, giving water driven by hurricanes an unobstructed path to the city." Judge Duval agreed with this argument. The government was expected to appeal the ruling.

MAJOR NATURAL DISASTERS OF 2006 AND 2007

Java Earthquake and Tsunami

Located in Indonesia, Java is a densely populated island, with more than 124 million people. Indonesia is situated on the Pacific Ring of Fire, and Java is part of a string of volcanic islands that run east to west. Southeastern Asia in general and Java in particular are prone to volcanic eruptions and earthquakes. If the earthquakes take place under the ocean, they can result in tsunamis.

The earthquake that hit Java on May 27, 2006, was the worst disaster to hit Indonesia since the 2004 tsunami. The earthquake directly affected the provinces of Yogyakarta and Central Java. Most of the people in the affected areas were poor, with annual incomes at about half the national average. The earthquake occurred in the early morning hours, when most people were asleep. Thus, many were trapped in their homes and were injured or killed when their homes collapsed. Peter Gelling reports in "Earthquake Reconstruction Will Cost $3 Billion, Indonesia Says" (*New York Times*, June 14, 2006) that the earthquake killed about 5,800 people, injured tens of thousands, and made hundreds of thousands homeless.

While recovering from the May earthquake, Java was hit with a tsunami two months later. According to the WHO, in "Central and West Java Earthquake and Tsunami: Situation Report #5" (July 21, 2006, http://www.searo.who.int/en/Section1257/Section2263/Section2337_12596.htm), an undersea earthquake about 100 miles (161 km) south of Java resulted in waves ranging from 6 to 23 feet (2 to 7 m) high. These waves traveled over 1 mile (about 2 km) inland, affecting many provinces including Yogyakarta and Central Java.

The article "Tsunami Death Toll Increases to 668" (*Los Angeles Times*, July 23, 2006) indicates that the earthquake was much smaller than the one that triggered the 2004 tsunami, so the 2006 tsunami was localized rather than widespread. Nonetheless, 668 people were reported dead and 287 missing. According to Shawn Donnan, in "Shelter Crisis after Indonesian Earthquake" (*Financial Times* [London], September 28, 2006), the UN reported that 1.2 million people were left homeless and that international and local aid was extremely slow to help those affected.

Indonesia was hit once again before the end of 2006. In December of that year the Indonesian province of Aceh, which was still recovering from the 2004 tsunami, experienced devastating floods. Bronwyn Curran explains in "After Aceh Floods, Relief Efforts Help Families Cope with Effects of 'Tsunami from the River'" (January 12, 2007, http://www .unicef.org/infobycountry/indonesia_38021.html) that seasonal floods are somewhat commonplace in this province, but the floods of December 2006 were much more severe than usual. Parts of the Aceh province that had not been affected by the 2004 tsunami were devastated by the floods, which killed around 70 people and affected 450,000 more.

Cyclone Sidr

On November 15, 2007, Cyclone Sidr made landfall on the coast of Bangladesh, which sits on the Bay of Bengal. Sidr brought with it sustained winds of 135 miles per hour (217 km/h). The damage that Bangladesh sustained was quite extensive. In "Hunger Threatens Three Million Bangladeshis" (*Sunday Tribune* [Dublin, Ireland], November 25, 2007), Andrew Buncombe states that 10 days after the cyclone hit, the death toll numbered 3,200. Buncombe also notes that Sidr was the most powerful cyclone to hit Bangladesh in more than a decade and that it destroyed between 50% and 90% of the region's rice crop.

Buncombe explains that the people most often killed in powerful storms are those living in poverty, because they have the least substantial housing and live in the most vulnerable areas. As mentioned previously in this chapter, poor countries and poor areas of countries are often without early warning systems, a situation that puts at-risk residents at even greater risk. However, Buncombe notes that before Sidr made landfall, the Bangladeshi government sent volunteers on bicycles with megaphones to ride through the villages in the path of the storm and tell the people to move to cyclone shelters. This low-tech system worked—2 million people were protected in the cyclone shelters by the time Sidr arrived. In addition, the storm hit at low tide, so the dikes built along the coast as protection provided some defense against the raging sea. Nevertheless, storm damage left 2 million people homeless.

The international community pledged more than $300 million. In addition, the Bangladeshi government promised enough rice to feed those left homeless from the storm for about four months. Within days of the storm, two U.S. ships delivered food and medical supplies to Bangladesh.

NATURAL DISASTERS OF 2008 AND 2009

Figure 8.1 and Figure 8.2 list the natural disasters that occurred in 2008 and 2009 as of December 11, 2009.

These figures show the funds that were raised internationally to help the victims of each devastating event. The two events that resulted in the highest level of funds to be raised for each year were Tropical Cyclone Nargis in Myanmar in May 2008 and the Sumatra Indonesia earthquake in September 2009.

Tropical Cyclone Nargis

Less than six months after Cyclone Sidr slammed into the coast of Bangladesh, another strong storm was brewing in the Bay of Bengal, just southeast of the country. This storm was not destined to hit Bangladesh, however, but would move into Burma (officially known as Myanmar), causing the worst natural disaster for that country in its recorded history. The storm track can be seen in Figure 8.3, with the formation of the storm shown on April 28, 2008, and its movement east by April 30, 2008. The U.S. Agency for International Development reports in "USAID Responds to Cyclone Nargis" (June 4, 2009, http://www.usaid.gov/locations/asia/countries/ burma/cyclone_nargis/) that the storm intensified to a category 4, also known as a very severe cyclonic storm, with a maximum sustained wind speed of approximately 132 miles per hour (212 km/hr) and a storm surge of 12 feet (3.7 m) when it when it made landfall on May 2, 2008, near the mouth of the Irrawaddy River and the surrounding Irrawaddy Delta. The cyclone's strength diminished somewhat as it moved over land, but it still hit Yangon (Rangoon) fiercely the next day. Yangon is the former capital of Burma and is the largest city in the country. According the article "Cyclone Nargis" (*New York Times*, April 30, 2009), both the delta area and the city were devastated.

The Irrawaddy Delta is a region with rivers, lakes, and rich soil. It is densely populated with rice farming and fishing communities. The article "Cyclone Nargis" notes that the storm surge was responsible for most of the destruction that occurred. The huge area of flooding can be seen in Figure 8.4. The article states, "It blew away 700,000 homes in the delta. It killed three-fourths of the livestock, sank half the fishing fleet and salted a million acres of rice paddies with its seawater surges." It killed nearly 85,000 people and left 54,000 missing.

The government in power at the time would not allow the French and American ships carrying relief supplies to dock, thinking that the devastation was less than it was and fearing a Western invasion. An international outcry ensued, and aid was eventually brought to the affected people. The Tripartite Core Group, which consists of the Association of Southeast Asian Nations, the government of Myanmar, and the UN Country Team, states in *Post Nargis Periodic Review III* (January 2010, https://aseanhtf.org/download_pr3report.html) that "food aid, health and sanitation assistance have largely reached the most affected townships. Positive impacts on health

FIGURE 8.1

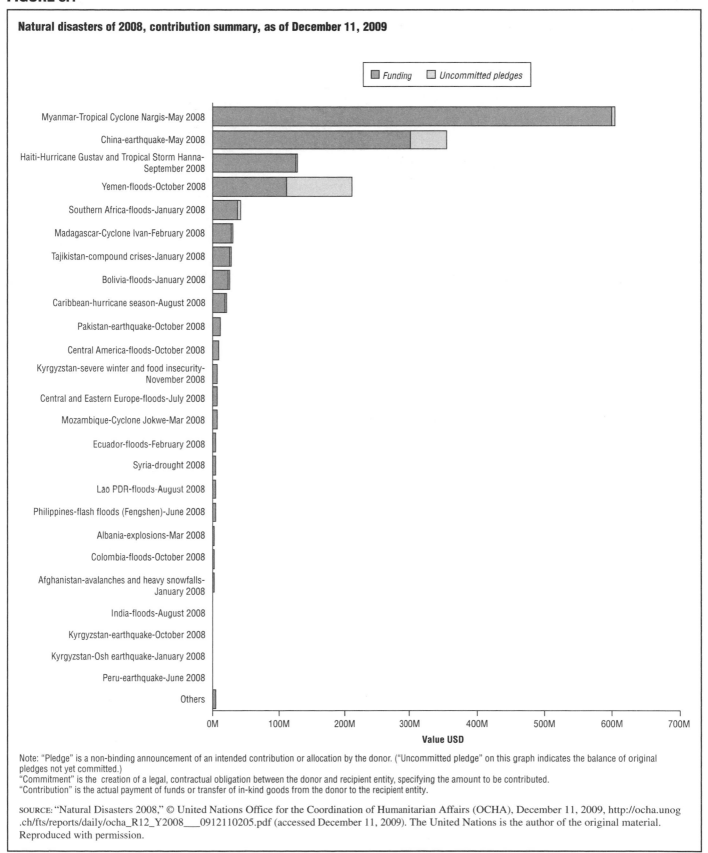

Natural disasters of 2008, contribution summary, as of December 11, 2009

Note: "Pledge" is a non-binding announcement of an intended contribution or allocation by the donor. ("Uncommitted pledge" on this graph indicates the balance of original pledges not yet committed.)
"Commitment" is the creation of a legal, contractual obligation between the donor and recipient entity, specifying the amount to be contributed.
"Contribution" is the actual payment of funds or transfer of in-kind goods from the donor to the recipient entity.

SOURCE: "Natural Disasters 2008," © United Nations Office for the Coordination of Humanitarian Affairs (OCHA), December 11, 2009, http://ocha.unog .ch/fts/reports/daily/ocha_R12_Y2008___0912110205.pdf (accessed December 11, 2009). The United Nations is the author of the original material. Reproduced with permission.

are visible, as measured by improvements in child mortality, child nutrition and the availability of health care and clean water. More than 90 per cent of the surveyed households reported that health personnel and medications were available in health care facilities all or some of the time in nearly 70 per cent of the sampled villages.

FIGURE 8.2

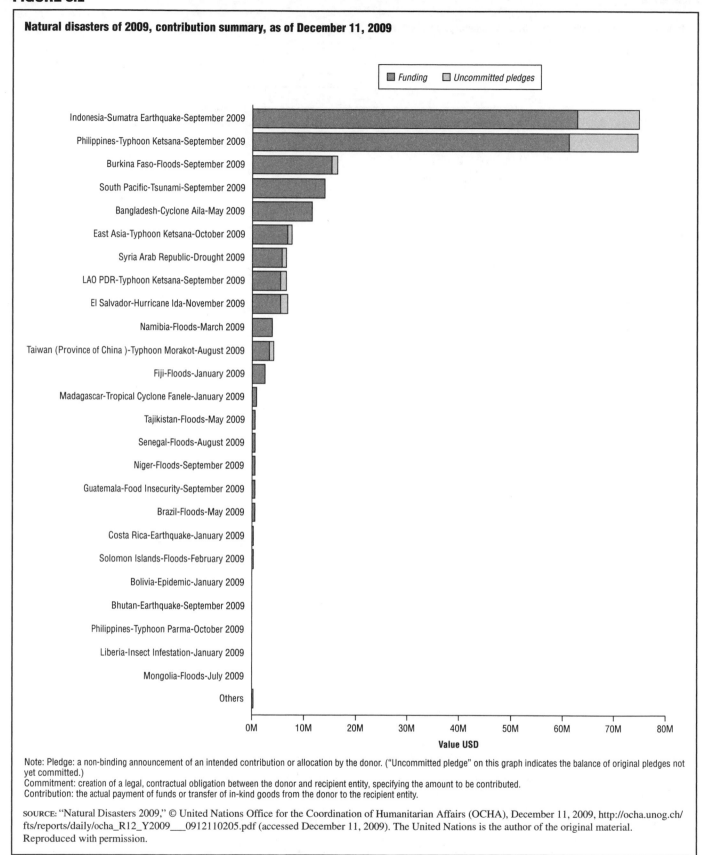

Natural disasters of 2009, contribution summary, as of December 11, 2009

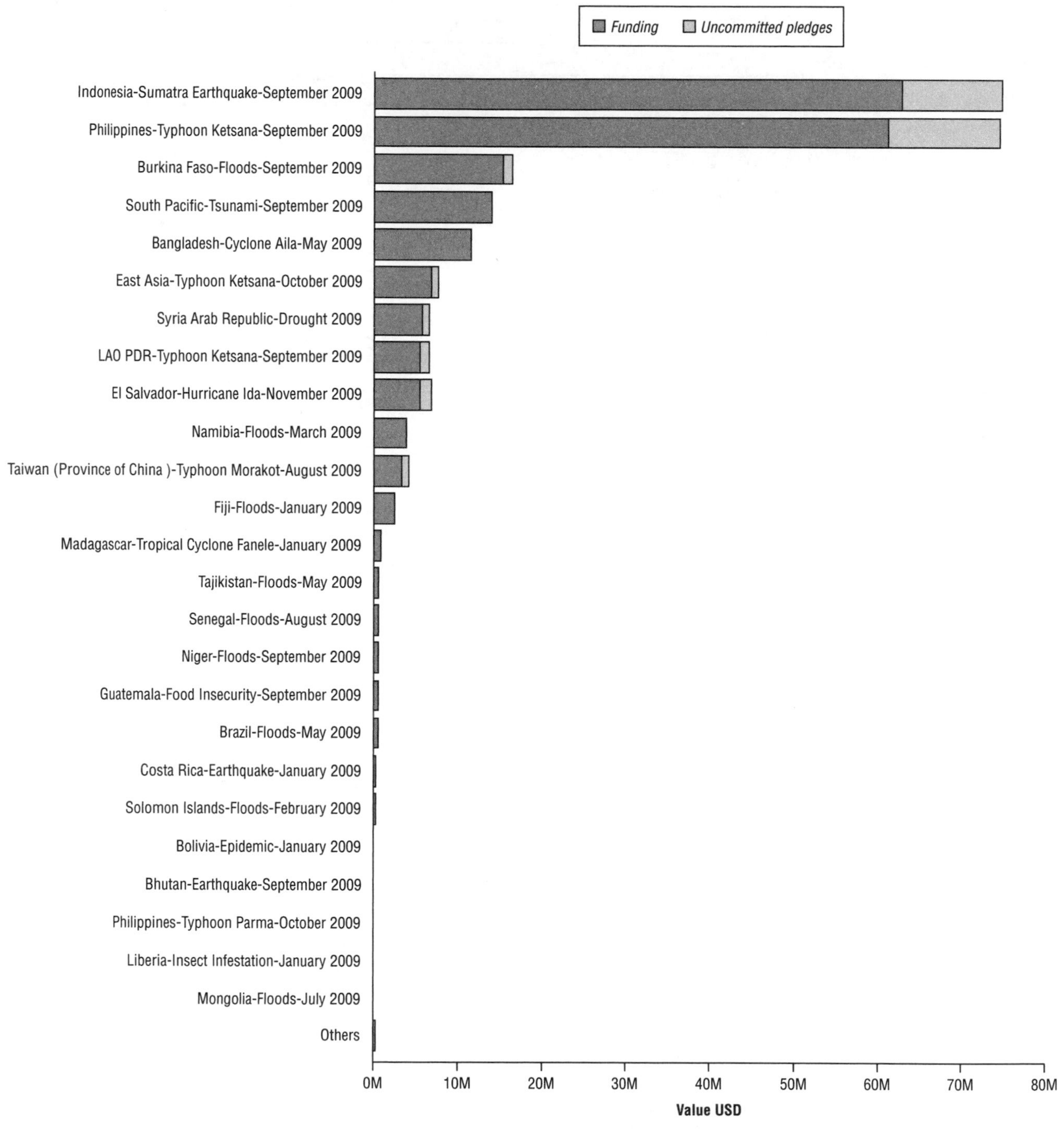
Funding
Uncommitted pledges
Indonesia-Sumatra Earthquake-September 2009
Philippines-Typhoon Ketsana-September 2009
Burkina Faso-Floods-September 2009
South Pacific-Tsunami-September 2009
Bangladesh-Cyclone Aila-May 2009
East Asia-Typhoon Ketsana-October 2009
Syria Arab Republic-Drought 2009
LAO PDR-Typhoon Ketsana-September 2009
El Salvador-Hurricane Ida-November 2009
Namibia-Floods-March 2009
Taiwan (Province of China)-Typhoon Morakot-August 2009
Fiji-Floods-January 2009
Madagascar-Tropical Cyclone Fanele-January 2009
Tajikistan-Floods-May 2009
Senegal-Floods-August 2009
Niger-Floods-September 2009
Guatemala-Food Insecurity-September 2009
Brazil-Floods-May 2009
Costa Rica-Earthquake-January 2009
Solomon Islands-Floods-February 2009
Bolivia-Epidemic-January 2009
Bhutan-Earthquake-September 2009
Philippines-Typhoon Parma-October 2009
Liberia-Insect Infestation-January 2009
Mongolia-Floods-July 2009
Others
0M
10M
20M
30M
40M
50M
60M
70M
80M
Value USD

Note: Pledge: a non-binding announcement of an intended contribution or allocation by the donor. ("Uncommitted pledge" on this graph indicates the balance of original pledges not yet committed.)
Commitment: creation of a legal, contractual obligation between the donor and recipient entity, specifying the amount to be contributed.
Contribution: the actual payment of funds or transfer of in-kind goods from the donor to the recipient entity.

SOURCE: "Natural Disasters 2009," © United Nations Office for the Coordination of Humanitarian Affairs (OCHA), December 11, 2009, http://ocha.unog.ch/fts/reports/daily/ocha_R12_Y2009___0912110205.pdf (accessed December 11, 2009). The United Nations is the author of the original material. Reproduced with permission.

Food security was reported as stable or improved over most of the affected area, with a few households relying on moderate to extreme coping practices."

Sumatra Earthquake

Figure 8.5 shows the island of Sumatra in western Indonesia, and Figure 8.6 shows an enlargement of the

FIGURE 8.3

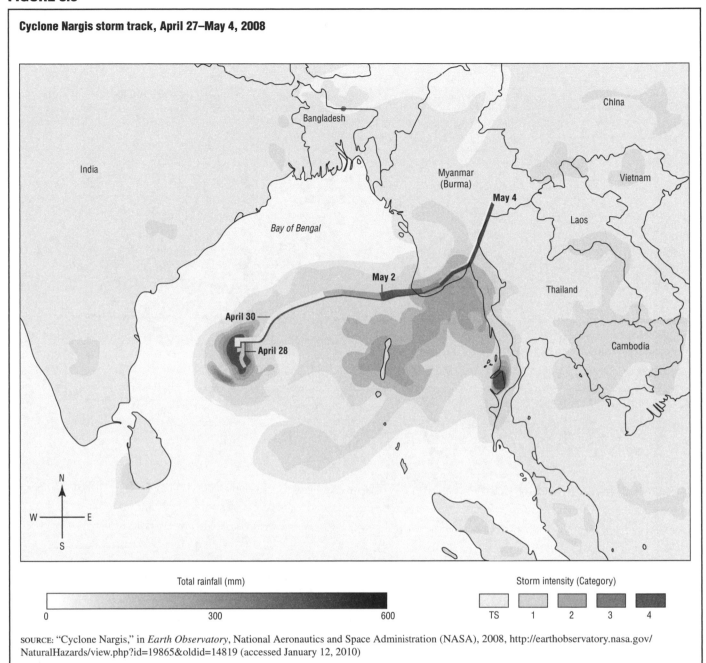

Cyclone Nargis storm track, April 27–May 4, 2008

Total rainfall (mm)

0   300   600

Storm intensity (Category)

TS   1   2   3   4

SOURCE: "Cyclone Nargis," in *Earth Observatory*, National Aeronautics and Space Administration (NASA), 2008, http://earthobservatory.nasa.gov/NaturalHazards/view.php?id=19865&oldid=14819 (accessed January 12, 2010)

southern coastline of Sumatra near Padang, a city that was close to the epicenter of a 7.6 magnitude earthquake that struck on September 30, 2009. The epicenter of a 5.5 magnitude aftershock is shown in the enlargement as well. The island and the city are located near the undersea fault between the Sunda Plate and the subducting Australia Plate, so they are prone to frequent earthquakes and volcanic activity. (See Figure 8.6.) The epicenter of this quake was just south of the epicenter of the much larger undersea quake that caused the Asian tsunami of 2004.

The article "Dozens Dead in Indonesian Quake" (BBC News, September 30, 2009) reports that the death toll in Padang and the surrounding areas was expected to be high

because many buildings, including schools and hotels, had collapsed during the violent shaking. Peter Gelling and Mark McDonald report in "Chaos and Panic after Sumatra Quakes" (*International Herald Tribune*, October 2, 2009) that the quake had collapsed Padang's three major hospitals and had damaged every building taller than three stories. According to Gelling and McDonald, there was chaos in the city because the people had no food, fuel, or money. Thousands tried to flee, but the roads were blocked with debris. The USGS notes in the press release "Earthquakes Cause over 1700 Deaths in 2009" (January 8, 2010, http://www.usgs.gov/newsroom/article.asp?ID=2378) that the final death toll was 1,117. It also indicates that the Sumatra quake was the deadliest for 2009.

FIGURE 8.4

Cyclone Nargis flooding, May 5, 2008

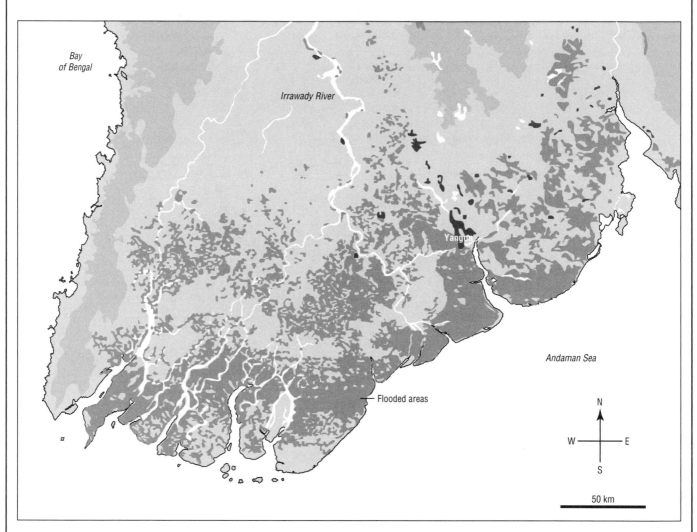

Bay
of Bengal

Irrawady River

Yangun

Andaman Sea

— Flooded areas

N
W — E
S

50 km

SOURCE: "Combination Satellite Image Gives Clearer Image of Cyclone Nargis Floods," in *Hurricanes/Tropical Cyclones*, National Aeronautics and Space Administration (NASA), May 20, 2008, http://www.nasa.gov/mission_pages/hurricanes/archives/2008/h2008_nargis.html (accessed January 12, 2010). Data from the Department of Geography, University of Maryland.

2010 BEGINS WITH DEVASTATING EARTHQUAKES IN HAITI AND CHILE

The Sumatra earthquake was soon overshadowed by a 7.0 earthquake that struck Haiti on January 12, 2010. The epicenter of the quake was only 10 miles (16 km) southwest of Port-au-Prince, the Haitian capital. Haiti is located on the Caribbean island of Hispaniola, which it shares with the Dominican Republic.

According to Simon Romero and Marc Lacey, in "Fierce Quake Devastates Haitian Capital" (*New York Times*, January 12, 2010), shortly after the quake the USGS seismologist David Wald predicted a "high number of casualties" because Port-au-Prince was "an area that is particularly vulnerable in terms of construction practice, and with a high population density." The poor quality of construction in Haiti existed not only with the city buildings

but also with the tin-roof shacks that were perched on the sides of steep ravines. Tens of thousands of Haitians lived in those shacks. As one of the poorest countries in the Western Hemisphere, Haiti had a human development rank of 149 out of 182 countries in 2009. (See Table 1.2 in Chapter 1.)

The article "Haiti Earthquake: Conflicting Death Tolls Lead to Confusion" (Associated Press, February 11, 2010) reports that at the time of the quake approximately 3 million people were in the capital city ready to leave schools and businesses for the day. About 250,000 houses and 30,000 commercial buildings were estimated to have collapsed, crushing their occupants. So many people died that their bodies were piled in the streets and then buried in mass graves; in some instances records were not kept. As a result, the death toll was in dispute, with estimates ranging from 170,000 to 230,000 killed.

FIGURE 8.5

Location of the island of Sumatra within Indonesia

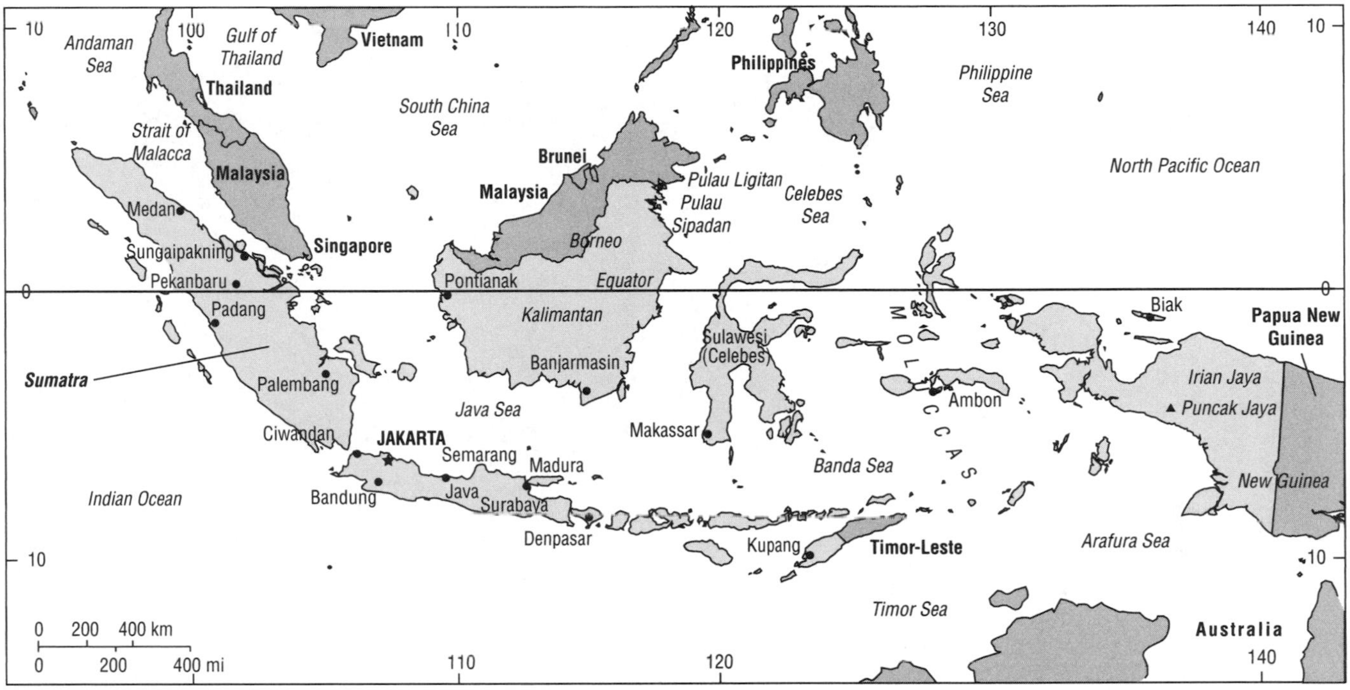

SOURCE: "Indonesia," in *The World Factbook*, Central Intelligence Agency (CIA), 2009, https://www.cia.gov/library/publications/the-world-factbook/geos/id.html (accessed January 12, 2010)

The worldwide reaction to the Haiti earthquake was immediate. Many countries sent rescue workers to find survivors in the rubble and to bring food, water, and medical aid. Damage to the airport, the seaport, and the roads made the rescue and relief mission extremely difficult.

While the world was still focused on the devastation in Haiti, a far more powerful earthquake and then a tsunami struck Chile. On February 27, 2010, an earthquake registering 8.8 on the Richter scale struck about 70 miles (113 km) west of Concepción, Chile's second-largest metropolitan area. Even though the Chilean earthquake was far stronger than the Haitian earthquake, the damage was expected to be less severe because of Chile's strict earthquake building codes, compared with the poor building construction in poverty-stricken Haiti. Nonetheless, four days after the earthquake shook Chile, 800 people were feared dead, most probably from the tsunami. The article "Tsunami May Prove Bigger Killer Than Chile Quake" (National Public Radio, March 3, 2010) reports that the tsunami "swamped towns small and large along a 435-mile [700-km] stretch of Chile's Pacific coast."

FIGURE 8.6

Location of Sumatra earthquake, September 2009

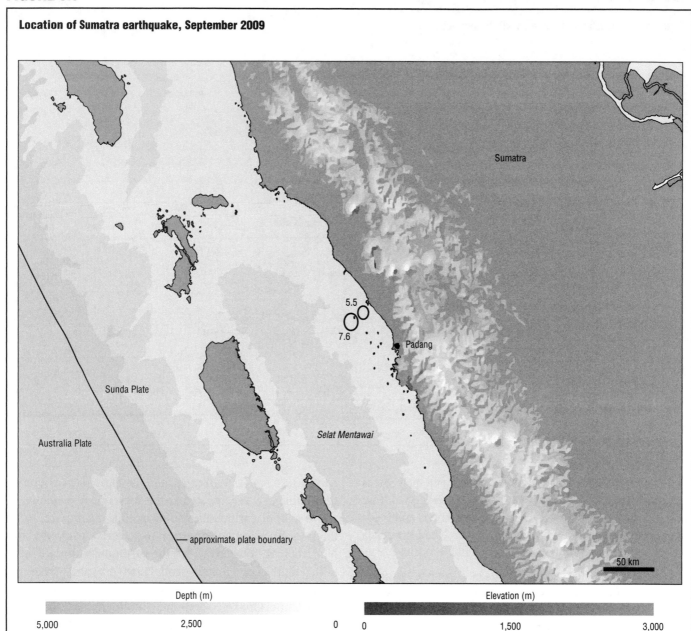

SOURCE: "7.6 Magnitude Earthquake off Sumatra," in *Earth Observatory*, National Aeronautics and Space Administration (NASA), September 2009, http://earthobservatory.nasa.gov/NaturalHazards/view.php?id=40537 (accessed January 12, 2010)

CHAPTER 9
POVERTY AND VIOLENT CONFLICT

The residents of countries engaged in conflict or warfare—whether the countries are developing, developed, or in transition—almost always experience some degree of economic hardship. For example, during World War II (1939–1945) much of Europe was reduced to near starvation, and even the United States—which did not engage in military action on its own soil except at Pearl Harbor—imposed strict rationing of goods on its citizens to divert more of its resources to the military effort. However, the United Nations Development Programme (UNDP) Oslo Governance Centre explains in "Governance and Conflict Prevention" (October 14, 2009, http://www.undp.org/oslocentre/overview/gover nance_conflict_prevention.html) that since the 1990s the most violent conflicts occurred in countries that were already poor and that experienced conditions far worse than rationing. More specifically, the Oslo Governance Centre states that "studies show that over half of the countries affected by conflict since 1990 were low income countries, an increase from one third in previous decades."

Punctuating this point, the Stockholm International Peace Research Institute (SIPRI) ranks countries by their relative state of peace in *SIPRI Yearbook 2009: Armaments, Disarmament and International Security* (2009, http://www .sipri.org/yearbook/2009/files/SIPRIYB09summary.pdf). The five least peaceful countries in 2009 were Iraq, Afghanistan, Somalia, Israel, and Sudan. Of these countries, Israel was the only one with a very high level of human development in 2009. Sudan had a medium level of human development and Afghanistan had a low level of human development. There were not enough data to rank Iraq and Somalia. On the Human Poverty Index Iraq was ranked at 75 out of 135 countries, Sudan at 104, and Afghanistan at 135—the most poverty-stricken of the countries ranked in 2009. (See Table 1.2 in Chapter 1.) In contrast, the five most peaceful countries in 2009 were New Zealand, Denmark, Norway, Iceland, and Austria. All these countries had a very high human development rank in 2009. (See Table 1.3 in Chapter 1.)

Conflict and warfare affects children in devastating ways. Figure 9.1 shows the child mortality–armed conflict link with data from the United Nations Children's Fund. The bar graph shows countries that had a high rate of child mortality from 1999 to 2005. Most of these countries, as shown by the lighter bars, experienced major armed conflict during this period. Those with the darker bars—a small proportion of the countries shown— did not experience armed conflict during this period.

Armed conflict in poor countries makes the dire situations of poor people even worse. The Oslo Governance Centre notes that "armed conflicts are now the leading cause of world hunger" and "are the biggest obstacles preventing adequate progress towards achieving the Millennium Development Goals."

VIOLENT CONFLICT AND ITS EFFECT ON HUMAN DEVELOPMENT

The Millennium Development Goals (MDGs; http://www.undp.org/mdg/basics.shtml) are a list of eight human development goals to be reached by 2015. (See Chapter 2.) These goals are a part of the Millennium Declaration (http://www.un.org/millennium/declaration/ares552e.htm), an agreement of 189 member countries of the United Nations (UN) signed on September 8, 2000, to increase the state of human development around the world. The MDGs focus on eradicating extreme poverty and hunger; achieving universal primary education; promoting gender equality and empowering women; reducing child mortality; improving maternal health; combating the human immunodeficiency virus (HIV), the acquired immunodeficiency syndrome (AIDS), malaria, and other diseases; ensuring environmental sustainability; and developing a global partnership for development. Achievement of the MDGs or progress toward their achievement has become a standard way to gauge levels of human development in all

FIGURE 9.1

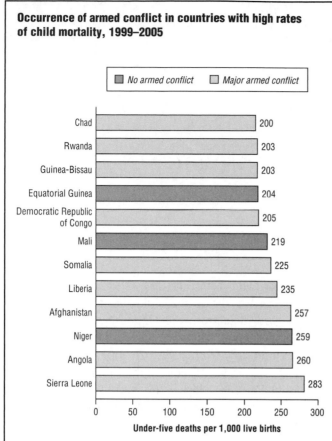

Occurrence of armed conflict in countries with high rates of child mortality, 1999–2005

■ No armed conflict   □ Major armed conflict

Country	Under-five deaths per 1,000 live births
Chad	200
Rwanda	203
Guinea-Bissau	203
Equatorial Guinea	204
Democratic Republic of Congo	205
Mali	219
Somalia	225
Liberia	235
Afghanistan	257
Niger	259
Angola	260
Sierra Leone	283

Under-five deaths per 1,000 live births

SOURCE: "Figure 2.3. Most of the Countries Where 1 in 5 Children Die before Five Have Experienced Major Armed Conflict since 1999," in *The State of the World's Children 2006: Excluded and Invisible,* United Nations Children's Fund, 2005, http://www.unicef.org/sowc06/pdfs/sowc0506_eps_charts.pdf (accessed April 8, 2006). Data on child mortality from: UNICEF, United Nations Population Division and United Nations Statistics Division; data on major armed conflicts from: Stockholm International Peace Research Institute and The Uppsala Conflict Data Program, *SIPRI Yearbook 2005: Armaments, Disarmament and International Security* (Oxford: Oxford University Press, 2005).

countries and regions of the world and contributes to countries' UNDP Human Development Index rank.

Civil war (a war between different factions within a country) affects a country's human development in many ways. According to Paul Collier, in *The Bottom Billion: Why the Poorest Countries Are Failing and What Can Be Done about It* (2007), civil wars typically last seven years, and each year economic growth drops by an average of 2.3%. Furthermore, refugees fleeing to neighboring countries, and the possibility of those countries being drawn into the fighting, can strain the entire region in which a conflict takes place.

In any type of war, the unbalanced gender ratio that usually results from violent conflict also affects a region's human development. With large numbers of men killed in the fighting, women are left to support and protect their families by themselves. This leaves them vulnerable to

attack and rape during conflict and to poverty and lowered levels of education and health care for themselves, their children, and future generations. In some cases the loss of an excessively large number of young men to fighting can bring about massive demographic changes and set back the security, education, and health of women for years. With fewer marriageable young men in the population, young women might become betrothed to elderly men or in some cases to relatives.

In addition, violent conflict increases the risk of a food crisis—especially in rural areas—because livestock, crops, and land fit for growing crops might be destroyed. However, it is not just the physical destruction of farms during war that leaves societies vulnerable to hunger. The displacement of farmers as refugees causes just as much harm to agricultural production.

Undernutrition during wars affects the health and strength of people, but the health of a population engaged in warfare decreases dramatically in other ways as well. People are not only killed during the fighting but also they die from things such as infectious diseases, which spread rapidly among refugees and quickly spill over from refugee camps into the populations surrounding them. Land mines are another consequence of war that kill and injure.

Land Mines

One of the most brutal tools of conflict affecting human health and security is the presence of land mines, which can damage and terrorize a population physically and psychologically for decades. Land mines are explosive devices that are usually buried underground or laid just above ground and triggered by vehicles or footsteps. Anti-tank land mines are, as their name suggests, designed to blow up tanks and large vehicles. Antipersonnel land mines (APLs) are designed so that they are triggered by even the lightest of footsteps. The International Campaign to Ban Landmines (ICBL) explains in "Arguments for a Ban" (February 2010, http://www.icbl.org/index.php/icbl/Problem/Landmines/Arguments-for-a-Ban) that APLs are by far the more devastating kind of land mine for two reasons. First, they are indiscriminate in blowing up both soldiers and civilians, and second, they exist in regions indefinitely after a war or conflict ends. Some APLs are designed to look like small, colorful toys, stones, or even butterflies, making them extremely dangerous to children.

The continuing presence of land mines after the end of a conflict limits development and increases poverty in affected regions. Areas known to contain land mines are unusable for farming, building, living, or commerce of any kind. According to the ICBL, in *Landmine Monitor Report 2009: Toward a Mine-Free World* (October 2009, http://lm.icbl.org/lm/2009/res/Landmines_Report_2009.pdf), in 2008 countries and areas in Africa, Europe, the Middle East, Asia and the Pacific, and Central and South America experienced 5,197 reported land mine–related deaths or injuries. Thirty-four percent of all recorded casualties were in two countries: Colombia and Afghanistan. The number of casualties reported in 2008 was less than in previous years.

Besides the human casualties, livestock and wild animals are frequently injured or killed by land mines. This situation not only harms regional environments but also destroys farming economies.

Refugees

In 1950 the Office of the UN High Commissioner for Refugees (UNHCR) was created, and in 1951 the UN Convention Relating to the Status of Refugees (http://www.unhcr.org/3b66c2aa10.html) was adopted. The two main tenets of the convention are that refugees are not to be returned to an area where they face persecution and that refugees are not to face discrimination in the country that accepts them. However, according to the UNHCR, in *State of the World's Refugees 2006: Human Displacement in the New Millennium* (April 2006, http://www.unhcr.org/4a4dc1a89.html), people seeking asylum as refugees are increasingly becoming the targets of xenophobes (those who have a fear of foreigners) and are being accused of terrorist activity.

In *Statistical Yearbook 2007: Trends in Displacement, Protection, and Solutions* (December 2008, http://www.unhcr.org/4981c4812.html), the UNHCR reports that as of January 1, 2008, there were an estimated 31.7 million "persons of concern": refugees, asylum seekers, internally displaced people (IDPs) protected/assisted by the UNHCR, stateless people (those without a country), returned refugees, returned IDPs, and others of concern. Of this group, 11.4 million (36%) were refugees and 740,000 (2%) were classified as asylum seekers—that is, they had applied for legal recognition in the country to which they had fled. Another 13.7 million (43%) were considered IDPs within their home nation, 2.9 million (9%) were stateless people, and 731,000 (2%) were returned refugees. These numbers reflect only those who received aid from the UNHCR. Among those not included in these figures are the estimated 4.6 million displaced Palestinians, who are counted by a related organization, the UN Relief and Works Agency for Palestine Refugees in the Near East (UNRWA). An unknown number of refugees and IDPs do not receive aid and therefore cannot be accurately counted.

Some people are forced to leave their homes and seek refuge in other countries because of natural disasters, but most become refugees because their homelands are torn by violent conflict or because human rights abuses are rampant. In situations of long-term conflict, groups of people may endure recurring periods of short-term displacement, or they may be displaced indefinitely. Many refugees find themselves relocated—by force or by choice—to countries that are hostile to their presence. Refugee camps are generally dangerous places because of violence both inside and outside of their boundaries. Refugees may be denied basic human rights, including the right to seek legal employment, which exacerbates their impoverished condition. Even when refugees are returned to their homelands, they sometimes encounter an unwelcoming environment because their houses, workplaces, farms, and possessions may have been destroyed, and the regime in control may react violently to their return.

Even though conditions for refugees are typically substandard in terms of housing, food, and other necessities, and even though they have the hardships of displacement to endure, those who cannot leave conflict regions because of extreme poverty or ill health are often the most vulnerable. Children and adolescents are a particularly vulnerable group as well. In regions of conflict children often become separated from their families and may become sexually or physically abused, forced into slavery, or forced to join armies. They may have no access to education, food, or physical care. The UNHCR states in *Statistical Yearbook 2007* that "children and adolescents represent the majority of people of concern in Africa and Asia. In the Central Africa and the Great Lakes as well as in the East and Horn of Africa regions, they constitute 55 and 54 per cent respectively of UNHCR's people of concern. The lowest proportion of children is found in countries covered by the Regional Bureau for Europe (18%)."

MILITARY SPENDING

The UNDP notes in *Human Development Report 2007/2008—Fighting Climate Change: Human Solidarity in a Divided World* (2007, http://hdr.undp.org/en/media/HDR_20072008_EN_Complete.pdf) that there are great differences in spending on health, education, and the military among countries that are and are not seriously involved in military conflict or located in volatile areas of the world. Countries with no armed conflicts on their soil, such as Canada, Japan, and the United Kingdom (UK), spend much less on military expenditures than on health and education. By contrast, countries involved in armed conflict or located in volatile areas, such as Israel, Oman, Saudi Arabia, Lebanon, and Iran, relegate a much higher share of their gross domestic product (GDP; the total value of all goods and services produced by a country in a year) to military expenditures.

Figure 9.2 shows the range of defense spending as a share of total budget among selected developed countries that are members of the Organization for Economic Cooperation and Development (OECD). The third band down from the top of each bar shows the proportion of that country's defense spending. The country with the

FIGURE 9.2

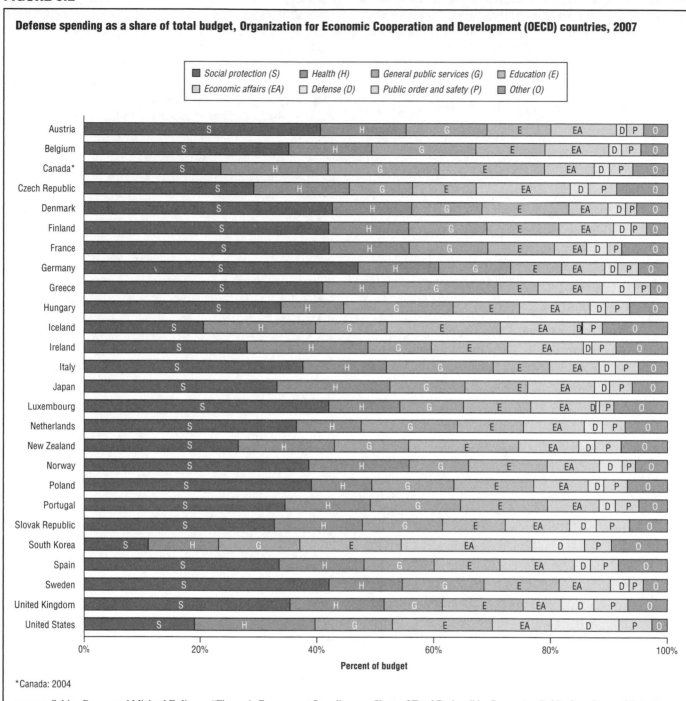

Defense spending as a share of total budget, Organization for Economic Cooperation and Development (OECD) countries, 2007

*Social protection (S)   Health (H)   General public services (G)   Education (E)
Economic affairs (EA)   Defense (D)   Public order and safety (P)   Other (O)*

Percent of budget

*Canada: 2004

SOURCE: Sabina Dewan and Michael Ettlinger, "Figure 4. Government Spending as a Share of Total Budget," in *Comparing Public Spending and Prioritiesa across OECD Countries*, Center for American Progress, October 2009, http://www.americanprogress.org/issues/2009/10/pdf/oecd_spending.pdf (accessed January 12, 2010). This figure was created by the Center for American Progress (www.americanprogress.org) with data from the OECD Economic Outlook

largest portion of its budget going to defense is the United States. In *Comparing Public Spending and Priorities across OECD Countries* (October 2009, http://www.americanprogress.org/issues/2009/10/pdf/oecd_spending.pdf), Sabina Dewan and Michael Ettlinger note that the United States spends about 12% of its annual budget on defense. Of the countries listed in the figure, South Korea spends the next highest percentage at 9% and Greece and the United Kingdom (UK) are next, each with 6%. The countries

spending the lowest percentage of their budget on defense are Iceland and Luxembourg, at less than 1% each. Austria, Belgium, Ireland, and Germany each spend about 2% of their budget on defense.

In *SIPRI Yearbook 2009*, the SIPRI reports that in 2008 world military expenditures totaled $1.2 trillion. (See Table 9.1.) Worldwide military spending increased 45% from 1999 to 2008. The SIPRI also notes that in

TABLE 9.1

World and regional military expenditure estimates, 1999–2008

Region	1999	2000	2001	2002	2003	2004	2005	2006	2007	2008	% change, 1999–2008
Africa	14.6	13.6	14.2	15.1	15.1	16.8	17.3	17.8	(18.6)	(20.4)	*+40*
North Africa	4.0	4.0	5.2	5.2	5.4	5.9	6.1	6.1	6.6	7.8	*+94*
Sub-Saharan Africa	10.6	9.5	9.1	9.9	9.7	10.9	11.2	11.7	(11.9)	(12 .6)	*+19*
Americas	368	383	388	430	482	523	549	559	576	603	*+64*
Caribbean	—	—	—	—	—	—	—	—	—	—	—
Central America	3.7	3.9	3.9	3.8	3.8	3.6	3.6	3.4	4.5	4.5	*+21*
North America	341	354	357	399	453	493	516	525	540	564	*+66*
South America	22.7	24.8	27.4	27.2	25.3	26.6	29.0	30.2	32.1	34.1	*+50*
Asia and Oceania	136	139	147	154	160	169	177	186	196	206	*+52*
Central Asia	0.5	—	—	—	—	—	—	—	—	—	
East Asia	101	104	110	116	122	127	133	140	149	157	*+56*
Oceania	12.3	12.2	12.7	13.2	13.5	14.0	14.5	15.4	16.2	16 .6	*+36*
South Asia	21.9	22.8	23.5	23.6	24.2	27.5	28.9	29.2	29.9	30.9	*+41*
Europe	281	287	289	298	302	303	303	309	314	320	*+14*
Eastern Europe	15.9	21.4	23.3	25.8	27.6	28.9	32.0	35.7	39.3	43.6	*+174*
West and Central	265	266	265	272	274	274	271	273	275	277	*+5*
Middle East	48.6	53.8	56.9	54.8	56.4	59.3	66.0	70.4	76.5	75.6	*+56*
World	847	877	895	952	1015	1071	1113	1142	1182	1226	***+45***
Annual change (%)		3.5	2.1	6.3	6.7	5.5	3.9	2.6	3.5	3.7	

*Some countries are excluded because of lack of data or of consistent time series data: Africa excludes Equatorial Guinea and Somalia; the Americas excludes Cuba, Guyana, Haiti and Trinidad and Tobago; Asia excludes North Korea and Myanmar; and the Middle East excludes Qatar. World totals exclude all these countries.
Notes: Figures are in US$ (United States dollars) billions, at constant (2005) prices and exchange rates.
Figures in italics are percentages. Figures may not add up because of the conventions of rounding.
( ) = total based on country data accounting for less than 90 percent of the regional total;
— = available data account for less than 60 percent of the regional total.

SOURCE: Sam Perlo-Freeman et al., "Table 5.1. World and Regional Military Expenditure Estimates, 1999–2008," in "Military Expenditure," *SIPRI Yearbook 2009: Armaments, Disarmament and International Security*, Stockholm International Peace Research Institute (SIPRI), 2009, http://www.sipri.org/yearbook/2009/files/SIPRIYB0 905.pdf (accessed January 12, 2010)

2008, 15 countries spent 81% of the world's total military spending, while the top five accounted for 60%. In order of amount spent, the top five were the United States, China, France, the UK, and Russia.

Besides being the leader in military spending, the United States also far surpasses other countries' spending. It is responsible for 41.5% of the world's total military spending, whereas the next four top countries are each responsible for 4% to 6%. The increase in U.S. military spending in Afghanistan and Iraq is the primary basis for the overall increase in military spending in the United States in recent years.

All regions and subregions of the world increased their military expenditures from 1999 to 2008, but western and central Europe increased the least at 5%. (See Table 9.1.) The SIPRI attributes this low level of military spending increase to the region's modest economic growth rates and a perceived lack of threat to its security. By contrast, eastern Europe had an extremely high level of increase in military spending (174%) from 1999 to 2008, largely due to increases in military spending by the Russian Federation, "whose military spending has been driven by high economic growth and the desire to re-establish its major power status." The SIPRI adds that "all countries in North Africa have made substantial increases [94%], but the majority of the subregional increase is due to Algeria, driven by strong economic growth, a growing regional political role and a worsening insurgency." China also increased its military spending, which is reflected in the 56% increase seen in East Asia in Table 9.1. This increase parallels China's economic growth and its aspirations to be a world power. The Middle East is another region that shows high increases in military spending (56%), and the SIPRI attributes this increase to ongoing conflicts.

POVERTY IN SOME OF THE MOST DANGEROUS PLACES ON EARTH

Darfur

Darfur is an enormous region in western Sudan, which is located in northeastern Africa. The Darfur region covers an area of about 125,000 square miles (324,000 sq km) and has a population of about 7 million people, most of whom are either subsistence farmers or nomadic herdsmen. The two main ethnic groups in the region are the Arabic Baggara (who are nomads) and the non-Arabic Fur (who are farmers). These groups are further divided into smaller ethnic groups. Tensions between the Baggara and the Fur have existed for centuries.

The Darfur region was a center of commercial activity during the slave trade, when native Africans were exported to Arabic countries. Since the mid-1950s the Sudanese government has been under Muslim control and in near constant conflict with non-Muslim opposition within the country. A combination of domination by ruling Muslims and competition for scarce resources caused tensions in Darfur to escalate in 2003, creating an immense humanitarian crisis in the region.

Early in 2003 Arabic Janjaweed militias began a campaign against the African rebel groups the Sudanese Liberation Army and the Justice and Equality Movement, who had taken up arms against the government. A major factor was the competition for water and land between the Arabic nomads and the non-Arabic farmers. However, the situation quickly degenerated into indiscriminate Janjaweed attacks on civilians. According to the article "Sudan: Killings Reported in South Darfur, Says UN" (IRINnews.org, November 11, 2005), the result was mass murder, rape, and the displacement of as many as 2 million people from their homes to refugee camps within Darfur and the neighboring country of Chad. All of this provoked international attention and led to the deployment in October 2005 of 7,000 African Union (AU) troops in an attempt to restore order, but the poorly funded and organized mission could do little to stop the atrocities. A number of temporary cease-fires were put in place, with no lasting success.

The Sudanese government was widely seen as supporting the actions of the Janjaweed, although it maintained that this was not the case. On September 8, 2004, U.S. Secretary of State Colin Powell (1937–) accused the Sudanese government and the Janjaweed militias of being responsible for a campaign of genocide in Darfur. According to the Human Rights Watch, in *World Report 2006* (January 2006, http://www.hrw.org/en/reports/2006/01/17/world-report-2006), the Sudanese government blocked the attempts of the AU troops to enforce a cease-fire agreement in April 2004 and supported Janjaweed attacks on AU forces and international aid workers. In addition, the Human Rights Watch reports that people living in internal displacement camps were subjected to many abuses, including arrests and detentions, and women reporting rape were humiliated and tried for adultery. Outside the camps civilians (particularly women and girls) were abducted, the livestock of the Fur farmers were stolen, and children were kidnapped or recruited to serve as soldiers.

In *To Save Darfur* (March 17, 2006, http://www.liberationafrique.org/IMG/pdf/To_save_darfur.pdf), the International Crisis Group (ICG) indicates that in 2005 an estimated 3.5 million people in the region were dependent on humanitarian aid for survival, although in some areas nongovernmental organizations were able to access only 45% to 70% of them. In West Darfur, where the fighting was most heavily concentrated, at least 140,000 people were left without assistance because nongovernmental organizations were forced to withdraw.

According to the U.S. embassy in Sudan, in the fact sheet "The Situation in Darfur: Darfur Peace Agreement" (May 8, 2006, http://sudan.usembassy.gov/dar_050806b.html), on May 5, 2006, a peace agreement was signed by the Sudanese government and the Sudan Liberation Movement. Because the treaty was not signed by all warring rebel factions, the ICG was not optimistic about the agreement's chances for success. In the policy briefing *Darfur's Fragile Peace Agreement* (June 20, 2006, http://www.crisisgroup.org/library/documents/africa/horn_of_africa/b039_darfur_s_fragile_peace_agreement.pdf), the ICG warned that without deployment of a "robust" UN peacekeeping force, sanctions against anyone who broke the cease-fire, and increased assistance to victims of the violence, the agreement had little chance of providing ongoing stability in the region.

By July 2006 violence in Darfur worsened, and the agreement was being ignored. In September the UN Security Council passed a resolution authorizing the creation of a UN peacekeeping force and in November the Sudanese government consented. Regardless, it was not until the end of 2007 that a joint UN-AU peacekeeping mission took over from the AU force. Ten days into the peacekeeping mission, Warren Hoge reported in "U.N. Official Warns of Darfur Failure" (*New York Times*, January 10, 2008) that "obstructionism by the Sudanese government, the failure of other countries to supply needed transportation equipment, and continued violence threatened to doom the mission." By March 2008 the situation had deteriorated once again, and, as Lydia Polgreen reported in "Scorched-Earth Strategy Returns to Darfur" (*New York Times*, March 2, 2008), "the janjaweed are back." Arab tribes and rebel groups began fighting among themselves, and according to Polgreen the situation was confusing, chaotic, and bloody. The UN continued to send in peacekeepers; by the end of October 2008 there were over 10,000 peacekeepers in Darfur.

In February 2009 judges at The Hague (an international court) took the unprecedented move of issuing an arrest warrant for a sitting head of state—President Omar al-Bashir (1944–) of Sudan—for war crimes and crimes against humanity. In response, Sudanese officials ordered aid workers, who provided support to millions of people in the country, to leave. Nonetheless, fighting in the country began to diminish as splintering occurred among opposition groups, so that by August 2009 the departing commander of the joint UN-AU forces declared that the war was over in Darfur. Neil MacFarquhar notes in "As Darfur Fighting Diminishes, U.N. Officials Focus on the South of Sudan" (*New York Times*, August 28, 2009) that the situation was still threatening and unpeaceful. According to Donald G. McNeil Jr., in "New Study Estimates That Disease Caused 80% of Deaths during Years of Darfur Strife" (*New York Times*, January 23, 2010), at the beginning of 2010 a fragile calm existed throughout the region. McNeil also notes the results of a recent study, which revealed that during the six years of fighting in the region approximately 300,000 people died, with disease killing at least 80% of them.

The conflict in Darfur left Sudan to be among the world's poorest countries. The Central Intelligence Agency (CIA) notes in *World Factbook: Sudan* (February 15, 2010, https://www.cia.gov/library/publications/the-world-factbook/geos/su.html) that the GDP per capita in Sudan was estimated to be $2,300 in 2009. The estimated average life expectancy at birth in 2009 was only 51.4 years and the infant mortality rate was 82.4 deaths per 1,000 live births. Sixty-one percent of Sudanese over the age of 15 were literate in 2003, and 40% of the population lived below the poverty line in 2004.

The Middle East

The Middle East is a geographic and political region encompassing countries in central and southwest Asia as well as North Africa. For the most part, these countries are historically Arabic and share many cultural similarities. The region is also the birthplace of three of the world's most prominent religions: Judaism, Christianity, and Islam. For many Westerners, the Middle East is associated with wealth because of the massive oil reserves located within the region. Nevertheless, according to the World Bank, in *Millennium Development Goals: Middle East and North Africa* (2006, http://ddp-ext.worldbank.org/ext/GMIS/gdmis.do?siteId=2&menuId=LNAV01REGSUB4), 17% of people in the region lived on less than US $2 per day in 2005. The World Bank refers to the infrastructure of the region as "well-developed," even though only 88% had access to improved water sources and 91% to electricity. Furthermore, the World Bank notes the long-time ongoing violence in the region has exacerbated poverty and diminished human development.

A HALF-CENTURY OF CONFLICT. The Middle East is at the heart of some of the worst tension and violence in the world, much of it in the form of terrorism. Some of this tension stems from ethnic and religious differences. Since the end of World War II there have been several major interstate conflicts—including the Arab-Israeli War (1948–1949), the Iran-Iraq War (1980–1988), and the Persian Gulf War (1990–1991)—as well as civil wars in Jordan and Lebanon and continuing tensions between various factions throughout the region. The Arab-Israeli War alone has led to four other wars since 1949. Iraq has been involved in six skirmishes, including the ongoing war with the U.S.-led coalition that began in 2003. Afghanistan is not always included as a Middle Eastern country, but its history, language, and culture are closely linked to those of Iran, so the U.S. invasion there, which began in late 2001, may also be considered a Middle Eastern conflict.

THE PALESTINIANS. The Israeli victory in the Arab-Israeli War resulted in the formation of the state of Israel on land that had been in the possession of the Palestinians. The war's other outcome was that at least 400,000 Palestinians were forced off their land and into neighboring areas, including Jordan, Syria, Lebanon, and Egypt, where they were placed into refugee camps. Following the Six-Day War (1967) between the Israelis and the Palestinians, Israel's territory expanded to include the regions known as the West Bank and the Gaza Strip, both of which were populated primarily by the Palestinians. After this war 300,000 Palestinians—many of them displaced for the second time after they had returned to their homes following the Arab-Israeli War—left the West Bank and the Gaza Strip for Syria, Lebanon, and Egypt. Most of the refugees were not permitted to return to their homes. In "The Palestinian Refugees" (August 10, 2008, http://www.mideastweb.org/refugees1.htm), the Mideast Web explains that this "Palestinian exodus," called the Nakba (disaster) by the Palestinians, resulted in generations of displaced people who numbered approximately 4.6 million in 2006.

The Palestinian refugees are stateless individuals. Most of them have not been granted citizenship in the countries in which they reside, nor are they allowed to return to Israel. Because so many of them are unable to work legally in their host countries, poverty is high among the refugees. The Palestinian refugees continue to hope that they will return to their land, and they therefore reject permanent resettlement in host countries. They also try to keep this hope alive in subsequent generations. However, as Ibrahim Hejoj states in "A Profile of Poverty for Palestinian Refugees in Jordan" (*Journal of Refugee Studies*, vol. 20, no. 1, 2007), "In the meantime the refugees are being forced to find ways of surviving harsh economic and political conditions and at the same time to realize that the 'return' will take longer than had been envisaged."

During elections that were held in January 2006 the political group Hamas—which is considered to be a terrorist organization by many international governments, including the United States—won control of the Palestinian National Authority (PNA), the transitional administrative organization for Palestinian territories in the West Bank and the Gaza Strip. Matthew Gutman reports in "Palestinians Fear Poverty If Foreign Aid Lifeline Is Severed" (*USA Today*, February 27, 2006) that in February 2006, in response to the election results, Israel decided to stop its monthly transfer of $50 million in tax revenue to the PNA. Furthermore, in April 2006 the Canadian, U.S., and European Union governments suspended all direct aid to the PNA because of the Hamas election victory, demanding that Hamas renounce terrorism. Altogether, Gutman estimates that the Palestinians stood to lose more than $1 billion annually in direct aid.

Gutman indicates that 90% of the PNA budget was spent on the salaries of its employees, who represented one-third of all Palestinians living in the West Bank and the Gaza Strip. Without the tax money and direct aid, the PNA risked not being able to continue operating and paying its employees. Many of the Palestinians who depended on the PNA for work and income were at risk of falling below the poverty line without it. The PNA was also responsible for funding, building, and maintaining the area's infrastructure. As a result, its financial troubles would leave Palestinians in the West Bank and the Gaza Strip with less access to utilities and other basic quality-of-life public services.

By mid-2007 Mahmoud Abbas (1935–), the president of the PNA, decreed an emergency government with no members from Hamas. In response, Israel resumed the monthly transfers of taxes to the PNA, and it slowly returned, in installments, the money that had been withheld since the previous year. Nonetheless, in late 2008 Hamas declared that the calm between Palestine and Israel was over and began rocket attacks on the country. Israel retaliated by closing key border crossings into Palestine and began air strikes on December 27, 2008. A special session of the UN Human Rights Council adopted a resolution that called for the Israeli attacks to end and for Israel to withdraw its occupying forces. The air strikes lasted through January 18, 2009, when the Israeli cabinet voted to end its three-week offensive. According to the editorial "A Year after the Gaza Offensive" (*Khaleej Times*, December 27, 2009), some Palestinians were still living in rubble because building materials were scarce, as were food, educational materials, and medicine. As of February 2010, severe socioeconomic and political challenges remained in the region.

Iraq

SANCTIONS WORSEN LIVING CONDITIONS. Under the rule of the dictator Saddam Hussein (1937–2006), Iraq invaded neighboring Kuwait in 1990, prompting the imposition of economic sanctions against Iraq by the UN Security Council. An international coalition led by the United States drove Iraq out of Kuwait in 1991. Sanctions and other restrictions on Iraq remained in place after the war ended. Because they had little effect on disarming Iraq—which was their stated goal—but instead caused a humanitarian crisis for Iraqi civilians, the sanctions were widely criticized. Regardless, the United States and the UK maintained that they would block any attempts to lift or soften the sanctions as long as Hussein remained in power.

In "A Hard Look at Iraq Sanctions" (*The Nation*, November 15, 2001), David Cortright estimates that from 1990 to 2000 an estimated 350,000 Iraqis died—mostly due to the sanctions but some resulting from bombing during the Persian Gulf War. Bombs destroyed essential infrastructure such as sanitation systems, and raw sewage then contaminated the sources of drinking water, which led to the spread of infectious disease among the civilian population. According to Cortright, the sanctions compounded the suffering by causing hunger and malnutrition and making it nearly impossible to treat disease. However, critics of Hussein contend that his own internal policies were more detrimental to the poor than international sanctions.

In 1991 the UN Security Council proposed an oil-for-food program in which Iraq would be allowed to sell limited amounts of oil on the open market in exchange for food and medicine for its impoverished citizens. Hussein rejected the plan on the grounds that it violated the country's sovereignty. In 1995 the UN countered with a plan that would increase Iraq's autonomy in distributing aid, but the Iraqi government again refused to participate. In the meantime, a full-scale humanitarian disaster was at hand. The United States was criticized for refusing to loosen sanctions, but foreign policy experts believe that Hussein and the Iraqi government were at least equally at fault. The UN continued negotiating a relief plan with Iraq; a deal was finally forged in 1996, and the first shipments of aid reached the Iraqis in 1997. Because the Iraqi government was allowed to administer aid in the southern and central regions of Iraq and the UN oversaw the relief in the north, the results of the oil-for-food program were uneven. For example, Mohamed M. Ali and Iqbal H. Shah indicate in "Sanctions and Childhood Mortality in Iraq" (*Lancet*, vol. 355, no. 9218, May 27, 2000) that child mortality decreased in the north, from 80 deaths per 1,000 live births to 72 deaths per 1,000 live births. By contrast, in southern and central Iraq the rates increased from 56 deaths per 1,000 live births from 1984 to 1989 to 131 deaths per 1,000 live births from 1994 to 1999, indicating a failure on the part of Iraqi officials to successfully provide humanitarian relief to their people.

POVERTY DURING AND AFTER THE U.S.-LED INVASION. A new coalition, once again led by the United States, invaded Iraq in 2003 and toppled Hussein's government. Sanctions were ended and the United States pledged to work to restore the Iraqi infrastructure and economy. Even though economic and living conditions had severely deteriorated since the beginning of the sanctions, hopes were high that the situation would improve. The UNDP indicates in "Iraq Living Conditions Survey 2004" (May 2005, http://www.reliefweb.int/rw/RWB.NSF/db900SID/KHII-6CC44A?OpenDocument) that in 2004, one year after the invasion began, 54% of families had access to safe drinking water, with 80% of families in rural areas using unsafe water, and only 37% of households were connected to sewer networks. Twelve percent of Iraqi children aged six months to five years were suffering from malnutrition, 8% of them in an acute condition (low weight for height) and 23% suffering a chronic condition (low weight for age). School enrollment for those aged six to 24 years was 55%, compared with a 62% average for Arab states overall during 2003. The literacy rate of people aged 15 to 25 years was 74%, compared with 81.3% in Arab states overall. In 2003 the average per capita annual income was $255; by the first half of 2004 it had fallen to $144.

In *Unsatisfied Basic Needs Mapping and Living Standards in Iraq 2006* (2006, http://www.iq.undp.org/UploadedFiles/Paragraphs/d15ca5bc-f2aa-45e4-a43a-fb88bf7a8f81.pdf), the UNDP notes that 5% of Iraqi households and 6% of Iraqi individuals were living in extreme poverty in 2004. The UNDP also indicates that chronic malnutrition was one of the worst human development problems in Iraq, with 18% of households having children under the age of five suffering from stunting (inadequate growth). Another major problem was sanita-

tion: 43% of households did not have healthy sanitation facilities.

Conflict in Iraq continued after the invasion defeated Hussein's government and conventional military. As of February 2010, the war in Iraq was characterized by sectarian and insurgent violence that impeded human development and infrastructure improvements in the country. Amnesty International reveals in "2009 Annual Report for Iraq" (February 2010, http://www.amnestyusa.org/annualreport.php?id=ar&yr=2009&c=IRQ) that even though violence in Iraq decreased during 2009, compared with previous years, thousands were killed. Life expectancy in the country was only 57.7 years, and the under-five mortality rate was 105 deaths per 1,000 children for boys and 98 deaths per 1,000 children for girls. In *World Factbook: Iraq* (February 18, 2010, https://www.cia.gov/library/publications/the-world-factbook/geos/iz.html), the CIA notes that 25% of Iraqi people lived below the poverty line.

CHAPTER 10
COMBATING POVERTY: MEASURING PROGRESS

We will spare no effort to free our fellow men, women and children from the abject and dehumanizing conditions of extreme poverty.

—United Nations Millennium Declaration, September 2000

How effective has the international community been in combating global poverty throughout and since the 20th century? The answers—for there are many—are varied. Some experts estimate that society is well on its way to achieving the United Nations' (UN) Millennium Development Goals (MDGs; http://www.undp.org/mdg/basics.shtml), which, among other things, strive to cut extreme poverty rates in half by 2015. Others believe that these estimates are overblown and that the reality is far more grim. During the first decade of the 21st century certain natural and human-made events—including earthquakes, hurricanes, and wars—put poverty at the forefront of international consciousness, and television and the Internet allowed everyone to witness the experiences of the poor like never before. New antipoverty campaigns were developed, some headed by renowned business people or celebrities. Charitable giving reached record highs, especially in the wake of the Asian tsunami in December 2004, Hurricane Katrina in August 2005, and the Haiti earthquake in January 2010. Nevertheless, poverty persists in every country in the world. As explained in Chapter 2, the reasons are complex, and the questions do not always have one correct answer. However, to fully understand the problem of poverty, it is best to examine the progress that has been made in decreasing poverty, hunger, and child mortality; increasing universal primary education and gender equality; and improving maternal health, safe water, and sanitation.

In 2002 heads of state and government met at the UN International Conference on Financing for Development held in Monterrey, Mexico. According to the UN secretary-general, in *Outcome of the International Conference on Financing for Development* (October 2002,

http://daccess-dds-ny.un.org/doc/UNDOC/GEN/N02/535/43/PDF/N0253543.pdf?OpenElement), during the conference developing countries officially accepted primary responsibility for achieving the MDGs, and developed countries officially accepted responsibility to help them via aid, trade, and debt relief. The development indicators presented in this chapter show the progress made by developing countries and those in transition.

POVERTY AND HUNGER
Progress in Reducing Extreme Poverty

Overall, the rates of global poverty dropped during the last decade of the 20th century and the first decade of the 21st century as measured by the international standard of percent of population living on less than US $1.25 per day (also called extreme poverty). In *World Development Indicators 2008: Poverty Data* (December 2008, http://siteresources.worldbank.org/DATASTATISTICS/Resources/WDI08supplement1216.pdf), the World Bank notes that from 1981 to 2005 the most notable decrease in the extreme poverty rate was in East Asia and the Pacific. In 1981 the extreme poverty rate in this region was 77.7%, and by 2005 it was 16.8%. The second-most dramatic drop in the extreme poverty rate was in South Asia. In 1981 the rate was 59.4%, and by 2005 it had dropped to 40.3%.

Even though poverty rates may drop in an area, the numbers of people in poverty in that area may rise due to an increase in the population over time. Figure 10.1 shows the number of people living in extreme poverty by region from 1981 to 2005. Each section of the figure represents a region of the world. In reading the figure, if the distance between the two lines defining that area becomes farther apart from 1981 to 2005, then the number of people in poverty in that area increased. If the distance between the two lines stays the same, then the number of people in poverty in that area stayed the same.

FIGURE 10.1

Number of people living in extreme poverty, by region, 1981–2005

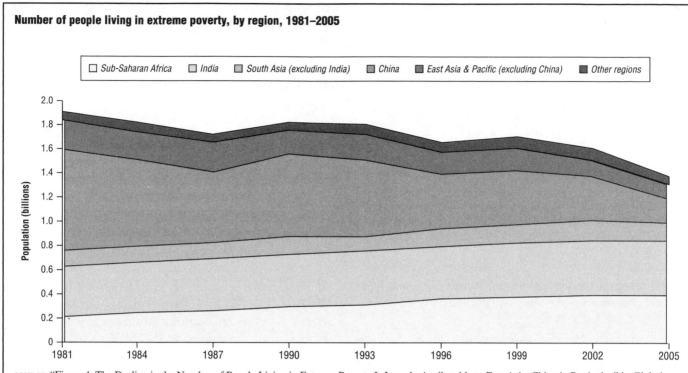

SOURCE: "Figure 4. The Decline in the Number of People Living in Extreme Poverty Is Largely Attributable to East Asia, China in Particular," in *Global Monitoring Report 2009: A Development Emergency*, The World Bank, 2009, http://siteresources.worldbank.org/INTGLOMONREP2009/Resources/5924349-1239742507025/GMR09_book.pdf (accessed December 10, 2009). Copyright © International Bank for Reconstruction and Development/The World Bank 2009.

If the distance narrows, then the number of people in poverty in that area decreased. As Figure 10.1 shows, the number of people living in extreme poverty dropped dramatically in China. It also dropped in East Asia and the Pacific, but not as dramatically as in China. Thus, in these areas both the percentage and the number of people living in extreme poverty fell. Such is not the case with South Asia. The percentage of those living in extreme poverty in the area dropped, but the number of people increased slightly in both South Asia excluding India and including India.

The World Bank also notes that extreme poverty rates in other regions dropped slightly from 1981 to 2005: in sub-Saharan Africa, from 53.4% to 50.9% (but the number of people living in poverty increased from 212 million to 388 million); in Latin America and the Caribbean, from 12.9% to 8.2% (the number of people living in poverty decreased from 47 million to 45 million); and in the Middle East and North Africa, from 7.9% to 3.6% (the number of people living in poverty decreased from 14 million to 11 million). The extreme poverty rate in the developing and transition countries of Europe and central Asia rose slightly. It was steady at about 1% throughout the 1980s, rose to 5% by the late 1990s, and then declined to 3.7% in 2005 (but the number of people living in extreme poverty increased dramatically from 7 million to 17 million).

The world has made strides in reducing poverty, but is it on track to meet MDG 1a of the first Millennium Development Goal? MDG 1 aims to eradicate extreme poverty and hunger. Target 1a under this goal focuses on reducing by half, from 1990 to 2015, the proportion of people living in extreme poverty. In *Global Monitoring Report 2009: A Development Emergency* (2009, http://siteresources.worldbank.org/INTGLOMONREP2009/Resources/5924349-1239742507025/GMR09_book.pdf), the World Bank helps answer this question by presenting estimates of a short-term extreme poverty outlook in Table 10.1 and a long-term extreme poverty outlook in Table 10.2.

In explaining its projections of short-term and long-term extreme poverty, the World Bank points out that recent food, fuel, and financial crises have slowed the pace of poverty reduction. The World Bank notes that grain prices "more than doubled between January 2006 and September 2008, including dramatic surges in staples such as wheat, rice, and soybean oil." In addition, oil prices began a sharp rise in 2007, peaked in June 2008, and then receded. A global financial crisis—considered the worst economic crisis since the Great Depression of the 1930s—took root in 2007. Worldwide, economic growth slowed; local, national, and global businesses failed; and unemployment rose. In light of these events, the World Bank concludes that 55 million to 90 million

TABLE 10.1

Number and percent of people living below the international poverty line of $1.25 per day, by world region, 2005–09

	Number of people (millions)		Change in number of people (millions)		% of population		Change (percentage points)	
	2008	2009	2005–08*	2009	2008	2009	2005–08*	2009
East Asia and the Pacific	222.5	203.0	−31.2	−19.5	11.5	10.4	−1.8	−1.1
Europe and Central Asia	15.1	15.5	−0.7	0.4	3.2	3.3	−0.2	0.1
Latin America and the Caribbean	37.6	40.3	−2.5	2.7	6.6	7.0	−0.5	0.4
Middle East and North Africa	8.6	8.3	−0.8	−0.3	2.7	2.5	−0.3	−0.2
South Asia	536.3	530.6	−19.8	−5.7	34.8	33.9	−1.8	−0.9
Sub-Saharan Africa	382.7	385.9	−1.9	3.2	46.7	46.0	−1.4	−0.7
Total	**1,202.8**	**1,183.6**	**−56.9**	**−19.2**	**21.3**	**20.7**	**−1.3**	**−0.6**
Low-income countries	952.3	947.8	−26.9	−4.5	38.0	37.2	−1.8	−0.8
Middle-income countries	262.1	247.2	−33.1	−14.9	8.3	7.8	−1.2	−0.5

*Simple annual average change for the three-year period 2005–08.

SOURCE: "Table 1.5. Short-term Poverty Outlook: People Living below the International Poverty Line of $1.25/Day (2005 PPP)," in *Global Monitoring Report 2009: A Development Emergency*, The World Bank, 2009, http://siteresources.worldbank.org/INTGLOMONREP2009/Resources/5924349-1239742507025/GM R09_book.pdf (accessed December 10, 2009). Copyright © International Bank for Reconstruction and Development/The World Bank 2009.

TABLE 10.2

Number and percent of people living below the international poverty line of $1.25 per day, by world region, 1990, 2005, and 2015

	Number of people (millions)			% of population			Over/under[a]
	1990	2005	2015	1990	2005	2015	MDG[b]
East Asia & Pacific	873.3	316.2	103.6	54.7	16.8	5.1	22.3
East Asia & Pacific, excluding China	190.1	108.5	43.5	41.3	18.7	6.7	14.0
Europe & Central Asia	9.1	17.3	12.8	2.0	3.7	2.7	−1.7
Latin America & the Caribbean	49.6	45.1	33.4	11.3	8.2	5.4	0.3
Middle East & North Africa	9.7	11.0	6.7	4.3	3.6	1.8	0.4
South Asia	579.2	595.6	416.1	51.7	40.3	24.5	1.4
South Asia, excluding India	143.7	139.8	97.7	53.1	36.6	21.2	5.4
Sub-Saharan Africa	295.7	388.4	352.6	57.6	50.9	36.6	−7.8
Total	**1,816.6**	**1,373.5**	**925.2**	**41.7**	**25.2**	**15.1**	**5.7**
Total, excluding China	**1,133.5**	**1,165.8**	**865.1**	**35.2**	**28.1**	**18.2**	**−0.6**
Low-income countries	920.4	1,032.9	789.3	52.8	43.5	28.0	−1.6
Middle-income countries	914.2	361.5	143.5	35.0	11.8	4.3	13.2

[a]The difference in percentage points between the MDG target and the projected poverty rate in 2015. Negative numbers indicate underperformance.
[b]Relates to MDG 1, target 1.A, which calls for halving, between 1990 and 2015, the proportion of people living below the poverty line.

SOURCE: "Table 1.6. Longer-term Poverty Outlook: People Living below the International Poverty Line of $1.25/Day (2005 PPP)," in *Global Monitoring Report 2009: A Development Emergency*, The World Bank, 2009, http://siteresources.worldbank.org/INTGLOMONREP2009/Resources/5924349-1239742507025/GMR09_book.pdf (accessed December 10, 2009). Copyright © International Bank for Reconstruction and Development/The World Bank 2009.

---

more people in developing countries would be living below the international poverty line of $1.25 per day in 2009 than was expected before these crises took hold.

Table 10.1 shows the World Bank's extreme poverty outlook from 2008 to 2009. East Asia and the Pacific saw the largest declines in numbers of people living on less than $1.25 per day: a decrease of 31.2 million in the three years preceding 2009, and a decrease of 19.5 million in 2009. Sub-Saharan Africa saw a decrease of 1.9 million extremely poor people from 2005 to 2008, but this number rose by 3.2 million people in 2009. Sub-Saharan Africa also had the highest proportion of its population living in extreme poverty: 46.7% in 2008 and 46% in 2009.

Overall, low-income countries showed less of a reduction than middle-income countries in the number of those living in extreme poverty from 2005 to 2008 and in 2009. (See Table 10.1.) However, middle-income countries showed less of a reduction than low-income countries in the percentage of those living in extreme poverty from 2005 to 2008 and in 2009. Nonetheless, middle-income countries had a far lower percentage of their population living in extreme poverty than did low-income countries. Globally, both numbers and percentages of those living in extreme poverty fell from 2005 to 2008 and in 2009. The World Bank concludes, "The MDG 1 for poverty reduction remains achievable at the global level, but the [global economic] crisis adds new risks.

In making its projections of extreme poverty to 2015, the World Bank assumes that developing countries will gradually recover economic growth by 2010, averaging a gross domestic product (the total value of all goods and services produced by a country in a year) per capita (per person) growth rate of 4.5% each year from 2011 to 2015. If these projections are correct, then the MDG target for extreme poverty reduction will be met globally with an overperformance of 5.7%. (See Table 10.2.) East Asia and the Pacific will exceed the target by 22.3%. Most other regions will reach the MDG target for extreme poverty reduction as well, except for Europe and central Asia, which will underperform by 1.7%, and sub-Saharan Africa, which will underperform by 7.8%. The World Bank concludes that "of all developing regions, Sub-Saharan Africa alone remains seriously off track to achieve the poverty reduction MDG."

Figure 10.2 shows how the developing countries as a whole are progressing toward achievement of the MDGs. For MDG 1a, 42% of developing countries did not have any data in 2007, 18% were seriously off track, 8% were off track, 17% were on track, and 13% had achieved MDG 1a. (Numbers do not add up to 100% due to estimation and rounding.)

In Figure 10.3 the World Bank distinguishes between middle-income countries, low-income countries, and fragile states with respect to their progress toward the MDGs. Fragile states are those that are extremely poor, may be experiencing conflict, and are hampered by difficult political and governance situations. The figure shows that 100% of middle-income countries had achieved MDG 1a in 2007. Slightly less than 40% of low-income countries had achieved their target. Only about 20% of fragile states had met their MDG 1a target.

Figure 10.4 shows progress toward the MDGs on the global level. In 2007, 80% of the world had met MDG 1a. This meant that the world as a whole was on track to meet this goal. This does not mean, however, that every region and country was on track, as shown in Figure 10.3 and Figure 10.2. Some countries will exceed their targets and reduce extreme poverty by more than half, which will statistically "make up for" the increases of other countries. In this way the world can achieve MDG 1a while individual countries do not.

ECONOMIC GROWTH AND POVERTY REDUCTION. Economic growth in a country does not necessarily mean that poverty in that country is reduced. The reduction of poverty depends on how income is distributed within a country. In some countries, when economic expansion occurs, those living in poverty do not benefit. Nevertheless, global output does provide a measure of the wealth of economies, which reflects the welfare of the region's residents and the prospects for the region's future growth.

Table 10.3 shows the annual percent change in the global output (gross world product) and in the output of selected countries and regions from 2002 to 2010. East Asia, and particularly China within this region, had the largest declines in extreme poverty from 2005 onward, as is shown in Table 10.1. Not coincidentally, East Asia and

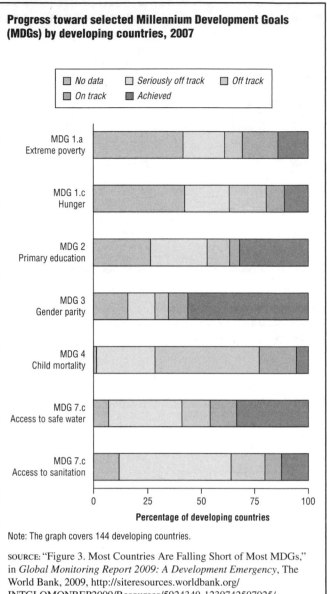

FIGURE 10.2

Progress toward selected Millennium Development Goals (MDGs) by developing countries, 2007

Note: The graph covers 144 developing countries.

SOURCE: "Figure 3. Most Countries Are Falling Short of Most MDGs," in *Global Monitoring Report 2009: A Development Emergency*, The World Bank, 2009, http://siteresources.worldbank.org/INTGLOMONREP2009/Resources/5924349-1239742507025/GMR09_book.pdf (accessed December 10, 2009). Copyright © International Bank for Reconstruction and Development/The World Bank 2009.

China, from 2005 to 2007, had the highest annual percentage growth in output of all the countries and regions listed in Table 10.3. In 2008 the downturn in all economies due to the global economic crisis that began in 2007 can be seen in diminished growth. Even though the crisis began in developed countries, it affected emerging markets and developing countries as well. The year of the steepest slowdown in growth and negative annual percent change was projected for 2009, and some recovery was projected for 2010.

Progress in Reducing Hunger

Target 1c of MDG 1 is to cut in half, from 1990 to 2015, the proportion of people who suffer from hunger. One of the progress indicators of this objective is the

FIGURE 10.3

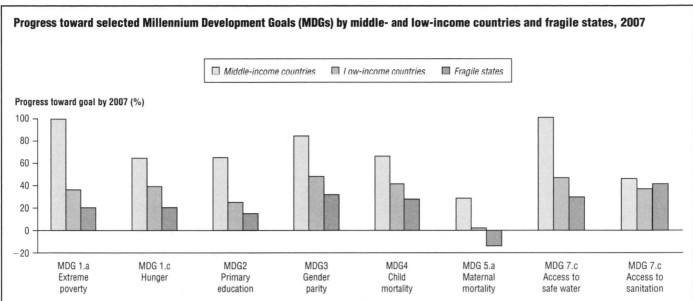

Progress toward selected Millennium Development Goals (MDGs) by middle- and low-income countries and fragile states, 2007

Note: According to the *Global Monitoring Report 2009*, Fragile states are those "wracked by conflict and hampered by weak governance and capacities. Fragile states present difficult political and governance contexts for effective delivery of development finance and services." More than half are in Sub-Saharan Africa.

SOURCE: "Figure 2. Fragile States Have Made the Least Progress toward the MDGs," in *Global Monitoring Report 2009: A Development Emergency*, The World Bank, 2009, http://siteresources.worldbank.org/INTGLOMONREP2009/Resources/5924349-1239742507025/GMR09_book.pdf (accessed December 10, 2009). Copyright © International Bank for Reconstruction and Development/The World Bank 2009.

FIGURE 10.4

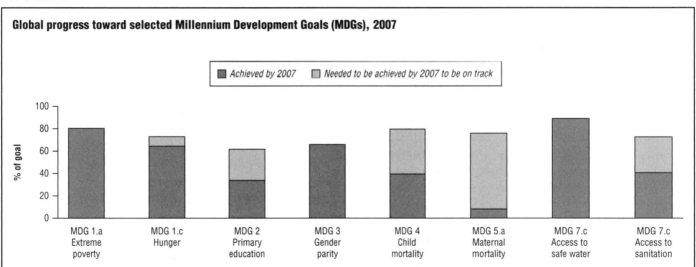

Global progress toward selected Millennium Development Goals (MDGs), 2007

Note: Calculations are based on the most recent year for which data are available. MDG 1.a: Poverty headcount ratio (PPP2005 US$1.25 a day); MDG 1.c: Underweight under-five children (U.S. child growth standards); MDG 2: Primary education completion rate; MDG 3: Gender parity in primary and secondary education; MDG 4: Under-five mortality rate; MDG 5.a: Maternal mortality ratio (modeled estimates); MDG 7.c: Access to improved water source; MDG 7.c: Access to improved sanitation facilities.

SOURCE: "Figure 1. MDGs at the Global Level: Serious Shortfalls Loom on Human Development Goals," in *Global Monitoring Report 2009: A Development Emergency*, The World Bank, 2009, http://siteresources.worldbank.org/INTGLOMONREP2009/Resources/5924349-1239742507025/GMR09_book.pdf (accessed December 10, 2009). Copyright © International Bank for Reconstruction and Development/The World Bank 2009.

prevalence of underweight in children under the age of five. Between 1990 and 2007 the prevalence of underweight in this age group decreased in almost all regions of the world. (See Figure 3.2 in Chapter 3.) However, in *Millennium Development Goals Report 2009* (2009, http://www.un.org/millenniumgoals/pdf/MDG_Report_2009_ENG.pdf), the UN calls the progress "scant" and notes that even this small amount of "progress on child nutri-

tion is likely to be eroded by high food prices and the state of the global economy."

Southern Asia had the highest percentage of underweight children under the age of five between 1990 and 2007. (See Figure 3.2 in Chapter 3.) In 1990, 54% of children under the age of five in this region were underweight, and in 2007 the percentage had dropped to 48%. Southern Asia is

TABLE 10.3

Annual percent change in world output by country and world region, 2002–10

	2002	2003	2004	2005	2006	2007	2008	Projections 2009	2010
World output	2.8	3.6	4.9	4.5	5.1	5.2	3.2	−1.3	1.9
Advanced economies of which	1.6	1.9	3.2	2.6	3.0	2.7	0.9	−3.8	0.0
United States	1.6	2.5	3.6	2.9	2.8	2.0	1.1	−2.8	0.0
Euro Area	0.9	0.8	2.2	1.7	2.9	2.7	0.9	−4.2	−0.4
Japan	0.3	1.4	2.7	1.9	2.0	2.4	−0.6	−6.2	0.5
Canada	2.9	1.9	3.1	2.9	3.1	2.7	0.5	−2.5	1.2
United Kingdom	2.1	2.8	2.8	2.1	2.8	3.0	0.7	−4.1	−0.4
Other advanced countries	3.9	2.5	4.8	4.0	4.6	4.7	1.6	−4.1	0.6
Emerging markets and developing countries	4.8	6.3	7.5	7.1	8.0	8.3	6.1	1.6	4.0
Emerging markets	4.6	6.3	7.5	7.1	8.0	8.3	6.1	1.5	3.9
Other developing countries	7.5	6.2	7.4	7.6	8.2	8.3	6.5	3.2	4.7
Africa of which	6.5	5.7	6.7	5.8	6.1	6.2	5.7	2.0	3.9
Sub-Saharan Africa	7.3	5.4	7.1	6.2	6.6	6.9	5.5	1.7	3.8
Central and Eastern Europe	4.4	4.9	7.3	6.0	6.6	5.4	2.9	−3.7	0.8
Commonwealth of Independent States	5.2	7.8	8.2	6.7	8.4	8.6	5.5	−5.1	1.2
Developing Asia	6.9	8.2	8.6	9.0	9.8	10.6	7.7	4.8	6.1
South Asia	4.4	6.5	7.6	8.7	9.1	8.7	7.0	4.3	5.3
East Asia	7.9	8.8	9.0	9.2	10.1	11.4	8.0	5.1	6.4
Middle East	3.8	7.0	6.0	5.8	5.7	6.3	5.9	2.5	3.5
Western Hemisphere	0.6	2.2	6.0	4.7	5.7	5.7	4.2	−1.5	1.6
Memorandum items:									
China	9.1	10.0	10.1	10.4	11.6	13.0	9.0	6.5	7.5
India	4.6	6.9	7.9	9.2	9.8	9.3	7.3	4.5	5.6

SOURCE: "Table 1.1. Summary of World Output: Annual Percent Change," in *Global Monitoring Report 2009: A Development Emergency*, The World Bank, 2009, http://siteresources.worldbank.org/INTGLOMONREP2009/Resources/5924349–1239742507025/GMR09_book.pdf (accessed December 10, 2009). Copyright © International Bank for Reconstruction and Development/The World Bank 2009. Data from International Monetary Fund.

not on track to reach the MDG 1c target in 2015, so it must step up its efforts to reduce the percentage of children in this age group who are underweight.

Three other world regions must also increase their efforts to reduce the percentage of underweight children under five years old to reach their targets: western Asia, sub-Saharan Africa, and Southeastern Asia. (See Figure 3.2 in Chapter 3.) Between 1990 and 2007 western Asia did not reduce its percentage of underweight children under the age of five; it held steady at 14%, whereas its target is 7%. Sub-Saharan Africa decreased its percentage of underweight children from 31% in 1990 to 28% in 2007; its target is 15.5%. Southeastern Asia reduced its percentage of underweight children the most of these three regions, from 37% in 1990 to 25% in 2007. However, its target is 18.5%, so this region still has considerable work to do.

There are three regions that are doing well in reaching their targets for MDG 1c. Eastern Asia decreased its percentage of underweight children from 17% in 1990 to 7% in 2007; its target is 8.5%. (See Figure 3.2 in Chapter 3.) Latin America and the Caribbean decreased its percentage from 11% in 1990 to 6% in 2007; its target is 5.5%. During this same period, northern Africa decreased from 11% to 7%, and its target is 5.5%.

Thus, progress has been made in reducing the percentage of underweight children in the developing regions of the world. Nonetheless, the overall progress is too slow. For instance, Figure 3.2 in Chapter 3 shows that develop-

ing regions as a whole have reduced the percentage of underweight children by only five percentage points since 1990, from 31% to 26%. The target for the region is 15.5%. Figure 10.2 shows another look at how the developing countries as a whole are progressing toward achievement of MDG 1c. About 43% of developing countries did not have any data in 2007, 21% were seriously off track, 18% were off track, 8% were on track, and 11% had achieved MDG 1c.

Figure 10.3 shows that the problem with reducing the percentage of underweight children extends to even the middle-income countries. In 2007 only 65% of middle-income countries had achieved MDG 1c. About 40% of low-income countries and only 20% of fragile states had met their MDG 1c target. On the global level, about 67% of the MDG 1c target was met worldwide in 2007. (See Figure 10.4.) To have been on track, approximately 75% of the target should have been achieved by 2007.

UNIVERSAL PRIMARY EDUCATION

MDG 2 aims to ensure that by 2015 children everywhere will be able to complete a full course of primary schooling. The World Bank states in "Millennium Development Goals 2: Achieve Universal Primary Education" (2004, http://ddp-ext.worldbank.org/ext/GMIS/gdmis.do?siteId=2&goalId=6&menuId=LNAV01GOAL2) that "education is the foundation of all societies and globally competitive economies. It is the basis for reducing poverty and inequality, improving health, enabling the use of new technologies, and creating and spreading knowledge. In an increasingly complex, knowledge-dependent world, primary education, as the gateway to higher levels of education, must be the first priority." Progress toward the goal of universal primary education is measured by the net enrollment ratio (NER) in primary education, the proportion of pupils starting grade one who graduate from the last grade of primary school (primary school completion rate), and the literacy rates of 15- to 24-year-olds. (The NER in primary education is the proportion of students of primary school age that are enrolled in primary school.)

Progress in the NER

Eastern Asia is a region that has been making great strides in reducing poverty and child underweight, buoyed in great part by progress in China. However, the UN Educational, Scientific, and Cultural Organization (UNESCO) indicates in *EFA Global Monitoring Report 2003/4* (March 2004, http://www.unesco.org/education/efa_report/zoom_regions_pdf/easiapac.pdf) that the region has been losing sight of the goal of universal primary education. UNESCO notes that in 1990 primary education was nearly universal in Eastern Asia with an NER of 97%, but by 2000 the NER of the region had fallen to 93%. In 2007 the NER in primary education in Eastern Asia was 95%. (See Figure 10.5.) UNESCO explains in *EFA Global Monitoring Report 2010* (2010, http://unesdoc.unesco.org/images/0018/001866/186606E.pdf) that the major reversals in child health and education resulted from the East Asian financial crisis of 1997. It also cites a problem of late entry into primary school as a problem in this region. However, Eastern Asia has made progress in shoring up its NER in primary education since 2000.

Even though huge strides have been made in achieving universal primary education worldwide, the UN reveals in *Millennium Development Goals Report 2009* that the 2015 target will likely not be met because "global numbers of out-of-school children are dropping too slowly and too unevenly." Figure 10.5 shows this uneven progress. Sub-Saharan Africa made enormous progress in increasing its primary school NER, from 58% in 2000 to 74% in 2007, an increase of 16 percentage points. Southern Asia also made great strides in raising its primary school NER, from 79% in 2000 to 90% in 2007, an increase of 11 percentage points. Northern Africa, the Commonwealth of Independent States, and western Asia all made modest gains of three to five percentage points, but western Asia was nevertheless far from its goal. Southeastern Asia did not make any progress between 2000 and 2007 and still had 6% of primary school students out of school. Worldwide, the primary school NER was 89% in 2007, which meant that 11% of primary school–aged children were out of school.

FIGURE 10.5

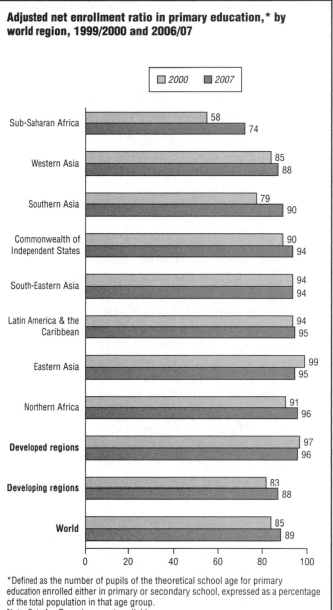

Adjusted net enrollment ratio in primary education,* by world region, 1999/2000 and 2006/07

*Defined as the number of pupils of the theoretical school age for primary education enrolled either in primary or secondary school, expressed as a percentage of the total population in that age group.
Note: Data for Oceania are not available.

SOURCE: "Adjusted Net Enrolment Ratio in Primary Education, 1999/2000 and 2006/2007 (Percentage)," in *The Millennium Development Goals Report 2009*, © United Nations, 2009, http://www.un.org/millenniumgoals/pdf/MDG_Report_2009_ENG.pdf (accessed December 5, 2009). The United Nations is the author of the original material. Reproduced with permission.

Progress in the Primary School Completion Rate

Figure 10.4 and Figure 10.3 reveal progress toward the goal of universal primary education by tracking the primary school completion rate. The 2015 goal is to have a 100% graduation rate of children of primary school age. Figure 10.4 shows that 60% of children of primary school age should have been graduating primary school in 2007 for the world to be on track to achieve universal primary education by 2015. Instead, less than 40% were graduating. Middle-income countries achieved the 60% mark in

2007. (See Figure 10.3.) Low-income countries had a primary school graduation rate of slightly more than 20% and fragile states had a rate of slightly more than 10%.

Figure 10.2 shows developing countries' progress toward meeting MDG 2 in both primary school NERs and completion rates. Among developing countries in 2007, 26% did not have any data, 26% were seriously off track, 11% were off track, 5% were on track, and 32% achieved the goal.

Achieving the goal of universal primary education requires sufficient classrooms, properly trained teachers, and the development of relevant curricula. In addition, barriers to attendance often exist, such as fees, inadequate transportation, and safety issues. Unless countries that are seriously off track accelerate their progress and address these obstacles to attendance, they will not reach the target before 2015, which will deprive several more generations of the benefits of education. In *Millennium Development Goals Report 2009*, the UN suggests that "the large number of out-of-school children is especially worrisome because of the impact it will have on the other MDGs. Evidence shows, for instance, that an increase in the share of mothers with a primary or secondary education is associated with a reduction in the child mortality rate, and that educated parents have better nourished children. Parental literacy also plays a role in whether children attend school. Education has been shown to have a positive effect on the success of HIV prevention and increases the probability of accessing decent employment."

Progress in Literacy

One of the progress indicators of MDG 2 is the literacy rate of 15- to 24-year-olds. As the World Bank notes in *World Development Indicators 2006* (April 2006, http://devdata.worldbank.org/wdi2006/contents/index2.htm), literacy rates are the only widely reported measure of educational outcomes. The World Bank also reports that the global literacy rate has risen from 75% in 1970 to 88% in 2000–04. According to the Central Intelligence Agency, in *World Factbook: World* (February 12, 2010, https://www.cia.gov/library/publications/the-world-factbook/geos/xx.html), the global literacy rate was 82% in 2005.

The World Bank notes that the overall literacy rate in developed and transition economies was nearly 100% by 2000–04 and that it was close to this percent even in 1970. In "Key Indicators: Regional Data from the WDI Database" (April 2009, http://siteresources.worldbank.org/DATASTATISTICS/Resources/reg_wdi.pdf), the World Bank lists literacy rates for both males and females aged 15 to 24 by region for 2007. Europe and central Asia had the highest literacy rates for both genders among the regions listed, at 99%. East Asia and the Pacific had the next highest literacy rate among male and female youth in 2007, at 98%. According to the World Bank, in *World Development Indicators 2006*, this region increased

its literacy rate from 85% in 1970. Latin America and the Caribbean did almost as well according to the "Key Indicators" list, achieving a literacy rate of 97% among youth in 2007, from about 82% in 1970. The Middle East and North Africa, South Asia, and sub-Saharan Africa have made exceptional strides in youth literacy since 1970 but still have much work to do. In 2007 the literacy rates for these regions were: Middle East and North Africa, 93% of males and 86% of females; South Asia, 84% of males and 74% of females; and sub-Saharan Africa, 77% of males and 67% of females.

GENDER EQUALITY
Progress in Eliminating Gender Disparity in Education

MDG 3 aims to eliminate gender disparity in primary and secondary education by 2005 and in all levels of education by 2015. In *Global Monitoring Report 2009*, the World Bank looks at gender parity in primary and secondary education worldwide and characterizes the progress as good. Figure 10.4 shows that the world is on target to meet the 2015 goal, in that over 60% of countries had reached gender parity in primary and secondary education in 2007. Figure 10.3 indicates that over 80% of middle-income countries, about 50% of low-income countries, and about 30% of fragile states had reached gender parity in 2007. According to Figure 10.2, 57% of developing countries reached gender parity at school in 2007, and an additional 9% were on track to reach gender parity at school by 2015. Seven percent were off track, 13% were seriously off track, and 16% of countries did not provide any data.

The UNESCO Institute for Statistics discusses in "Gender Parity in Education: Not There Yet" (March 2008, http://www.uis.unesco.org/template/pdf/EducGeneral/UIS Factsheet_2008_No%201_EN.pdf) the progress made in various regions of the world in gender parity in primary and secondary schooling. In primary schooling, UNESCO determines the Gender Parity Index (GPI) for enrollment in the first grade. The GPI is derived by subtracting the relative excess or deficit of boys over girls (as a percent) in primary and secondary school from 100%, and then converting to a decimal format. Thus, if 10% more boys than girls are in school, the GPI for this country would be 90% (100% minus 10%), or 0.90; and if 5% more girls than boys are in school, the GPI would be 105% (100% minus [-5%]), or 1.05. The lower the number (below 1.0) means the greater the gender disparity that is favoring boys; whereas the higher the number (above 1.0) means the greater the gender parity with the advantage to girls. UNESCO considers gender parity to be reached when the GPI is within the range of 0.97 (more boys than girls) to 1.03 (more girls than boys). The regions that achieved gender parity in first-grade enrollments by 2005 were central Asia, East Asia and the Pacific, North America and western Europe, and central and eastern Europe. The regions that had not yet reached gender parity were sub-Saharan Africa (0.88 in 1999 to 0.92 in 2005), the Arab states (0.93 in 1999 to 0.95 in 2005), South and West Asia (0.83 in 1999 to 0.92 in 2005), and Latin America and the Caribbean (0.95 in 1999 to 0.93 in 2005). Thus, gender disparity in first-grade enrollments favored boys in all instances.

UNESCO also reports on gender disparity in secondary and tertiary (postsecondary) school enrollments. Developed countries and countries in transition have both reached gender parity in secondary education enrollments. Interestingly, in 1991 in countries in transition, the GPI was 1.03. By 1999 the GPI had dropped to 0.99, and in 2005 it dropped further to 0.98. Developing countries have not yet reached gender parity in secondary school enrollments, but they have made enormous progress. In 1991 the GPI for secondary school enrollments was 0.75. By 1999 it rose to 0.88, and by 2005 to 0.94. UNESCO notes that gender parity is rare in tertiary education. In developed countries and countries in transition girls far outnumber boys in tertiary school enrollments. In developed countries in 2005 the GPI was 1.28 and in countries in transition it was 1.29. In developing countries the GPI is 0.91, up from 0.78 in 1999.

CHILD MORTALITY

Under-Five Mortality Rate

MDG 4 focuses on reducing the under-five mortality rate (U5MR) by two-thirds from 1990 to 2015. The UN reports in *Millennium Development Goals Report 2009* that developed regions of the world were close to meeting their U5MR of 4 deaths per 1,000 live births, having reduced the rate from 11 deaths per 1,000 live births in 1990 to 6 deaths per 1,000 live births in 2007. (See Figure 10.6.) Developing regions are far from their goal of 34 deaths per 1,000 live births, however. The U5MR in developing regions was 103 deaths per 1,000 live births in 1990, and it was reduced to 74 deaths per 1,000 live births in 2007. The UN expects continued progress to be made in reducing U5MRs in the developing world because of interventions that "include vitamin A supplementation, the use of insecticide-treated bed nets (to prevent malaria), exclusive breastfeeding and immunization. In addition, there has been wider coverage of critical HIV interventions in most sub-Saharan countries where HIV prevalence is high. This includes antiretroviral treatment for pregnant mothers who are HIV-positive, to prevent transmission of the virus to their babies." The UN points out that the areas of greatest concern are sub-Saharan Africa and southern Asia, where the U5MRs were 145 deaths per 1,000 live births and 77 deaths per 1,000 live births, respectively, in 2007.

MATERNAL HEALTH

Maternal Mortality Ratio

Maternal mortality refers to the death of a woman during or shortly after pregnancy. The maternal mortality ratio (MMR) is the number of maternal deaths per 100,000 live births. The MMR can be viewed as a measure of the quality of a country's health care system.

MDG 5a aims to reduce the MMR by three-quarters from 1990 to 2015. The UN Population Fund presents MMRs for the world and its regions in Table 7.3 in Chapter 7. In addition, the UN analyzes in *Millennium Development Goals Report 2009* progress toward reducing the MMR. Developed regions had an MMR of 11 deaths per 100,000 live births in 1990, and they reduced that to 9 deaths per 100,000 live births in 2005. Their goal is 3 deaths per 100,000 live births, so developed regions still have progress to make. In developing regions some progress has been made in lowering maternal deaths, but so much more progress must be made because, as the UN points out, "almost all of these deaths (99 per cent) occur in developing countries." The MMR in developing regions was 480 deaths per 100,000 live births in 1990, and it was reduced to 450 deaths per 100,000 live births in 2005. The target is 120 deaths per 100,000 live births. Little progress has been made in sub-Saharan Africa, where the MMR in 1990 was 920 deaths per 100,000 live births, and in 2005 it was still extremely high at 900 deaths per 100,000 live births.

Figure 10.4 shows that the world is far off target to meet the 2015 goal with only 10% of the target reached in 2007. Figure 10.3 indicates that about 30% of middle-income countries and about 2% of low-income countries had reached their maternal mortality goals in 2007. Fragile states had lost ground, regressing about 15% toward the maternal mortality goal.

Another progress indicator for this target is the proportion of births attended by skilled health personnel. Inadequate health care during pregnancy and delivery is one cause of maternal mortality. Thus, an increase in the proportion of births attended by skilled health personnel generally results in a lowering of the MMR.

Figure 7.3 in Chapter 7 shows the proportion of women attended four or more times during pregnancy by skilled health personnel from 2003 to 2008. Only 36% of pregnant women in southern Asia and only 42% in sub-Saharan Africa received regular health care. The UN states in *Millennium Development Goals Report 2009* that "many health problems among pregnant women are preventable, detectable or treatable through visits with trained health workers before birth." In addition "these [visits] enable women to receive important services, such as tetanus vaccinations and screening and treatment for infections, as well as potentially life-saving information on warning signs during pregnancy."

FIGURE 10.6

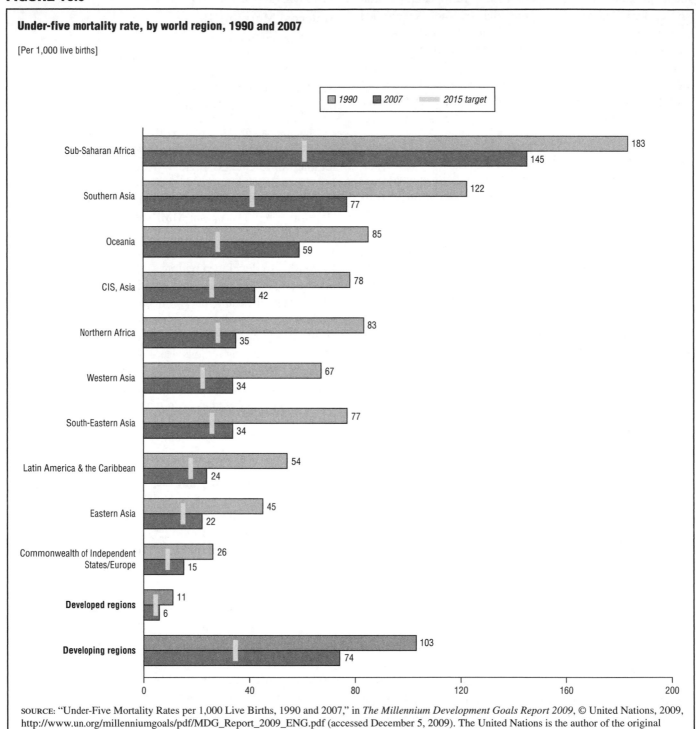

Under-five mortality rate, by world region, 1990 and 2007

[Per 1,000 live births]

Legend: ■ 1990 ■ 2007 ▨ 2015 target

- Sub-Saharan Africa: 183 (1990), 145 (2007)
- Southern Asia: 122 (1990), 77 (2007)
- Oceania: 85 (1990), 59 (2007)
- CIS, Asia: 78 (1990), 42 (2007)
- Northern Africa: 83 (1990), 35 (2007)
- Western Asia: 67 (1990), 34 (2007)
- South-Eastern Asia: 77 (1990), 34 (2007)
- Latin America & the Caribbean: 54 (1990), 24 (2007)
- Eastern Asia: 45 (1990), 22 (2007)
- Commonwealth of Independent States/Europe: 26 (1990), 15 (2007)
- Developed regions: 11 (1990), 6 (2007)
- Developing regions: 103 (1990), 74 (2007)

SOURCE: "Under-Five Mortality Rates per 1,000 Live Births, 1990 and 2007," in *The Millennium Development Goals Report 2009*, © United Nations, 2009, http://www.un.org/millenniumgoals/pdf/MDG_Report_2009_ENG.pdf (accessed December 5, 2009). The United Nations is the author of the original material. Reproduced with permission.

SAFE WATER AND SANITATION
Safe Drinking Water and Basic Sanitation

MDG 7c focuses on cutting in half, by 2015, the proportion of people without sustainable access to safe drinking water and basic sanitation. In *Human Development Report 2006—Beyond Scarcity: Power, Poverty, and the Global Water Crisis* (2006, http://hdr.undp.org/en/media/HDR06-complete.pdf), Kevin Watkins of the UN Development Programme considers access to safe drinking water and basic sanitation a fundamental human right, and adds, "Clean water and sanitation would save the lives of countless children, support progress in education and liberate people from the illnesses that keep them in poverty." The World Bank agrees, and adds in *Global Monitoring Report 2009* that "indirectly, infrastructure [which includes clean water and improved sanitation] influences the achievement of most MDGs, be they health, education, gender equality, or income poverty,

TABLE 10.4

Percent of people with access to selected types of infrastructure, by world region, 2000 and 2006

Type of infrastructure	East Asia & Pacific		Europe & Central Asia		Latin America & Caribbean		Middle East & North Africa		South Asia		Sub-Saharan Africa	
	2000	2006	2000	2006	2000	2006	2000	2006	2000	2006	2000	2006
Access to electricity	87	89	—	99	87	90	—	78	41	52	23	26
Access to improved water supply	80	87	93	95	89	91	89	89	81	87	55	58
Urban	95	96	98	99	96	97	96	95	93	94	81	81
Rural	72	81	85	88	69	73	80	81	77	84	42	46
Access to improved sanitation	60	66	89	89	75	78	74	75	27	33	29	31
Urban	71	75	94	94	85	86	86	89	54	57	41	42
Rural	52	59	79	79	47	51	58	59	17	23	22	24
Access to rural transport	—	90	—	82	—	59	—	59	—	57	—	34
Mainline telephone density (per 100 people)	0.0	3.0	—	3.0	0.0	2.6	—	—	0.0	0.2	—	—

Notes: — = Not available. China is included in data for East Asia and the Pacific. North African countries are excluded from data for the Middle East and North Africa.

SOURCE: "Table 2.2. Access to Infrastructure Is Improving but Still Lags Seriously in Some Regions," in *Global Monitoring Report 2009: A Development Emergency*, The World Bank, 2009, http://siteresources.worldbank.org/INTGLOMONREP2009/Resources/5924349–1239742507025/GMR09_ book.pdf (accessed December 10, 2009). Copyright © International Bank for Reconstruction and Development/The World Bank 2009.

through its effect on household opportunities." Chapter 7 highlights the importance of having clean water and basic sanitation and of having both easily accessible.

Table 10.4 shows progress in access to an improved water supply and improved sanitation between 2000 and 2006 in developing regions and regions in transition. In all regions, access is more widespread in urban areas than in rural areas. In all regions except sub-Saharan Africa, well over 90% of urban populations had access to clean water in both 2000 and 2006. In sub-Saharan Africa only 81% of urban populations had access to clean water in both 2000 and 2006. Less than half of rural populations in sub-Saharan Africa had access to clean water, although progress was made, from 42% in 2000 to 46% in 2006. In all other regions, between 73% and 88% of rural populations had access to clean water in 2006, with all having made progress since 2000. Figure 10.4 shows that the MDG 7c goal of access to safe water will likely be achieved globally by 2015.

Not as much progress has been made in access to improved sanitation in developing regions and regions in transition. The highest proportion of urban populations having access to improved sanitation was in Europe and central Asia at 94% in both 2000 and 2006, but this region did not make any progress during this period. The lowest proportion of urban populations having access to improved sanitation in 2006 was in sub-Saharan Africa (42%), but South Asia (57%) was doing poorly as well. Rural populations in South Asia and sub-Saharan Africa also had low levels of access to improved sanitation (23% and 24%, respectively).

Figure 10.7 shows the progress that must be made in access to improved sanitation to meet the MDG 7c goal by 2015. The figure shows the numbers of people who had gained access by 2006 and the numbers that must gain access by 2015. The trajectories of most regions are in line to make the target. However, in spite of making notable gains thus far, southern Asia and sub-Saharan Africa must step up their rate of progress to achieve MDG 7c. Figure 10.4 shows that the MDG 7c goal of access to improved sanitation will not likely be achieved globally by 2015.

THE MDG CALL TO ACTION

In September 2000 the UN established the MDGs in hopes of achieving eight world-changing goals by 2015. It is clear from the analysis in this chapter and throughout this book that much has been done, yet much is left to be achieved. Some areas of the world, such as China, are moving forward quickly toward achieving the MDGs, but some, such as sub-Saharan Africa, are struggling and falling behind.

In July 2007 the British prime minister Gordon Brown (1951–) and the UN secretary-general Ban Ki-Moon (1944–) launched the MDG Call to Action—a reenergizing of efforts in the international community to meet the promise of achieving the eight MDGs. Specifically, the Call to Action challenges the technology sector, medical and academic professions, nongovernmental organizations, faith groups, and cities to employ their knowledge and resources into meeting the MDGs. A series of meetings was scheduled to develop specific Call to Action programs throughout 2008, including a conference bringing together private-sector support in May 2008, an economic summit in Japan in July 2008, and a UN meeting on the MDGs in late 2008.

FIGURE 10.7

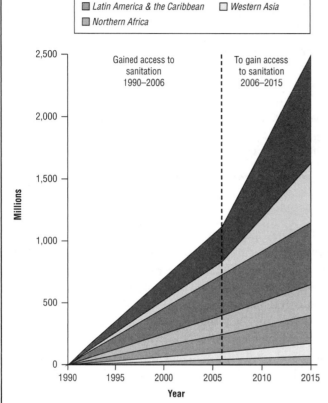

Progress toward the Millennium Development Goal (MDG) for sanitation (millions who gained access to improved sanitation), by world region, 1990–2006, with targets to 2015

Legend:
- Southern Asia
- Eastern Asia
- Latin America & the Caribbean
- Northern Africa
- Sub-Saharan Africa
- South-Eastern Asia
- Western Asia

Gained access to sanitation 1990–2006

To gain access to sanitation 2006–2015

(Y-axis: Millions; X-axis: Year 1990–2015)

SOURCE: "Population That Gained Access to an Improved Sanitation Facility 1990–2006 (Millions) and Population That Needs to Gain Access to an Improved Sanitation Facility to Meet the MDG Target, 2006–2015 (Millions)," in *The Millennium Development Goals Report 2009*, © United Nations, 2009, http://www.un.org/millenniumgoals/pdf/MDG_Report_2009_ENG.pdf (accessed December 5, 2009). The United Nations is the author of the original material. Reproduced with permission.

In his speech before the UN General Assembly on July 31, 2007, Brown declared:

We cannot allow our promises that became pledges to descend into just aspirations, and then wishful thinking, and then only words that symbolise broken promises.

We did not make the commitment to the Millennium Development Goals only for us to be remembered as the generation that betrayed promises rather than honoured them and undermined trust that promises can ever be kept.

So it is time to call it what it is: a development emergency which needs emergency action.

If 30,000 children died needlessly and avoidably every day in America or Britain we would call it an emergency. And an emergency is what it is.

So when the need is pressing, when it is our generation that has made historic commitments, when the time to meet them is now short, the simple questions that—to paraphrase the words of an American president—we must ask are:

If not now, when?

If not us, who?

If not together, how?

And I believe the scale of the challenge is such that we cannot now leave it to some other time and some other people but must act now, working together....

Today we have the science, technology, medicine and wealth: what we now need is the unity and strength of purpose to employ the ingenuity and resources we have—and to employ them well—to help those who need it.

IMPORTANT NAMES
AND ADDRESSES

Amnesty International
One Easton St.
London, WC1X 0DW United Kingdom
011-44-20-7-413-5500
FAX: 011-44-20-7-956-1157
URL: http://www.amnesty.org/

Asian Development Bank
Six ADB Ave.
Mandaluyong City, 1550 Philippines
011-632-632-4444
FAX: 011-632-636-2444
URL: http://www.adb.org/

Brookings Institution
1775 Massachusetts Ave. NW
Washington, DC 20036
(202) 797-6000
URL: http://www.brookings.edu/

Center for Economic and Policy Research
1611 Connecticut Ave. NW, Ste. 400
Washington, DC 20009
(202) 293-5380
FAX: (202) 588-1356
E-mail: cepr@cepr.net
URL: http://www.cepr.net/

Chronic Poverty Research Center
Institute for Development Policy and
Management
School of Environment and Development
University of Manchester
Humanities Bridgeford St.
Manchester, M13 9PL United Kingdom
011-44-161-275-2810
FAX: 011-44-161-273-8829
URL: http://www.chronicpoverty.org/

Food First/Institute for Food and
Development Policy
398 60th St.
Oakland, CA 94618
(510) 654-4400
FAX: (510) 654-4551

E-mail: info@foodfirst.org
URL: http://www.foodfirst.org/

Global Policy Forum
777 United Nations Plaza, Ste. 3D
New York, NY 10017
(212) 557-3161
FAX: (212) 557-3165
E-mail: gpf@globalpolicy.org
URL: http://www.globalpolicy.org/

Human Rights Watch
350 Fifth Ave., 34th Floor
New York, NY 10118-3299
(212) 290-4700
FAX: (212) 736-1300
E-mail: hrwnyc@hrw.org
URL: http://www.hrw.org/

Institute for Economic Democracy
13851 N. 103 Ave.
Sun City, AZ 85351
1-888-533-1020
E-mail: ied@ied.info
URL: http://www.ied.info/

International Committee of the Red Cross
19 Avenue de la Paix
Geneva, CH 1202 Switzerland
011-41-22-734-6001
FAX: 011-41-22-733-2057
URL: http://www.icrc.org/

International Crisis Group
149 Avenue Louise, Level 24
Brussels, B-1050 Belgium
011-32-2-502-9038
FAX: 011-32-2-502-5038
URL: http://www.crisisgroup.org/

International Forum on Globalization
1009 General Kennedy Ave., Ste. 2
San Francisco, CA 94129
(415) 561-7650
FAX: (415) 561-7651
E-mail: ifg@ifg.org
URL: http://www.ifg.org/

International Labour Office
4 Route des Morillons
Geneva 22, CH 1211 Switzerland
011-41-22-799-6111
FAX: 011-41-22-798-8685
E-mail: ilo@ilo.org
URL: http://www.ilo.org/

MADRE
121 W. 27th St., Ste. 301
New York, NY 10001
(212) 627-0444
FAX: (212) 675-3704
E-mail: madre@madre.org
URL: http://www.MADRE.org/

National Center for Children in Poverty
Columbia University
Mailman School of Public Health
215 W. 125th St., Third Floor
New York, NY 10027
(646) 284-9600
FAX: (646) 284-9623
E-mail: info@nccp.org
URL: http://www.nccp.org/

New Economics Foundation
Three Jonathan St.
London, SE11 5NH United Kingdom
011-44-20-7820-6300
FAX: 011-44-20-7820-6301
E-mail: info@neweconomics.org
URL: http://www.neweconomics.org/

Oxfam International
226 Causeway St., Fifth Floor
Boston, MA 02114-2206
(617) 482-1211
FAX: (617) 728-2594
E-mail: info@oxfamamerica.org
URL: http://www.oxfam.org/

Social Watch
18 de Julio 1077/902
Montevideo, 11100 Uruguay

011-598-2-902-0490
URL: http://www.socialwatch.org/

UN Children's Fund
Three United Nations Plaza
New York, NY 10017
(212) 326-7000
FAX: (212) 887-7465
URL: http://www.unicef.org/

UN Development Fund for Women
304 E. 45th St., 15th Floor
New York, NY 10017
(212) 906-6400
FAX: (212) 906-6705
URL: http://www.unifem.org/

UN Development Programme
One United Nations Plaza
New York, NY 10017
(212) 906-5000
FAX: (212) 906-5001
URL: http://www.undp.org/

UN Educational, Scientific, and Cultural Organization
Seven Place de Fontenoy
Paris 07 SP, 75352 France

011-33-1-4568-1000
FAX: 011-33-1-4567-1690
E-mail: bpi@unesco.org
URL: http://www.unesco.org/

UN Population Fund
220 E. 42nd St.
New York, NY 10017
(212) 297-5000
FAX: (212)370-0201
E-mail: hq@unfpa.org
URL: http://www.unfpa.org/

U.S. Bureau of Labor Statistics
Second Massachusetts Ave. NE
Washington, DC 20212-0001
(202) 691-5200
URL: http://www.bls.gov/

U.S. Census Bureau
4600 Silver Hill Rd.
Washington, DC 20233
(301) 763-4636
URL: http://www.census.gov/

U.S. Department of Agriculture
1400 Independence Ave. SW
Washington, DC 20250
(202) 720-2791
URL: http://www.usda.gov/

Women's Environment and Development Organization
355 Lexington Ave., Third Floor
New York, NY 10017
(212) 973-0325
FAX: (212) 973-0335
URL: http://www.wedo.org/

World Bank
1818 H St. NW
Washington, DC 20433
(202) 473-1000
FAX: (202) 477-6391
URL: http://www.worldbank.org/

World Food Programme
Via C. G. Viola 68
Parco dei Medici
Rome, 00148 Italy
011-39-06-65131
FAX: 011-39-06-659-0632
URL: http://www.wfp.org/

World Health Organization
Avenue Appia 20
Geneva 27, 1211 Switzerland
011-41-22-791-2111
FAX: 011-41-22-791-3111
E-mail: info@who.int
URL: http://www.who.int/

RESOURCES

The United Nations Development Programme (UNDP) publishes the annual *Human Development Report,* which focuses on a different aspect of human development each year. In addition, it publishes regional and national reports on poverty and development.

Other United Nations (UN) programs focus on specific facets of human development. The UN Children's Fund (UNICEF), which is devoted to the rights and needs of children, publishes the annual *State of the World's Children.* Programs within UNICEF address children's health—most notably children with the human immunodeficiency virus (IIIV) and the acquired immunodeficiency syndrome (AIDS)—and education. UNICEF's Innocenti Research Centre publishes a variety of papers on topics such as child poverty, child work and labor, and conflict and displacement. The UN Development Fund for Women publishes reports and papers on topics such as ending violence against women, ending the spread of HIV/AIDS among girls and women, and achieving gender equity. Part of the mission of the UN Educational, Scientific, and Cultural Organization (UNESCO) is to monitor and report on the state of education in developing countries. Through its Education for All program, UNESCO publishes the annual *EFA Global Monitoring Report.* The Food and Agriculture Department of the UN publishes the annual *State of Food Insecurity in the World.* Another UN agency, the International Labour Office, is dedicated to policing and reporting on human and labor rights around the world, particularly on poverty-related issues such as low wages, the informal economy, and human trafficking. The UN Population Fund (UNFPA) focuses on improving the living conditions—especially reproductive health—of women in developing countries. The UNFPA publishes the annual *State of World Population.* The World Health Organization (WHO) is the arm of the UN devoted to tracking and promoting health issues, many of which affect the poor, including HIV/AIDS, malaria, infectious disease, and child mortality. The WHO publishes the annual *World Health Report.* IRINnews.org is an online news source run by the UN Office for the Coordination of Humanitarian Affairs; it publishes news stories on events in sub-Saharan Africa, the Middle East, and central Asia.

Like the UNDP, the World Bank is an international organization of member countries concerned about poverty and human development. Besides its primary function of offering low-interest loans and lines of credit to underdeveloped and developing countries, the World Bank publishes numerous reports on the economic and development status of regions and individual nations. It also publishes reports on topical issues affecting the poor, such as natural disasters.

The Asian Development Bank is similar to the World Bank in its structure and goals, but it is focused exclusively on ending poverty in Asian countries. It publishes the annual *Asian Development Outlook.*

The U.S. Census Bureau provides valuable information on how poverty is measured and defined. The U.S. Department of Agriculture provides reports on regional and local poverty—particularly in rural areas—as well as information on food security and food assistance programs in the United States. The U.S. Bureau of Labor Statistics tracks historical and recent patterns of wages, unemployment, and careers. Its information is available in published reports and online.

Many nongovernmental organizations, think tanks, and watchdog groups provide invaluable insight and information on poverty and the poor. Among them are Amnesty International, the Brookings Institution, the Chronic Poverty Research Center, Global Policy Forum, Human Rights Watch, the International Committee of the Red Cross, the International Forum on Globalization, the Institute for Economic Democracy, the National Center for Children in Poverty, Oxfam International, Social Watch, and Women's Environment and Development Organization.

INDEX

Page references in italics refer to photographs.
References with the letter t *following them*
indicate the presence of a table. The letter f
indicates a figure. If more than one table or
figure appears on a particular page, the exact
item number for the table or figure being
referenced is provided.

A

Abbas, Mahmoud, 144
Absolute poverty, 1, 87
Adolescents
    birth rates, 111, 114(*f* 7.7)
    psychosocial effects of poverty, 87–88
Afghanistan, 47–49, 48*t*
Africa
    life expectancy, 37*f*
    regions, 33–34
    See also Sub-Saharan Africa
African Americans, 128–129
African Union, 142
Agriculture
    Afghanistan, 49
    famine, 124–125
    subsidies and aid, 26–27
Aid
    Darfur, 142
    famine, 125–127
    food, 26–27
    Iraq, 144
    Korea, North, 84–85
    natural disaster aid funding, 131*f*, 132*f*
    Palestinians, 143–144
AIDS. *See* HIV/AIDS
Alcoholism, 103
Alkatiri, Mari, 50
Antipersonnel land mines, 138–139
Arab-Israeli War, 143
Asia
    Afghanistan, 47–49
    child and infant mortality rates, 63*t*

China, People's Republic of, 58–62
    developing countries, 53–58, 54*t*
    drinking water, 66*t*
    education, 57*t*, 58*t*
    India, 62–68
    malnutrition, 65*t*
    maternal mortality, 61*t*
    percent of people living on less than $1.25
        per day, by region and country, 56*t*
    population and diversity, 46–47
    sanitation, 67*t*
    skilled health professionals attending
        childbirth, 62*t*
    Timor-Leste, 49–51
    tsunami, 127
    underweight children, 64*t*, 151–152
    See also Central Asian republics
Automobiles, 60

B

Band Aid (concert), 126
Bangladesh, 130
Bashir, Omar al-, 142
Beijing Declaration, 104, 112
Berdymukhammedov, Gurbanguly, 81
Birth rates, 111, 113(*f* 7.6), 114(*f* 7.7)
BLS (U.S. Bureau of Labor Statistics), 15,
    17–18
Bono, 126
Brown, Gordon, 157–158
Buerk, Michael, 126
Burma, 130–132, 133*f*, 134*f*
Bush, George W., 118, 128

C

Caloric intake, 35, 36(*f*3.4), 37
Canada, 107
Caste system (India), 65–66, 67
CCP (Chinese Communist Party), 59
Census Bureau, U.S., 88

Central American Free Trade Agreement, 29
Central and Eastern Europe, 75(*f* 5.3)
Central Asian republics
    child mortality, 75–76, 75(*f*5.4),
        75(*f*5.5)
    developing countries, 54
    extreme poverty among children,
        75(*f*5.3)
    history, 74
    hunger and malnutrition, 76(*f*5.6)
    Kazakhstan, 77–79
    Kyrgyzstan/Kyrgyz Republic, 77–79
    Tajikistan, 80–81
    Turkmenistan, 81–82
    Uzbekistan, 82–83
    water, clean, 76–77, 77*f*
Child labor, 19, 120–121, 122*f*
Child mortality
    Afghanistan, 48
    Asia and the Pacific, 63*t*
    causes of deaths, 120*f*
    Central and Eastern Europe and the
        Commonwealth of Independent States,
        75–76, 75(*f*5.4)
    China, 61
    India compared with China, 68
    international comparisons, 119–120,
        121*f*
    Iraq, 144, 145
    Kazakhstan, 79
    Millennium Development Goals,
        150*f*, 151*f*
    progress in reducing, 45*t*–46*t*, 48*t*, 155,
        156*f*
    Tajikistan, 81
    Turkmenistan, 82
    Uzbekistan, 83
    violent conflict, 138*f*
Childbirth
    Asia and the Pacific, 62*t*
    early childbearing, 114(*f*7.8)

obstetric fistula, 111–112
skilled health professionals attending, 62*t*, 110, 110*f*, 155
Children
child labor, 19, 122*f*
China, 61–62
Convention on the Rights of the Child, 103
extreme poverty among children, central and Eastern Europe and the Commonwealth of Independent States, 75(*f*5.3)
health, 118–119
hunger and malnutrition, United States, 95
hunger and malnutrition in sub-Saharan Africa, 35
immunizations, Afghanistan, 49
immunizations, Timor-Leste, 51
insecticide-treated mosquito nets, use of, 41*f*, 42*f*
labor, 120–121
mortality, 119–120
poverty rates, 93*f*, 97–98, 99*f*, 118
psychosocial effects of poverty, 87–88
refugees, 139
violent conflict, effects of, 137
Chile, 135
China, People's Republic of, 59–62, 68
Chinese Communist Party (CCP), 59
Civil war, 138
Classification
economic development levels, 12–13
underdeveloped countries, 33
Clinton, Bill, 60
Cognitive function, 87–88
Cold War, 12–13
Colonialism
India, 65
Latin America and the Caribbean, 71
Communications, 51
Communism, 59
Composite poverty indicators, 4, 5*t*–9*t*, 10–11, 10*t*
Contraception
family planning, 112*f*
Kazakhstan, 78*t*
Kyrgyz Republic, 79*t*
Russian Federation, 100*t*
Tajikistan, 81*t*
Turkmenistan, 82*t*
Uzbekistan, 83*t*
women, 109, 110–111, 113(*f*7.5)
Convention on the Rights of the Child, 103
Corporatist welfare model, 97
Crimes against humanity, 142–143
Cyclone Nargis, 130–132, 133*f*, 134*f*
Cyclone Sidr, 130

D
Dalits (in India's caste system), 65–66
Darfur, 141–143
Debt, 29–30, 30*t*, 31*t*
Demographic characteristics
hunger and malnutrition, United States, 95
United States poverty rates, 90*t*–91*t*
Developed countries
absolute *vs.* relative poverty, 87
child poverty, by immigrant or native status, 99*f*
Germany, 98–99
human poverty and income poverty, 10–11, 10*t*
international comparisons of poverty rates, 88*f*
military spending, 139–141, 140*f*
overcrowded housing, 98*f*
psychosocial effects of poverty in, 87–88
Russian Federation, 99–102
United Kingdom, 97–98
United States, 88–96
western Europe, 97
Developing countries
Asia, 53–58, 54*t*
central Asian republics, 74–83
extreme poverty among children, Central and Eastern Europe and the Commonwealth of Independent States, 75(*f*5.3)
hunger and malnutrition, 22, 23, 26–27, 28(*f*2.10)
informal economy, 18–20
Kazakhstan, 77–79
Korea, North, 83–85
Kyrgyzstan/Kyrgyz Republic, 79–80
Latin America and the Caribbean, 69–74
Tajikistan, 80–81
Turkmenistan, 81–82
Uzbekistan, 82–83
Development indicators
Kazakhstan, 78*t*
Kyrgyzstan/Kyrgyz Republic, 79*t*
Russian Federation, 100*t*
Tajikistan, 81*t*
Turkmenistan, 82*t*
Uzbekistan, 83*t*
Discrimination, 65–66
Dodd, Christopher J., 93

E
Earthquakes, 127–130, 132–135, 136*f*
East Asia, 54–55
East Timor. *See* Timor-Leste
Eastern Europe, 99–102
Economic growth, 12–13, 150, 152*t*
Economic reform, 100
Economic sanctions, 144

Education
Afghanistan, 49
Asia and the Pacific, 57*t*, 58*t*
attainment, 21–22, 22(*t*2.5)
child labor, 120–121
China, 62
East Asia, 55
gender parity, 115*t*
health education, 28
HIV/AIDS in sub-Saharan Africa, effect of, 46*f*
homelessness, United States, 95–96
Iraq, 145
Kazakhstan, 78–79, 78*t*
Kyrgyzstan/Kyrgyz Republic, 79*t*, 80
Latin America and the Caribbean, 73–74, 74*f*
literacy and illiteracy, 20–21, 20*f*
Millennium Development Goals, 150*f*, 151*f*
postsecondary education, 117(*f*7.12)
primary school enrollment, 116(*f*7.9), 153*f*
progress, 45*t*–46*t*, 48*t*, 152–154
Russian Federation, 100*t*, 102
secondary education, 116(*f*7.10), 117(*f*7.11)
South Asia, 56–57
sub-Saharan Africa, 43–45
Tajikistan, 81–82, 81*t*
Timor-Leste, 51
Turkmenistan, 82, 82*t*
Uzbekistan, 83, 83*t*
women and girls, 112–116, 154–155
Elderly persons, 88–89
Electricity, 77
Emergency housing, 129
Emerging and transitional economies
China, People's Republic of, 59–62
India, 62–68
Employment
child labor, 120–121, 122*f*
global trends, 16(*f*2.2)
poverty in the United States, 90*t*–91*t*
women's earnings in select occupations, 106*f*
See also Working poor
Environmental hazards, 123–127
See also Natural disasters
Environmental sustainability progress, 45*t*–46*t*, 48*t*
Ethiopia, 125–126
European Union, 107
Extreme poverty
Central and Eastern Europe and the Commonwealth of Independent States, 75, 75(*f*5.3)
progress toward eradicating, 45*t*–46*t*, 147–150, 150*f*, 151*f*
by world region, 148*f*

F

Fair trade, 29
Family planning, 112f
Family status, 89, 90t–91t
Famine, 124–127, 125t
FAO (Food and Agriculture Organization),
    22–24, 126
Federal Emergency Management Agency
    (FEMA), 129
FEMA (Federal Emergency Management
    Agency), 129
Fertility rates
    education, 114
    Kazakhstan, 78t
    Kyrgyz Republic, 79t
    Russian Federation, 100t
    Tajikistan, 81t
    Turkmenistan, 82t
    Uzbekistan, 83t
Flooding. See Natural disasters
Food aid, 26–27, 125–127, 144
Food and Agriculture Organization (FAO),
    22–24, 126
Food insecurity. See Hunger and
    malnutrition
Forced labor, 19f
Formaldehyde, 129
Fourth World Conference on Women, UN,
    103
Free trade, 29

G

GDP. See Gross domestic product
Geldof, Bob, 126
Gender
    balance, 138
    education, 114–116, 115t
    Gender-Related Development Index, 47,
        104–105, 105t
    literacy and illiteracy, 21, 112–113
    Millennium Development Goals
        progress, 45t–46t, 48t, 150f, 151f,
        154–155
    postsecondary education, 117(f7.12)
    primary school enrollment, 116(f7.9)
    secondary school attendance, 116(f7.10)
    secondary school enrollment, 117(f7.11)
    unemployment, 108t
    working poor, 17, 18t
Genocide, 142
Germany, 98–99
Gini coefficients
    Asia, 53, 54
    Latin America and the Caribbean, 71
Globalization, 28–30
Gorbachev, Mikhail, 99
Gross domestic product (GDP)
    Afghanistan, 47
    Asia, 55t

child mortality, 76(f5.5)
    China, 60
    Darfur, 143
    developing countries in Asia, 53–54
    India, 68
    Kazakhstan, 78t
    Kyrgyz Republic, 79t
    Russian Federation, 100t
    sub-Saharan Africa, 39t
    Tajikistan, 81t
    Turkmenistan, 82t
    Uzbekistan, 83t
Gulf Coast, 128–129

H

Haiti, 134–135
Hamas, 143
Health
    Afghanistan, 47–49
    children, 118–120
    China, People's Republic of, 61–62
    India, 68
    India compared with China, 68
    Kazakhstan, 79
    Latin America and the Caribbean,
        71–73
    Russian Federation, 102–103
    sub-Saharan Africa, 34–35, 37–43, 40t
    Tajikistan, 81
    Timor-Leste, 50–51
    Turkmenistan, 82
    Uzbekistan, 83
    See also Specific issues
Health care
    access to, in sub-Saharan Africa, 39t
    Afghanistan, 48
    skilled health professionals attending
        childbirth, 62t
    Timor-Leste, 50
Health education, 28
Heavily Indebted Poor Countries Initiative,
    29–30
Higher education, 116
Hinduism, 65
HIV/AIDS
    Africa, 37f
    Kazakhstan, 78t
    Kyrgyz Republic, 79t
    malaria susceptibility, 40
    progress in combating, 45t–46t, 48t
    Russian Federation, 100t, 102–103
    sub-Saharan Africa, 37–39, 38f, 39t,
        46f
    Tajikistan, 81t
    Turkmenistan, 82t
    Uzbekistan, 83t
Homelessness
    United States, 95–96
    violence against women, 118

Housing
    Hurricane Katrina, 129
    overcrowded housing, 98f
    United Kingdom, 98
Human Development Index
    Afghanistan, 47
    China, 60
    countries ranked by, 5t–9t
    developed countries, 10t
    human development effects, 138
    Kazakhstan, 77
    sub-Saharan Africa, 34
    trends, by region, 34f
    Uzbekistan, 83
Human Poverty Index
    China, 60–61
    country rankings, 5t–9t
    developed countries, 10t
    international comparisons, 4, 5t–9t,
        10–11, 10t
Human rights
    Beijing Declaration and Platform for
        Action, 104, 112
    Dalits, 65–66
    Darfur, 141–143
Human Suffering Index, 11
Hunger and malnutrition
    Commonwealth of Independent States,
        76, 76(f5.6)
    dietary energy consumption, 36(f3.4)
    famine, 124–127, 125t
    international comparisons, 22–28, 23f,
        24f, 27f, 28(f2.10)
    Iraq, 144–145
    Kazakhstan, 78t
    Korea, North, 84–85
    Kyrgyz Republic, 79t
    Latin America and the Caribbean,
        71–72, 73f
    Millennium Development Goals
        progress, 150f, 151f
    progress in eradicating, 45t–46t
    progress in reducing, 150–152
    Russian Federation, 100t
    sub-Saharan Africa, 34–35, 36(f3.3), 37
    Tajikistan, 81, 81t
    Turkmenistan, 82t
    United States, 94–95, 96t, 97f
    Uzbekistan, 83t
    violent conflict, effects of, 137, 138
    See also Underweight children
Hurricane Katrina, 128–129
Hussein, Saddam, 144–145

I

Illiteracy. See Literacy and illiteracy
Immigrants
    child poverty in select developed
        countries, 99f
    poverty in the United States, 88

Immunizations
    Afghanistan, 49
    Timor-Leste, 51
Income
    China, 60
    Germany, 99
    Iraq, 145
    as a measure of poverty, 1–4, 5t–9t, 10t
    Russian Federation, 101
    Tajikistan, 80
    women, 105–107, 106f
India, 62–68
Indigenous peoples, 71
Infant mortality
    Asia and the Pacific, 63t
    Darfur, 143
    international comparisons, 119, 119t
    Latin America and the Caribbean,
       71, 72t
    Turkmenistan, 82
Informal economy, 18–20, 106
Insecticide-treated mosquito nets, 40–42
Internally displaced people, 139
International Conference on Financing for
    Development, United Nations, 147
International Labour Office,
    United Nations
    unemployment, 15
    working poor in the informal economy,
       18–20
International Monetary Fund, 29–30,
    30t, 31t
Iraq, 144–145
Israel, 143–144

J

Jackson, Michael, 126
Janjaweed, 142
Java, 129–130

K

Kazakhstan, 78t
Kim Il-Sung, 83–84
Kim Jong-Il, 84
Korea, North, 83–85
Korea, Republic of (South Korea), 55
Korean War, 83
Kuwait, 144
Kyrgyzstan/Kyrgyz Republic, 79–80

L

Land mines, 138–139
Latin America and the Caribbean, 69–74,
    70t, 72t, 73f, 74f
Least developed countries. See
    Underdeveloped countries
Legislation
    Measuring American Poverty Act
       (proposed), 12, 93

Less-developed countries
    Human Development Index ranking,
       5t–9t
    human poverty and income poverty, 4,
       5t–9t, 10
Liberal welfare model, 97
Life expectancy
    Afghanistan, 47–48
    Africa, 37f
    Darfur, 143
    international comparisons, 24, 28(f2.12)
    Iraq, 145
    Kazakhstan, 78t, 79
    Kyrgyzstan/Kyrgyz Republic, 79t, 80
    Russian Federation, 100t, 102
    sub-Saharan Africa, 37–39
    Tajikistan, 81, 81t
    Turkmenistan, 82, 82t
    Uzbekistan, 83, 83t
Literacy and illiteracy
    Afghanistan, 49
    Darfur, 143
    developed countries, 10t
    international comparisons, 5t–9t, 20–22,
       20f, 21t, 22(t2.4)
    Iraq, 145
    Kazakhstan, 79
    Kyrgyzstan/Kyrgyz Republic, 80
    progress, 154
    sub-Saharan Africa, 44–45
    Turkmenistan, 82
    Uzbekistan, 83
    women, 112–113
Live Aid, 126

M

Malaria, 39–42, 48
Malnutrition. See Hunger and malnutrition
Mao Zedong, 59
Maternal health, 45t–46t, 48t
Maternal mortality
    Asia and the Pacific, 61t
    China, 61
    India compared with China, 68
    international comparisons, 109–110,
       109t
    Kazakhstan, 79
    Kyrgyzstan/Kyrgyz Republic, 80
    progress in reducing, 155
McDermott, Jim, 92
MDGs. See Millennium Development Goals
MDRI (Multilateral Debt Relief Initiative),
    29–30, 30t, 31t
Measurement
    composite poverty indicators, 4, 10–11
    National Academy of Sciences, 12
    poverty lines, United States, 11–12
    United States poverty thresholds, 11t,
       92–93

    weaknesses in, 12
    World Bank poverty line standards, 2–4
Measuring American Poverty Act
    (proposed), 93
Middle class, 60
Middle East, 143–144
Military spending, 139–141, 140f, 141t
Millennium Development Goals (MDGs)
    Afghanistan, progress in, 45t–46t
    Call to Action, 157–158
    child mortality, progress in reducing,
       155, 156f
    clean water and sanitation progress,
       156–157, 157t
    gender parity, progress in, 154–155
    goals and targets, 25t–26t
    hunger and malnutrition, eradicating,
       22–24, 150–152
    literacy progress, 154
    maternal mortality, progress in reducing,
       155
    primary education progress, 150–152
    progress, 147, 148–150, 150f, 151f
    sanitation progress, 158f
    sub-Saharan Africa, progress in, 45t–46t
    violent conflict, 137
    women and children, 104–105
Mongolia, 55
Mortality
    Afghanistan, 47–49
    Africa, 37f
    Asia and the Pacific, 61t, 63t
    child, 28(f2.11)
    China, 61
    HIV/AIDS, 37–39
    hunger, 24, 26
    Kazakhstan, 78t
    Kyrgyz Republic, 79t
    life expectancy, 28(f2.12)
    malaria, 40
    Russian Federation, 100t
    Tajikistan, 81t
    ten most common causes of death in sub-
       Saharan Africa, 40t
    Turkmenistan, 82t
    Uzbekistan, 83t
    See also Child mortality; Infant
       mortality; Maternal mortality
Mosquito nets, 40–42
Multilateral Debt Relief Initiative (MDRI),
    29–30, 30t, 31t

N

National Academy of Sciences, 12
National poverty lines, 2
Natural disasters
    aid funding, 131f, 132f
    antipoverty campaigns, 147
    Asian tsunami, 127

Chile earthquake, 135
Cyclone Nargis, 133*f*, 134*f*
Cyclone Sidr, 130
Haiti earthquake, 134–135
hunger and malnutrition, causes of, 27–28
Hurricane Katrina, 128–129
Java earthquake and tsunami, 129–130
Pakistan earthquake, 127–128
Sumatra earthquake, 132–133, 136*f*
Tropical Cyclone Nargis, 130–132
underdeveloped and developing countries, 123–124
Natural resources, 49
Net enrollment ratio, 153
Nixon, Richard M., 59
Niyazov, Saparmurad, 81
North American Free Trade Agreement, 29

O

Obstetric fistula, 111–112
Occupations, 106*f*, 107
Oil (petroleum)
oil-for-food program, 144
Timor-Leste, 50
Overcrowded housing, 98, 98*f*

P

Pakistan, 127–128
Palestinians, 143–144
People's Republic of China. *See* China, People's Republic of
Pharmaceutical drugs, 40
Platform for Action, 104
Politics
agricultural subsidies, trade, and food aid, 26–27
Ethiopia, 125
Postsecondary education, 116, 117(*f*7.12), 155
Poverty lines, 2–4, 11–12, 11*t*, 12*t*, 92–93
Poverty rates
children in poverty, United States, 93*f*
developed countries, 10*t*
extreme poverty, 147–150, 148*f*
Germany, 99
international comparisons, 88, 88*f*
Kazakhstan, 77
Kyrgyzstan/Kyrgyz Republic, 79–80
less developed countries, 5*t*–9*t*
Russian Federation, 100, 102
Tajikistan, 80
trends and projections, 149*t*
Turkmenistan, 82
United States, 94*f*
United States, by age, 91*f*
United States, by demographic characteristics, 90*t*–91*t*
Uzbekistan, 83

Poverty thresholds. *See* Poverty lines
Powell, Colin, 142
Prenatal care, 110, 111*f*, 155
Prices, food, 23
Primary education
enrollment, by region, 153*f*
girls, 155
international comparisons, 115, 116(*f*7.9)
Kazakhstan, 78*t*
Kyrgyz Republic, 79*t*
Millennium Development Goals, 150*f*, 151*f*
progress, 45*t*–46*t*, 48*t*, 152–154
Russian Federation, 100*t*
Tajikistan, 81*t*
Turkmenistan, 82*t*
Uzbekistan, 83*t*
Psychosocial effects of poverty in wealthy countries, 87–88
Purchasing power parity, 3–4, 47

R

Race/ethnicity
poverty in the United States, 88, 90*t*–91*t*
working poor, 17–18, 18*t*
Ramos-Horta, José, 50
Reform, 81–82
Refugees
Palestinians, 143
violent conflict, 139
Relative poverty
definition, 1
developed countries, 10–11, 87
United States, 94
Religious conflict, 143–144
Repression, government, 81–82
Reproductive health, 108–112, 155
Ritchie, Lionel, 126
Rural areas
Central and Eastern Europe and the Commonwealth of Independent States, 76–77
India, 68
Kazakhstan, 77–78
Latin America and the Caribbean, 69
poverty in the Russian Federation, 100
Russian Federation, 99–102, 100*t*

S

Sanctions, economic, 144
Sanitation
China, 62
India compared with China, 68
international comparisons, 43*f*
Iraq, 145
Millennium Development Goals, 150*f*, 151*f*
progress, 156–157, 157*t*, 158*f*

sub-Saharan Africa, 42–43
Timor-Leste, 51
use of sanitation facilities, by region, 43*f*
SAPs (structural adjustment programs), 29
Secondary education, 115–116, 116(*f*7.10), 117(*f*7.11), 155
Sexual exploitation, 113
Slave labor, 120
Social democratic welfare model, 97
South Korea. *See* Korea, Republic of
Southern Asia, 55–56, 151–152
Soviet Union, dissolution of, 74, 99–100
Stalinism, 81
State poverty rates, 92*t*
Statistical information
birth rate for women aged 15–19, 114(*f*7.7)
child and infant mortality rates, Asia and the Pacific, 63*t*
child labor, 122*f*
child mortality, Central and Eastern Europe and the Commonwealth of Independent States, 75(*f*5.4), 76(*f*5.5)
child mortality, international comparisons, 28(*f*2.11), 121*f*
child mortality, progress in reducing, 156*f*
childbearing, by household wealth, 113(*f*7.6)
childhood deaths, causes of, 120*f*
children in poverty, United States, 93*f*
clean water, access to, Central and Eastern Europe and the Commonwealth of Independent States, 77*f*
clean water and sanitation progress, 157*t*
contraception, 113(*f*7.5)
dietary energy consumption, 36(*f*3.4)
drinking water, 44*f*
drinking water, Asia and the Pacific, 66*t*
economic growth, 152*t*
educational attainment, 22(*t*2.5)
employment, global trends in, 16(*f*2.2)
extreme poverty, 148*f*
extreme poverty among children, Central and Eastern Europe and the Commonwealth of Independent States, 75(*f*5.3)
family planning, 112*f*
food-insecure people, Commonwealth of Independent States, 76(*f*5.6)
food-insecure people, Latin America and the Caribbean, 73(*f*5.2)
food-insecure people, sub-Saharan Africa, 36(*f*3.3)
forced labor, 19*f*
GDP, 55*t*
gross domestic product, HIV prevalence, and access to health care, sub-Saharan Africa, 39*t*

HIV/AIDS in sub-Saharan Africa, 38*f*

human development index trends, by region, 34*f*

human poverty and income poverty in developed countries, 10*t*

human poverty and income poverty in less developed countries, 5*t*–9*t*

hunger and malnutrition, developing countries, 28(*f*2.10)

hunger and malnutrition, United States, 97*f*

illiteracy, 20*f*, 21*t*

infant mortality, international comparisons, 119*f*

infant mortality, Latin America and the Caribbean, 72*t*

insecticide-treated mosquito nets, children's use of, 41*f*, 42*f*

international comparisons of poverty rates, 88*f*

life expectancy, international comparisons, 28(*f*2.12)

life expectancy in Africa, 37*f*

literacy, international comparisons, 22(*t*2.4)

malnutrition, Asia and the Pacific, 65*t*

malnutrition, Latin America and the Caribbean, 73(*f*5.1)

maternal mortality, Asia and the Pacific, 61*t*

maternal mortality, international comparisons, 109*t*

military spending, international comparisons, 141*t*

military spending for developed countries, 140*f*

Millennium Development Goals progress, 150*f*

Multilateral Debt Relief Initiative, 31*t*

natural disaster aid funding, 131*f*, 132*f*

overcrowded housing in selected developed countries, 98*f*

people living on less than $1.25 per day, Asia and the Pacific, 56*t*

percent child poverty in select developed countries, by immigrant or native status, 99*f*

postsecondary education, international comparisons, 117(*f*7.12)

poverty in the United States, by age, 91*f*

poverty rates, by state, 92*t*

poverty rates, trends and projections, 149*t*

poverty rates, United States, 94*f*

prenatal care, international comparisons, 111*f*

primary education enrollment, by region, 153*f*

primary enrollment, Asia and the Pacific, 57*t*

primary school completion, Asia and the Pacific, 58*t*

primary school enrollment, international comparisons, 116(*f*7.9)

sanitation, Asia and the Pacific, 67*t*

sanitation, international comparisons, 43*f*

sanitation facility use, by region, 43*f*

sanitation progress, international comparisons, 158*f*

school enrollment, Latin America and the Caribbean, 74*f*

secondary school attendance, by urban/rural residence and household wealth, 116(*f*7.10)

secondary school enrollment, international comparisons, 117(*f*7.11)

skilled health professionals attending childbirth, Asia and the Pacific, 62*t*

sub-Saharan Africa's progress in reaching Millennium Development Goals, 45*t*–46*t*

ten most common causes of death in sub-Saharan Africa, 40*t*

undernourished people, by selected regions, 27(*f*2.9)

undernourished people worldwide, 27(*f*2.8)

underweight children, Asia and the Pacific, 64*t*

underweight children, by world region, 35*f*

unemployment, by sex, 108*t*

unemployment, global trends in, 16(*f*2.1)

United States poverty guidelines, 12*t*

United States poverty rates, by demographic characteristics, 90*t*–91*t*

United States poverty thresholds, 11*t*

violent conflict and child mortality rates, 138*f*

women's earnings in select occupations, 106*f*

working poor in the United States, 17*f*, 17*t*

working poor in the United States, by age, sex, and race/ethnicity, 18*t*

working poor trends, by region, 3*t*

world development indicators, Kazakhstan, 78*t*

world development indicators, Kyrgyz Republic, 79*t*

world development indicators, Russian Federation, 100*t*

world development indicators, Tajikistan, 81*t*

world development indicators, Turkmenistan, 82*t*

world development indicators, Uzbekistan, 83*t*

Structural adjustment programs (SAPs), 29

Sub-Saharan Africa

economic well-being, 45–46

HIV/AIDS, 38*f*

HIV/AIDS and access to health care, 39*t*

hunger and malnutrition, 34–35, 36(*f*3.3), 37

insecticide-treated mosquito nets, children's use of, 41*f*, 42*f*

malaria, 39–42

Millennium Development Goals, 45*t*–46*t*

ten most common causes of death, 40*t*

Subsidies, food, 84

Sudan, 141–143

Sumatra, 135*f*

Sumatra earthquake, 132–133, 136*f*

T

Tajikistan, 80–81, 81*t*

Timor-Leste, 49–51

Trade, 26–27, 29

Transportation, 60

Treaties and international agreements

Beijing Declaration, 104, 112

Convention on the Rights of the Child, 103

free trade agreements, 29

Millennium Declaration, 22–24, 25*t*–26*t*

Platform for Action, 104

Tropical Cyclone Nargis, 130–132, 133*f*, 134*f*

Tsunamis, 129–130

Tuberculosis, 48–49, 102

Turkmenistan, 81–82, 82*t*

U

Underdeveloped countries

criteria for identifying, 33

Human Development Index ranking, 5*t*–9*t*

United Nations list of, 34*t*

See also Asia; Sub-Saharan Africa

Underweight children

Asia and the Pacific, 64*t*

China, 61–62

India compared with China, 68

international comparisons, 5*t*–9*t*, 119

Iraq, 145

Latin America and the Caribbean, 73

trends, 151–152

by world region, 35*f*

See also Hunger and malnutrition

UNDP (United Nations Development Programme), 4

Unemployment

developed countries, 10*t*

gender, 108*t*

Germany, 98–99

global trends, 16(*f*2.1)

international comparisons, 15

Russian Federation, 100

women, 108

UNESCO (United Nations Educational, Scientific, and Cultural Organization), 20–22, 20*f*, 21*t*, 22*t*
UNIFEM (United Nations Development Fund for Women), 105–106
United Nations
    Call to Action, 157–158
    Convention on the Rights of the Child, 103
    Darfur peacekeeping mission, 142
    Food and Agriculture Organization, 126
    Fourth World Conference on Women, 103
    International Conference on Financing for Development, 147
    Iraq War, 144
    Millennium Declaration, 22–24, 25*t*–26*t*
    underdeveloped countries list, 34*t*
    World Food Programme, 127
    See also Food and Agriculture Organization (FAO); International Labour Office, United Nations; United Nations Educational, Scientific, and Cultural Organization (UNESCO)
United Nations Development Fund for Women (UNIFEM), 105–106
United Nations Development Programme (UNDP), 4
United Nations Educational, Scientific, and Cultural Organization (UNESCO), 20–22, 20*f*, 21*t*, 22*t*
United States
    children in poverty, 93*f*
    Convention on the Rights of the Child, ratification of, 103
    homelessness, 95–96
    hunger and malnutrition, 96*t*, 97*f*
    Hurricane Katrina, 128–129
    international comparisons with, 88
    Iraq, invasion of, 144–145
    military spending, 141
    poverty guidelines, 12*t*
    poverty rates, 88–90, 92, 94*f*
    poverty rates, by demographic characteristics, 90*t*–91*t*
    poverty rates, by state, 92*t*
    poverty thresholds, 11–12, 11*t*, 12*t*, 92–93
    relative poverty, 94
    violence against women, 118
    women's earnings, 107
    working poor, 15, 17–18, 17*f*, 17*t*

working poor, by age, sex, and race/ethnicity, 18*t*
Universal primary education, 152–154
Urban areas
    Kazakhstan, 77–78
    Latin America and the Caribbean, 69
    poverty in the Russian Federation, 100–101
Ure, James, 126
U.S. Bureau of Labor Statistics (BLS), 15, 17–18
Utilities, 77–78
Uzbekistan, 82–83, 83*t*

V

VAWA (Violence against Women Act), 118
Violence against women, 117–118
Violence against Women Act (VAWA), 118
Violent conflict
    Afghanistan, 49
    child mortality rates, 138*f*
    Darfur, 141–143
    Ethiopia, 125
    human development effects, 137–138
    Iraq, 144–145
    Korean War, 83
    land mines, 138–139
    Middle East, 143–144

W

Wages. *See* Income
War. *See* Violent conflict
War crimes, 142–143
Wastewater, 42
Water, clean
    Afghanistan, 49
    Central and Eastern Europe and the Commonwealth of Independent States, 76–77, 77*f*
    China, 62
    India compared with china, 68
    international comparisons, 5*t*–9*t*, 42–43, 44*f*
    Iraq, 144
    Millennium Development Goals, 150*f*, 151*f*
    progress, 156–157, 157*t*
    by region, 44*f*
    sub-Saharan Africa, 42–43
    Timor-Leste, 51

Welfare
    models of social welfare programs, 97
    United Kingdom, 98
West Bank and Gaza Strip, 143–144
Western Europe, 97–99
WHO (World Health Organization), 117–118
Women
    average number of children, by household wealth, 113(*f*7.6)
    Beijing Declaration and *Platform for Action*, 104, 112
    birth rates, 114(*f*7.7)
    contraception, 113(*f*7.5)
    education, 112–116
    family planning, 112*f*
    gender parity, progress in, 154–155
    Gender-Related Development Index, 104–105, 105*t*
    maternal health, 45*t*–46*t*, 48*t*
    Millennium Development goals, 104
    prenatal care, 111*f*
    reproductive health, 108–112
    unemployment, 108
    violence against, 117–118
    wages and income, 105–107, 106*f*
    See also Maternal mortality
Working conditions, 19–20
Working poor
    informal economy, workers in the, 18–20
    trends, by region, 3*t*
    United States, 15, 17–18, 17*f*, 17*t*, 18*t*
World Bank
    lending and debt relief, 29–30
    measurement of poverty, 1–4
    Multilateral Debt Relief Initiative, 30*t*, 31*t*
    poverty definition, 4
    poverty trends, 147–150
World Food Programme, 127
World Health Organization (WHO), 117–118
World Trade Organization (WTO), 60
WTO (World Trade Organization), 60

Y

Yeltsin, Boris, 99–101
Youth. *See* Adolescents